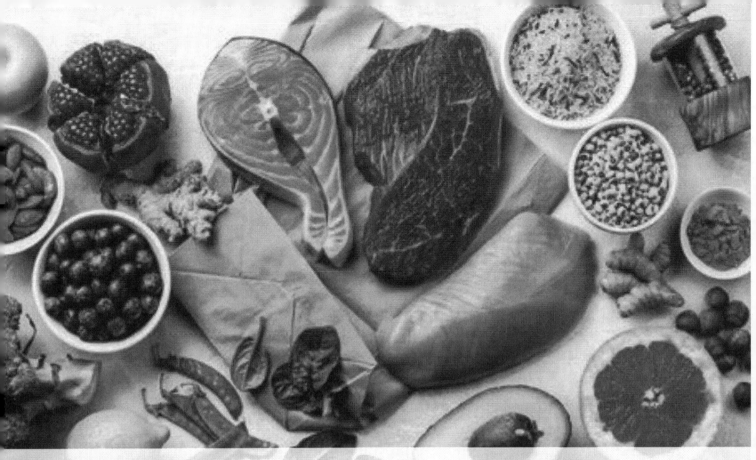

Introduction

Diabetes and Symptoms

Diabetes

Before we start with the recipes, we want to talk about the illness itself. You are a victim from this illness especially because it came out of nowhere. I think that you deserve to know everything there is about it and calm yourself because it can be treated, and you can be healthy while having it.

Diabetes Mellitus is the collective term for various disorders of the human metabolism, the main characteristic of which is chronic hyperglycaemia (high blood sugar). This is why one speaks of "diabetes." However, it is not always just the carbohydrate metabolism that is disturbed in diabetes. It can be proven again and again that fat and protein metabolism are also out of balance.

Insulin, a vital metabolic hormone that controls the carbohydrate, fat and protein metabolism, plays a crucial role in the development of diabetes. The causes of diabetes lie in various disorders of the release of insulin from the so-called beta cells of the pancreas up to an absolute insulin deficiency.

Triggers can also be gradually very different disorders of the action of insulin in important organs such as the brain, liver, muscles and adipose tissue.

Symptoms

The classic symptoms such as as weight loss, noticeable thirst and increased urine flow are mainly observed in younger people with the onset of type 1 diabetes. These complaints are rather untypical in older people. It, therefore, makes sense to have the fasting glucose level checked as part of preventive medical check-ups (e.g., a doctor's check-up).

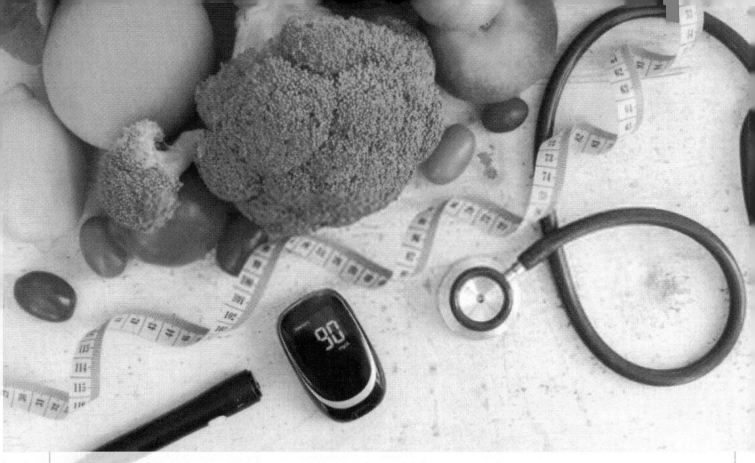

How to Manage Diabetes If You Have Just Been Diagnosed

Type 1 and Type 2 – the difference ● ● ●

Type 2 diabetes

About 90% of those affected have type 2 diabetes.

A characteristic of this form of diabetes is that the effect of insulin in the body›s cells is reduced (= insulin resistance), always coupled with an insulin deficiency.

Type 2 diabetes is extremely complex and manifests itself in different degrees of insulin resistance and insulin deficiency.

Type 2 diabetes or its precursors (increased fasting plasma glucose and / or impaired glucose tolerance = prediabetes) are often linked to other problems of the metabolic syndrome. Over 80% of this type of diabetes is associated with obesity.

Type 2 diabetes is the most common form of diabetes.

Symptoms

- Fatigue, poor performance, lack of drive
- Depressive moods
- Disturbances in memory and concentration
- Hunger, polyphagia (pathologically increased appetite / pathologically increased food intake)
- General tendency to infection (skin, mucous membranes, urinary tract)
- Itching
- Complications of diabetes

Type 1 diabetes

Type 1 diabetes is an autoimmune disease in which the insulin-producing cells in the so-called islets of Langerhans in the pancreas are destroyed by the body's defense system.

The body no longer produces insulin. There is an absolute insulin deficiency with the result that the fuels contained in the food (e.g., grape sugar = glucose) can no longer be adequately channeled into the body cells and metabolized.

People with type 1 diabetes therefore have to inject insulin several times a day throughout their life and adjust the insulin dose again and again to keep blood glucose as stable and normal as possible. In this way, serious secondary disease of blood vessels and nerves can largely be prevented or significantly delayed.

Classic type 1 diabetes occurs primarily in children, adolescents and young adults and affects 0.3 to 0.4% of the population.

Symptoms

- Excessive thirst
- Frequent urination
- Tiredness / exhaustion
- General weakness
- Hunger or loss of appetite
- Sudden weight loss
- Badly healing wounds
- Increased susceptibility to infection
- "Blurred vision"

The difference

Doctors differentiate between two types of diabetes: In type 1 diabetes - formerly also called juvenile diabetes - the insulin-producing cells of the pancreas are destroyed. In type 2 or adult diabetes, on the one hand, the insulin does not work fully; the cells are not sensitive enough to the hormone through an autoimmune reaction of the body. You can only absorb and burn a little glucose. On the other hand, the pancreas does not release enough insulin. In the course of type 2 diabetes, the formation of insulin also decreases.

How the sugar metabolism works

With the intake of food, the glucose enters the bloodstream. The pancreas constantly measures blood sugar - if it is high, it releases insulin. Insulin ensures that glucose is absorbed by the body's cells and that sugar stores are built up in the liver.

If the blood sugar is low, the hormone glucagon is released, which releases glucose from the existing sugar stores.

The exact causes have not yet been clarified

The exact causes of the disease are still not fully understood. Doctors suspect a combination of genetic factors, viral infection and autoimmune disease in type 1 diabetes. In type 2 diabetes, there is an innate or acquired insulin resistance of the cells, which is coupled with a reduced release of insulin. Overeating increases the insulin resistance. As a result, the pancreas must first make more insulin. In the long term, the insulin-producing cells are overburdened. The consequence of these complex processes is the picture of diabetes.

Which food is good against diabetes?

Diet is important in diabetes. This applies to both type 2 diabetes - the most common form of the disease - and type 1 diabetes. However, nutrition plays different roles in the treatment of the two forms of diabetes.

Type 2 Diabetes: Lose Weight

Being very overweight, especially on the abdomen, is one of the most important causes of type 2 diabetes. The nutritional recommendations for people with type 2 diabetes are therefore aimed at reducing excess weight along with other lifestyle changes and thus improving metabolic control.

Type 1 diabetes: Correctly assess carbohydrates

In type 1 diabetes, proper nutrition cannot improve the disease. People with type 1 diabetes need to know how many carbohydrates are in their food. This is the only way to correctly calculate the amount of insulin required to correct blood sugar to avoid excessively high values or hypoglycaemia. The same goes for all type 2 diabetics who depend on insulin.

People with diabetes learn how to correctly assess carbohydrates in food as part of a training course at the beginning of therapy.

Meal Prep

People with diabetes should eat a balanced diet and make sure that there is a good mix of carbohydrates, fats and proteins. Above all, it is crucial to get these nutrients from good food sources. The most important tips at a glance:

Carbohydrates:

Foods with complex carbohydrates prevent blood sugar spikes after eating: Complex carbohydrates pass more slowly from the intestine into the blood and do not cause the sugar levels to rise as quickly. At the same time, they keep you full longer - ideal for losing weight. Complex carbohydrates can be found in legumes, bread and pasta made from whole grains, for example. On the other hand, if possible, avoid foods with carbohydrates that quickly get into the blood - such as pasta, pizza and bread made from white flour - and go for the whole grain variant.

Fats:

Unsaturated fatty acids are preferable here, especially the so-called omega-3 fatty acids. Omega-6 fatty acids, which can promote inflammation in the body, should, on the other hand, be contained in rather small amounts in food. Flax and rapeseed oil, linseed and some nuts have a good ratio of omega-3 and omega-6 fatty acids. Sea fish is also a good source of omega-3s. Eat fats from animal sources in moderation. The quality of the meat also plays a role here: Meat from animals raised on pasture, for example, contains more omega-3 fatty acids.

If possible, people with diabetes should avoid foods that are high in trans fats. Trans fats can increase the level of harmful LDL cholesterol in the blood and lower the level of beneficial HDL cholesterol. Trans fats are mainly found in industrially processed foods such as chips, baked goods, fast food and sausages.

Proteins: In the case of kidney damage - a typical long-term consequence of permanently high blood sugar levels - too high a protein intake can be harmful. Patients with damaged kidneys should always seek individual advice on how much protein they can eat.

Sources of protein are, on the one hand, animal foods: i.e., meat and fish, eggs and dairy products. But many plant-based foods also contain valuable protein: legumes, for example, whole grains, some vegetables or potatoes. So, if you want to do without animal products every now and then, you usually don't have to worry about your protein supply.

Eat lots of fiber

Dietary fibers are carbohydrates that the human digestive system can hardly or not at all process. This slows down the processing of carbohydrates in the intestines, so that they pass more slowly into the blood. They also improve insulin sensitivity and ensure a more prolonged feeling of satiety. People with type 2 diabetes should therefore eat around 40 grams of fiber per day. Whole grain foods, legumes, nuts and many types of fruit and vegetables are particularly rich in fiber.

Avoid sugar - especially in beverages

People with diabetes should avoid sugar whenever possible. This is especially true for sugar in beverages, as these are empty calories. This means that they hardly contribute to the feeling of satiety, but that excess energy promotes the build-up of body fat. In addition, the sugar from them passes into the blood very quickly, which can lead to blood sugar spikes. Especially if you want to watch your weight, you should avoid soda, cola and juice. Better alternatives are water, tea, coffee and fruit spritzers.

Recommendation

Many prejudices persist about the right diet in diabetes. So, the most important message first: people with diabetes can in principle eat anything. This applies to both type 1 and type 2. Sugar is not taboo either but should be eaten or drunk as little as possible. Special foods are also not necessary. The earlier label "Suitable for diabetics" on food packaging no longer exists.

For people with diabetes, by and large, the same dietary recommendations apply as for healthy people. That means:

- Lots of fresh fruits and vegetables - three servings of vegetables and two servings of fruit should be taken daily
- Avoid sugar whenever possible. Sugar drives up blood sugar and thus also insulin levels. Insulin fills the fat cells and prevents fat from being broken down
- Rely on the whole grain variant for rice, pasta, bread and other grain product
- Eat meat, sausage, cheese and other animal foods in moderation
- Prefer certain fats from plants - for example olive and rapeseed oil as well as nuts and seeds are good
- Use salt sparingly - this is especially true if you have high blood pressure.

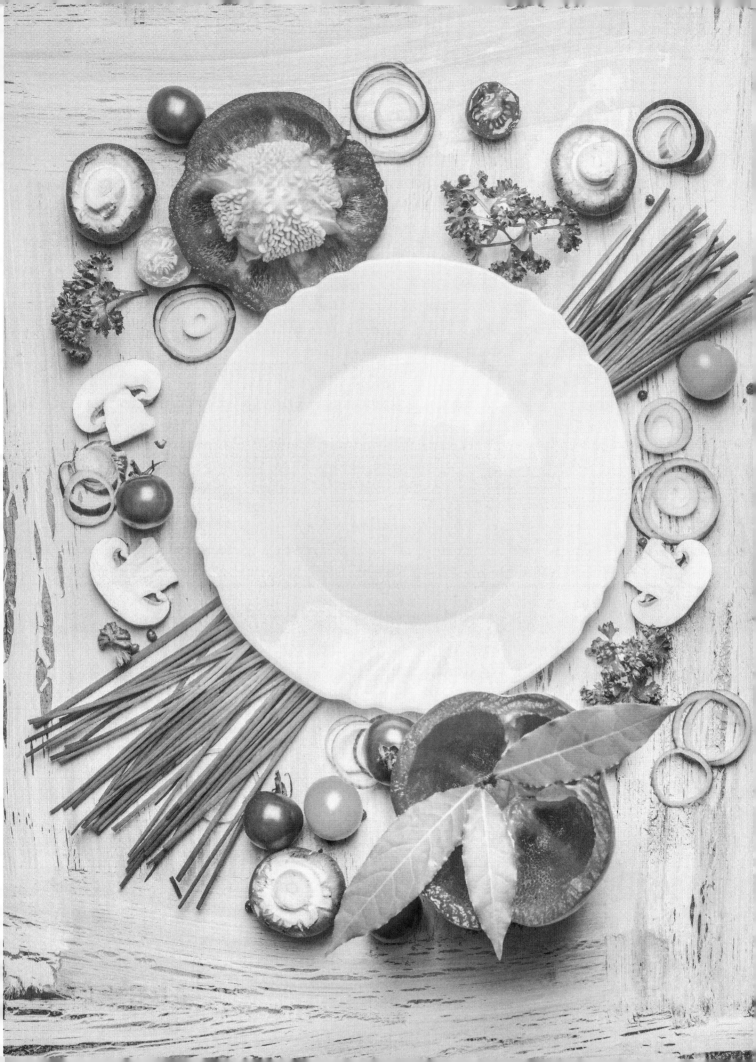

Recipes

BREAKFAST

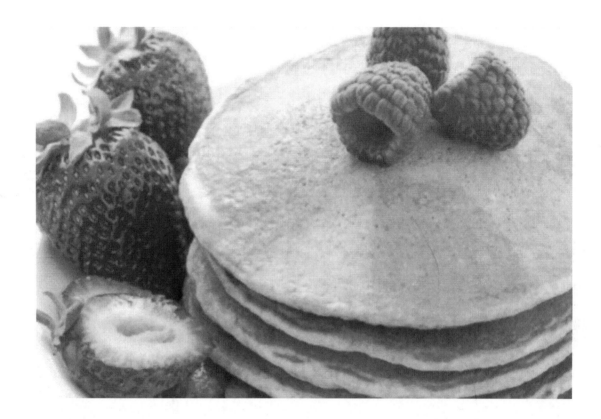

1) *Reduced Carb Berry Parfaits*

Ingredients:

- *For The Nut Granola:*
- *2 cups mixed nuts*
- *1 tbsp. flaxseed*
- *1 tbsp. sesame seeds*
- *1 tbsp. chia seeds*
- *2 tbsp. pumpkin seeds*
- *2 tbsp. coconut oil melted*
- *2 tbsp. honey or low carb sweetener to taste (optional)*

For The Blueberry Sauce:

- *2 cups frozen blueberries*
- *3 tbsp. Xylitol or (sugar alternative)*
- *1 tbsp. water*
- *For The Parfait:*
- *Plain Greek yogurt*
- *Fresh raspberries or other fruit of your choice*
- *Pinch of salt*

Direction: Preparation Time: 7 minutes Cooking Time: 23 minutes Servings: 4

✓ *To prepare the granola, heat the oven to about 175°C and cover a baking tray with baking parchment.*

✓ *Mix all the granola ingredients, put them in the oven, and then drop them onto the baking tray.*

✓ *Leave it to bake until the nuts are golden brown for 5–10 minutes. Regularly inspect the granola since it will quickly melt.*

✓ *Allow cooling after you have removed it from the oven.*
Combine all the ingredients in a shallow saucepan to make the blueberry sauce and get it to a boil. Allow the berries to cook for 5–10 minutes until their juice is released. Remove from the oven and allow for few minutes to cool.

✓ *Lay the yogurt with granola, fresh fruit, and sauce in your preferred bowl to make the parfaits. If the parfait is made in a pot, close the lid and place it overnight in the fridge before serving.*

Nutrition:Calories: 2171 Protein: 65g Fat: 168g

2) *Healthy Avocado Toast*

Ingredients:

- *1 avocado peeled and seeded*
- *2 tbsp. chopped cilantro*
- *Half lime, juiced*
- *½ tbsp. red pepper flakes optional*
Salt and pepper to taste

- *1 slice of wholegrain bread or bread of your choice*
- *2 eggs fried, scrambled (optional)*

Direction: Preparation Time: 5 minutes Cooking Time: 13 minutes Servings: 4

✓ *Toast 2 wholegrain slices in an oven until they are crispy and golden.*

✓ *Mix and crush the avocado, lime, cilantro, and salt, and pepper in a shallow bowl to taste.*
Spread on all the toasted bread slices with half of the combination.

✓ *Top with fried poached or scrambled egg, if wished.*

Nutrition: Calories: 501 Fat: 28g Protein: 16g

3) *Whole Egg Baked Sweet Potatoes*

Ingredients:

- *For the Potatoes:*
- *4 medium sweet potatoes*
- *2 heads garlic*
- *2 tsp. extra virgin olive oil*
- *½ tbsp. taco Seasoning*
- *¼ cup fresh cilantro, plus additional for garnish Salt and pepper*
- *4 eggs*
- *For the Sauce:*
- *½ cup avocado, about 1 medium avocado 1 tbsp. fresh lime juice*
- *1 tsp. Lime zest Salt and pepper*
- *2 tbsp. water*

Direction: Preparation Time: 30 minutes Cooking Time: 60 minutes Servings: 4

✓ *Preheat the oven to 395°F, cover with a baking sheet and tinfoil then place the potatoes on it.*

✓ *Rip off the garlic tips, keep the head intact, and softly rub in the olive oil on top of the uncovered cloves. Create 2 layers of tinfoil in a small packet, wrap the garlic in it, and then put it in the pan.*

✓ *Bake the garlic for about 40 minutes, until it is tender. Remove from the pan and cook the potatoes for additional 25–35 minutes, until fork-tender and soft.*

✓ *When the potatoes are tender, set them aside for about 10 minutes until they're cool enough to treat. In addition, decrease the temperature of the oven to 375°F.*

✓ *Break the potatoes down the middle and softly peel the skin back, leaving the skin intact on the sides. In a wide cup, carefully scoop out*

✓ *the skin, leaving a little amount on the sides of the potato to help maintain its form.*

✓ *Mash the flesh of the sweet potato and then cut half*

of it from the bowl (you will not use this flesh, so use it at a later date in another meal!) Add in the taco seasoning, cilantro and season with salt and pepper to taste into the mashed flesh. Finally, from the roasted heads, squeeze in all the fluffy garlic. Blend well.

✓ *Divide the flesh between the 4 sweet potatoes, spreading it softly to fill the meat, leaving a large hole in the middle of each potato.*

✓ *Back on the baking sheet, put the sweet potatoes and crack an egg into each hole and spray it with pepper and salt. Bake to your taste until the egg is well fried. For a good runny yolk, it usually takes about 10–15 minutes and blend until smooth.*

✓ *Then, with the food processor running, pour in the water and combine until well mixed. Sprinkle with salt and pepper to taste.*

✓ *Break the avocado sauce between them until the potatoes are cooked, spreading it out on top.*

✓ *Garnish with sliced tomatoes and cilantro in addition. And enjoy!*

Nutrition: Calories: 399 Fat: 32g Protein: 18g

4)   Black Bean Tacos Breakfast

Ingredients:

- ½ cup red onion, diced
- 86-inch white soft corn tortillas, warmed
- 1 garlic clove, minced
- 1 tsp. avocado oil
- ¼ cup chopped fresh cilantro
- 1(15 oz.) can black beans, rinsed and drained
- 1 small avocado, diced
- ¼ tsp. ground chipotle powder
- ½ cup fresh or your favorite jarred salsa
- 4 eggs

Direction: Preparation Time: 9 minutes Cooking Time: 13 minutes Servings: 4

✓ *Scramble the Eggs. You know how it can be done. Make them as you would usually make them. Here's a guide if you need a reminder, maybe!*

✓ *Sauté the beans: Heat the avocado oil over moderate heat in a large skillet. Sauté the onion for about 3 minutes until it is tender.*

✓ *Add the garlic and beans and heat until fully cooked, about 2–5 minutes.
Blister the tortillas or heat them in a dry skillet over an open fire on the range. Put aside, wrapped to keep them warm, in a cloth napkin.*

✓ *Layer the beans, then slice each tortilla with the eggs. Maintain to only*

✓ *¼ cup beans per taco. You may be tempted, but try not to overstuff the tortillas. Top up as needed with salsa, avocado, and cilantro.*

Nutrition: Calories: 349 Protein: 11.5g Fat: 15g

5)   Strawberry Coconut Bake

Ingredients:

- ½ cup chopped walnuts
- cups unsweetened coconut flakes
- 1 tsp. cinnamon
- ¼ cup chia seeds
- 2 cups diced strawberries
- 1 ripe banana mashed
- 1 tsp. baking soda 4 large eggs
- ¼ tsp. salt
- 1 cup unsweetened nut milk
- 2 tbsp. coconut oil, melted

Direction: Preparation Time: 11 minutes Cooking Time: 41 minutes Servings: 2

✓ *Preheat your oven to 375°F. Grease a square 8-inch pan and set it aside.*

✓ *Combine the dried ingredients in a big bowl: walnuts, chia seeds, cinnamon, salt, and baking soda.*

✓ *Whisk the eggs and milk together in a smaller dish. Now, add mashed banana and coconut oil to the mixture. To dry, add the wet ingredients and blend properly. Fold the strawberries in.*

✓ *Bake for about 40 minutes, or until the top is golden and solid.*

✓ *And serve hot!*

Nutrition: Calories: 395 Fat: 40g Protein: 7.5g

6)   Paleo Breakfast Hash

Ingredients:

- Eight oz. white mushroom, quartered
- 1 lb. Brussels sprout, quartered Everything bagel seasoning
- 1 tbsp. olive oil or avocado oil
- 3 garlic cloves, minced
- 1 small onion diced
  Crushed red pepper, optional
- Eight slices of nitrate-free bacon sugar-free, for Whole 30, cut into pieces
- Sea salt and pepper to taste 6 large eggs

Direction: Preparation Time: 7 minutes Cooking Time: 33 minutes Servings: 5

✓ *Preheat to 425°F in your oven. Arrange the mushrooms and Brussels sprouts in a single layer on a sheet tray, drizzle with the olive oil and add salt and pepper. Sprinkle the onions on the end and place the strips of bacon equally over the vegetables.*

✓ *Roast for 15 mins in the preheated oven, then sprinkle with the garlic and stir gently. Roast for 10*

mins or until the bacon and vegetables are crisp and fluffy. Extract from the stove.
For each egg, make tiny gaps in the hash, gently smash one at a time into a space, careful not to 'split' the yolk. Sprinkle all the bagel seasoning and crushed red pepper over the bacon, eggs, and vegetables as you wished.

✓ *Return the baking tray to the oven and bake for another 5–10 minutes or until the eggs are ideally fried. For me, for solid whites and light yolks, it was 7 minutes. Remove from the oven and quickly serve. Enjoy!*

Nutrition: Calories: 250 Protein: 14g Fat: 18g

7)   *Omelet with Chickpea Flour*

Ingredients:

* ½ tsp. Onion powder
* ¼ tsp. black pepper 1 cup, chickpea flour
* ½ tsp. garlic powder
* ½ tsp. baking soda
* ¼ tsp. white pepper
* 1/3 cup nutritional yeast
* 3 finely chopped green onions
* 4 oz. sautéed mushrooms

Direction: Preparation Time: 10 minutes Cooking Time: 20 minutes Servings: 1

✓ *Combine the onion powder, white pepper, chickpea flour, garlic powder, black and white pepper, baking soda, and nutritional yeast.*

✓ *Add 1 cup water and create a smooth batter. On medium heat, put a frying pan and add the batter just like the way you would cook pancakes.*
On the batter, sprinkle some green onion and mushrooms. Flip the omelet and cook evenly on both sides.

✓ *Once both sides are cooked, serve the omelet with spinach, tomatoes, hot sauce, and salsa.*

Nutrition: Calories: 150 Fats: 1.9g Carbohydrates: 24.4g Proteins:10.2g

8)   *White Sandwich Bread*

Ingredients:

* 1 cup warm water
* 2 tbsp. active dry yeast
* 4 tbsp. oil
* 2 ½ tsp. salt
* 2 tbsp. raw sugar or 4 tbsp. maple syrup/agave nectar
* cup warm almond milk or any other non-dairy milk of your choice
* 6 cups all-purpose flour

Direction: Preparation Time: 10 minutes Cooking

Time: 20 minutes Servings: 16

✓ *Add warm water, yeast, and sugar into a bowl and stir. Set aside for 5 minutes or until lots of tiny bubbles are formed, sort of bubbly.*

✓ *Add flour and salt into a mixing bowl and stir. Pour the oil, yeast mix, and milk and mix into the dough. If the dough is too hard, add a little water, a tbsp. at a time and mix well each time. If the dough is too sticky, add more flour, a tbsp at a time. Knead the dough until soft and supple. Use hands or hook attachment of the stand mixer.*

✓ *Now spray some water on top of the dough. Keep the bowl covered with a towel. Let it rest until it doubles in size.*

✓ *Remove the dough from the bowl and place it on your countertop. Punch the dough.*
Line a loaf pan with parchment paper. You can also grease with some oil if you prefer.

✓ *Place the dough in the loaf pan. Now spray some more water on top of the dough. Keep the loaf pan covered with a towel. Let it rest until the dough doubles in size.*

✓ *Bake in a preheated oven at 370°F for about 40–50 minutes.*

✓ *Let it cool to room temperature. Cut into 16 equal slices and use as required. Store in a breadbox at room temperature.*

Nutrition: Cal: 209 Fat: 4g Carbs: 35g Protein: 1g

9)   *Sprouted Toast with Creamy Avocado and Sprouts*

Ingredients:

* 2 tiny sized bread sprouts
* 1 cup finely cut tomatoes
* 2 moderate size avocados
* 1 small cup alfalfa
* Pure sea salt and bell pepper

Direction: Preparation Time: 10 minutes Cooking Time: 15 minutes Servings: 3

✓ *Add the avocado, alfalfa, and tomatoes to the bread and season to taste with pure sea salt and pepper.*
. Have a sumptuous breakfast with any freshly extracted juice of your choice.

Nutrition: Calories: 82 Fiber: 15g Protein: 30g Sugar: 7g

10)   *Scrambled Turmeric Tofu*

Ingredients:

* 1 crumbled serve of tofu
* 1 small cup finely chopped onions
* 1 tsp. the fresh parsley
* 1 tsp. coconut oil

- *1 cup soft spinach*
- *small tsp. Turmeric*
- *avocado serves 75g tomatoes*
- *1 small spoon roasted paprika*

Direction: Preparation Time: 5 minutes Cooking Time: 15 minutes Servings: 4

✓ *Make tofu crumbs with your hands and keep them separately. Sauté diced onions in oil till it softens. Put your tofu, tomatoes, and other seasonings and combine till tofu is well prepared. Add veggies and stir. Serve in a bowl alongside some avocado.*

Nutrition: Calories: 91 Fiber: 12g Protein: 30g Sugar: 8g

11) *Breakfast Salad*

Ingredients:

- *1 cup finely diced kale*
- *1 cup cabbage, red and Chinese*
- *2 tbsp. coconut oil*
- *1 cup spinach*
- *2 moderate avocados*
- *1.2kg chickpeas sprout*
- *tbsp. sunflower seed sprouts Pure sea salt (seasoning)*
- *Bell pepper (seasoning)*
- *Lemon juice (seasoning)*

Direction: Preparation Time: 5 minutes Cooking Time: 15 minutes Servings: 3

✓ *Add spinach, Chinese and red cabbage, kale, coconut oil, to a container*
  Add seasoning to taste and mix adequately.

✓ *Add other ingredients ad mix.*

Nutrition: Calories: 112 Protein: 28g Fiber: 10g Sugar: 1g

12) *Green Goddess Bowl with Avocado Cumin Dressing*

Ingredients:

- *heaping cups finely sliced kale*
- *1 small cup diced broccoli florets*
- *½ cup zucchini spiralized noodles*
- *½ cup soaked Kelp noodles*
- *3 cups tomatoes*
- *2 tbsp. hemp seeds*
- *1 tbsp. olive oil Bell pepper*
- *1 tbsp. powdered cumin*
- *Tahini dressing ingredients:*
- *1 small cup sesame butter*
- *1 cup alkaline water*

- *cup freshly extracted lemon*
- *1 garlic, finely chopped clove*
- *¾ tbsp. pure sea salt*
- *1 tbsp. olive oil Bell pepper*
- *Avocado Dressing Ingredients:*
- *1 big avocado*
- *freshly extracted lime 1 cup alkaline water*

Direction: Preparation Time: 10 minutes Cooking Time: 20 minutes Servings: 4

✓ *Simmer veggies—kale and broccoli for about 4 minutes.*

✓ *Combine noodles and add avocado cumin dressing. Toss for a while. Add tomatoes and combine well.*

✓ *Put the cooked kale and broccoli on a plate, add Tahini dressing, add noodles and tomatoes.*

✓ *Add a couple of hemp seeds to the whole dish and enjoy it.*

Nutrition: Calories: 109 Protein: 25g Fiber: 17g Sugar: 8g

13) *Quinoa Burrito*

Ingredients:

- *1 cup quinoa*
- *2 cups black beans*
- *4 finely chopped onions, green*
- *4 finely chopped garlic*
- *2 freshly cut limes*
- *1 big tbsp. cumin*
- *2 beautifully diced avocado*
- *1 small cup beautifully diced cilantro*

Direction: Preparation Time: 15 minutes Cooking Time: 10 minutes Servings: 1

✓ *Boil quinoa. During this process, put the beans in low heat.*

✓ *Add other ingredients to the bean pot and let it mix well for about 15 minutes.*

✓ *Serve quinoa and add the prepared beans.*

Nutrition: Calories: 117 Protein: 27g Fiber: 10g

14) *Baked Banana-Nut Oatmeal Cups*

Ingredients:

- *3 cups rolled oats.*
- *1 ½ cups low-fat milk*
- *2 ripe bananas*
- *¼ cup packed brown sugar*
- *2 larges lightly beaten eggs.*
- *1 tsp. Baking powder*
- *tsp. ground cinnamon*

- *1 tsp. vanilla extract*
- *½ tsp. salt*
- *½ cup toasted chopped pecans*

Direction: Preparation Time: 17 minutes Cooking Time: 40 minutes Servings: 4

✓ *Preheat the cooking appliance to 375°F. Coat a gem tin with a change of state spray.*

✓ *Combine oats, milk, bananas, refined sugar, eggs, leaven, cinnamon, vanilla, and salt during a giant bowl. Fold in pecans. Divide the mixture among the gem cups (about ¹/₃ cup each). Bake till a pick inserted within the center comes out clean, within twenty-five minutes.*

✓ *Cool within the pan for ten minutes, then end up on a wire rack.*

✓ *Serve heat or at temperature.*

Nutrition: Calories: 178 Protein: 5.3g Fat 6.3g

15)   *Veggie Breakfast Wrap*

Ingredients:

- *tsp. olive oil or other*
- *1 cup sliced mushrooms*
- *2 eggs*
- *½ cup egg white or egg replacement*
- *1 cup firmly packed spinach or other greens*
- *2 tbsp. sliced scallions*
- *cooking nonstick spray*
- *whole wheat and low-carb flour tortillas*
- *2 tbsp. salsa*

Direction: Preparation Time: 12 minutes Cooking Time: 13 minutes Servings: 2

✓ *Add oil to the frying pan over medium heat. Add mushrooms and sauté till nicely brown at edges (about 3 minutes), set aside.*

✓ *Beat eggs with egg whites or egg substitute in a medium-sized bowl, employing a mixer or by hand, till emulsified. Stir in cut spinach, and scallions. you'll additionally further recent or dried herbs like basil or parsley for Moe flavor. Begin heating medium/large frying pan over medium-low heat—coat pan munificently with a change of state spray. Pour in the egg mixture and still scramble the mixture because it cooks employing a spatula. once eggs area unit broiled to your feeling, close up the warmth and stir in mushrooms.*

✓ *Unfold ½ the egg mixture down the middle of every battercake. high every with 1 tbsp. recent condiment or alternative e sauce of your alternative. Garnish with additional toppings like avocado slices, bell pepper, or tomato if desired, then roll it up to form a wrap.*

Nutrition: Calories: 220 Fat: 11g Protein: 19g

16)   *Breakfast Egg and Ham Burrito*

Ingredients:

- *4 eggs*
- *egg whites*
- *1 dash hot pepper sauce*
- *¼ tsp. black pepper*
- *2 tbsp. cheddar cheese*
- *2 tbsp. margarine*
- *4 slices deli*
- *¼ cup sliced onion*
- *¼ cup diced green pepper.*
- *4 heated corn tortilla Salsa*

Direction: Preparation Time: 21 minutes Cooking Time: 13 minutes Servings: 3

✓ *Using a medium bowl, whisk along the eggs, egg whites, hot Poivrade, black pepper, and cheese. Heat the spread during a medium non-stick pan over medium heat. Add the ham and sauté for 2–3 minutes. Take away the ham from the pan.*

✓ *Add the onions and fresh peppers to the recent pan, and cook for 5 minutes. Add the ham back to the pan.*

✓ *Scale back the warmth to low and add the eggs to the pan. Gently stir the eggs with a spoon or spatula and gently change the state over low heat until the eggs area unit is broiled and set.*

✓ *Equally, divide the egg mixture into 4 servings. Spoon every portion of the egg mixture into a battercake and high every with 1 tsp. Salsa. Fold the battercake to shut.*

Nutrition: Calories: 210 Fat: 9g Carbohydrate: 16g

17)   *Breakfast Cups for Meat Lover*

Ingredients:

- *1 tbsp. light sour cream*
- *2 pre-cooked defrosted and diced turkey breakfast sausage patties*
- *1 clove of minced garlic*
- *2 tbsp. thinly sliced onion*
- *1 ½ cup frozen hash browns*
- *1 tsp. canola oil*
- *¼ tsp. salt*
- *A pinch of black pepper*
- *1 cup egg substitute*
- *2 tbsp. turkey bacon*
- *2 tbsp. Monterey jack cheese*

Direction: Preparation Time: 12 minutes Cooking Time: 13 minutes Servings: 4

✓ *Heat the kitchen appliance to 400°F. Coat a 6-cup quick bread tin with sloppy preparation spray.*

Equally, divide the hash browns among the quick bread cups and press firmly into the lowest and up the perimeters of every cup.

✓ In an exceedingly giant frying pan, heat the oil over medium heat. Sauté the onion till tender. Add the garlic and sausage; cook for 1 minute additional. Take away the frying pan from the heat; stir within the soured cream.

✓ In an exceedingly medium bowl, beat the egg substitute with the salt and black pepper, then pour it equally into the potato-lined quick bread cups. High every cup with a number of the sausage mixture, bacon, and cheese.

✓ Bake 15 to 19 minutes, or till the eggs area is set. Serve instantly, or freeze for later.

Nutrition: Calories: 120 Fat 4g Carbohydrate: 10g

18)   Breakfast Quesadilla

Ingredients:

- 1 cooking spray
- ¼ cup canned green chiles
- 4 beaten eggs
- ¼ tsp. black pepper
- 2 10-inch of whole wheat flour tortillas
- 1 ½ cup cheddar cheese (reduced fat)
- 4 slices of turkey bacon (cooked crisp and crumbled)

Direction: Preparation Time: 13 minutes Cooking Time: 16 minutes Servings: 4

✓ Lightly brush a small skillet with cooking oil.

✓ Sauté the green chilies over medium-low heat for 1–2 minutes. Attach beaten eggs and cook until scrambled and set, stirring. Season with some pepper.

✓ Lightly brush a second large skillet with cooking oil. Place 1 tortilla in the skillet and cook over medium heat for about 1 minute, until the air bubbles begin to form. Flip the tortilla and cook for another 1 minute (don't let the tortilla get crispy).

✓ Layer half of the cheese thinly over the tortilla, protecting the corners.

✓ Reduce heat to minimum temperatures. Arrange half of the fried bacon and half of the egg mixture over the cheese quickly. Cook until the cheese begins to melt for about 1 minute.

✓ To make a half-moon shape, fold the tortilla in half. Flip the folded tortilla over and cook for 1–2 minutes, until lightly toasted and the cheese filling is fully melted.

Nutrition: Calories: 160 Fat: 19g Carbohydrate: 8g

19)   Toasts with Egg and Avocado

Ingredients:

- 4 eggs
- 4 slices hearty wholegrain bread
- 1 avocado (mashed)
- ½ tsp. salt (optional)
- ¼ tsp. black pepper
- ¼ cup Greek yogurt (nonfat)

Direction: Preparation Time: 17 minutes Cooking Time: 0 minutes Servings: 4

✓ To poach each egg, fill ½ cup water with a 1 cup microwaveable bowl or teacup. Crack an egg into the water softly, make sure it's fully submerged. Cover on high for around 1 minute with a saucer and microwave, or before the white is set and the yolk starts to set, but still fluffy (not runny).

✓ Toast the bread and use ¼ of the mashed avocado to scatter each slice.

✓ Sprinkle the salt with avocado (optional) and pepper. Top with a poached egg on each piece. Top the egg with 1 tbsp. Greek yogurt.

Nutrition: Calories: 230 Fat: 13g Carbohydrate: 26g

20)   Turkey Sausages and Egg Casserole

Ingredients:

- ½ cup green chopped onions
- 2 cups nonfat milk
- 1 nonstick cooking spray
- ½ tsp. mustard powder
- ¼ tsp. salt
- ¼ tsp. black pepper egg substitute
- 4 slices of whole wheat bread (cut into ½–inch cubes)
- 3 precooked (diced turkey breakfast sausage patties
- ¼ cup cheddar cheese (reduced-fat, shredded)

Direction: Preparation Time: 13 minutes Cooking Time: 13 minutes Servings: 5

✓ Preheat oven to 350°F. Coat a 9x13 baking dish with cooking spray.

✓ In a medium bowl, whisk together nonfat milk, green onions, dry mustard, salt (optional), pepper, and egg substitute.

✓ Place bread cubes and sausage on the bottom of the baking dish, pour egg mixture evenly over bread and sausage. Top with cheddar cheese.

✓ Cover pan with aluminum foil and bake for 20 minutes. Remove foil and bake for an additional 40 minutes.

Nutrition: Calories: 120 Fat: 3g Carbohydrate: 9g

21)   Apple-Walnut French Toast

Ingredients:

- *4 slices multigrain Italian bread 6 oz.*
- *1 cup egg substitute*
- *4 tsp. pure maple syrup*
- *1 cup diced apple*
- *walnuts (chopped)*

Direction: Preparation Time: 12 minutes Cooking Time: 14 minutes Servings: 4

✓ *Preheat your oven to 450°F. Meanwhile, put the bread in a baking pan of 13 to 9 inches, pour over all the egg substitutes, and turn several times until the bread slices are thoroughly coated and the egg mixture is used. (Stand in the baking pan when preheating the oven.) Put bread slices coated with cooking spray on the baking sheet.*
Bake for 6 minutes, turn, and bake for 5 minutes or until the bottom is golden. Serve with similar proportions of syrup, apples, and nuts in the mixture.

Nutrition: Calories: 276 Fat: 12g Carbohydrate: 33.56

22)   Summer Smoothie Fruit

Ingredients:

- *1 cup fresh blueberries*
- *1 cup fresh strawberries, chopped*
- *2 peaches, peeled, seeded, and chopped*
- *Peach flavored Greek-style yogurt (nonfat)*
- *1 cup unsweetened almond milk*
- *2 tbsp. ground flax seed*
- *½ cup ice*

Direction: Preparation Time: 12 minutes Cooking Time: 0 minutes Servings: 4

✓ *Combine in a blender and puree all ingredients until creamy.*
✓ *Serve*

Nutrition: Calories: 130 Fat: 4g Carbohydrate: 23g

23)   Chicken and Egg Salad

Ingredients:

- *2 cooked chicken breasts*
- *3 hard-boiled eggs*
- *2 tbsp. fat-free mayo*
- *1 tbsp. curry powder*
- *Chives or basil (optional)*
- *Salt (optional)*

Direction: Preparation Time: 5 minutes Cooking Time: 25 minutes Servings: 2

✓ *.Bake the chicken for maybe 15 minutes in the oven around 360°F (confirm with just a knife that now the meat is cooked all the through).*
✓ *For 8 minutes, cook the eggs. Cut the eggs and chicken into a small- sized piece.*
✓ *Combine the cream cheese with curry powder In a large bowl, combine everything and mix.*
✓ *Allow a minimum of 10 minutes to chill in the refrigerator (it gets even better if you leave it overnight in the refrigerator).*
✓ *Serve with chives on toast or muffins and a bit of salt on top.*

Nutrition: Calories: 139 Fat 9g Carbohydrate: 23g

24)   Nicoise Salad Tuna

Ingredients:

- *4 oz. Ahi tuna steak*
- *1 whole egg*
- *2 cups baby spinach (3oz)*
- *2 oz. green beans*
- *1 ½ oz. broccoli*
- *Half red bell peppers*
- *3 and a half oz. cucumber*
- *1 radish*
- *3 large black olives*
- *Handful of parsley*
- *1 tsp. olive oil*
- *1 tsp. balsamic vinegar*
- *½ tsp. Dijon mustard*
- *½ tsp. pepper*

Direction: Preparation Time: 12 minutes Cooking Time: 5 minutes Servings: 1

✓ *Cook the egg, and place it aside to cool.*
✓ *Steam beans and broccoli, then set aside. 2–3 mins of a little water in the microwave or 3 minutes in a kettle of hot water does the trick.*
✓ *In a tub, heat a bit of oil over high heat.*
✓ *On all sides, season the seafood using pepper, then place it there in the heat and stir on each edge for about 2 minutes.*
✓ *To the salad bowl or pan, add the spinach Chopped the red pepper, grapefruit as well as egg into pieces that are bite-sized. Add the spinach on top.*
✓ *Cut the radish into slices and mix the broccoli, beans, and olives. Add the spinach salad on top.*
✓ *Break the tuna into strips and add it to the salad.*
✓ *Toss the olive oil, balsamic vinegar, mustard, salt, and pepper together.*
✓ *The parsley is chopped and added to the vinaigrette.*

✓ *For drizzling the vinaigrette over a salad, use a spoon.*

Nutrition: Calories: 149 Fat: 6g Carbohydrate: 21g

25) Rolls with Spinach

Ingredients:

- *16 oz. frozen spinach leaves*
- *3 eggs*
- *2 ½ oz. onion*
- *2 oz. carrot*
- *1 oz. low-fat mozzarella cheese*
- *4 oz. fat-free cottage cheese*
- *1 garlic clove*
- *1 tsp. curry powder*
- *¼ tsp. chili flakes Salt*
- *1 tsp. pepper Cooking spray*
- *½ cup parsley*

Direction: Preparation Time: 15 minutes Cooking Time: 40 minutes Servings: 4

✓ *Preheat the oven to 200ºC (400º F).*

✓ *Thaw the spinach and squeeze the water out (you can use a filter). In order to accelerate the thawing process, you can microwave the spinach for a few minutes.*

✓ *Mix the spinach, 2 eggs, mozzarella, ginger, half the salt, and pepper together in a baking bowl.*

✓ *Place parchment paper on a baking sheet and coat it with cooking spray. Move the spinach mixture, about half an inch thick and about 10 to 12 inches in height, to the sheet and press it down.*

✓ *Bake for 15 minutes and then set aside to cool on a rack. Don't turn the oven off.*

✓ *Finely chop the onion and parsley. Grate the carrots.*
In a pan with a bit of cooking oil, fry the onions for about a minute. Add the carrots and parsley to the pan and let it cook for about 2 minutes.

✓ *Add cottage cheese, curry, chili, salt, and pepper to the other half. Briefly mix.*

✓ *Remove the fire from the pan, add an egg, and mix it all together.*

✓ *Spread the filling over the spinach that has been cooled. Do not stretch it all the way to the corners or as you fold it out, it will fall out.*

✓ *Roll the spinach mat carefully and fill it, then bake for 25 minutes.*

✓ *Take out the roll once the time is up, and let it cool for 5–10 minutes before cutting it into slices and serving.*

Nutrition: Calories: 149 Fat: 11g Carbohydrate: 26g

26) Balanced Turkey Meatballs

Ingredients:

- *20 oz. ground turkey*
- *3 ½ fresh or frozen spinach*
- *¼ cup oats*
- *2 egg whites*
- *Celery sticks*
- *3 garlic cloves*
- *½ green bell peppers*
- *Half red onion*
- *½ cup parsley*
- *½ tsp. cumin*
- *1 tsp. mustard powder*
- *1 tsp. thyme*
- *½ tsp. turmeric*
- *½ tsp. chipotle pepper*
- *1 tsp. salt*
- *A pinch pepper*

Direction: Preparation Time: 12 minutes Cooking Time: 26 minutes Servings: 2

✓ *Preheat the oven to 350ºF (175ºC).*

✓ *Chop the onion, garlic, and celery very finely (or use a food processor), and add to a large mixing cup.*

✓ *In the dish, add the ham, egg whites, oats, and spices and combine well. Make sure the mix contains no pockets of spices or oats.*

✓ *Spinach, green peppers (stalked and seeded), and parsley are chopped. The bits need to be about a dime's size.*
To the tub, add the vegetables and mix them until well-combined.

✓ *Line the parchment paper with a baking sheet.*

✓ *Roll the turkey mixture (about the size of golf balls) into 15 balls and put them on the baking sheet.*

✓ *Bake for 25 minutes, until fully baked.*

Nutrition: Calories: 129 Fat: 9g Carbohydrate: 22g

27) Curried Chicken with Apples

Ingredients:

- *1lb. cooked, diced chicken breast*
- *1 Granny Smith diced apple*
- *celery stalks, diced*
- *2 green onions, diced*
- *½ cup sliced cashew*
- *1 cup plain Greek yogurt*
- *1 tbsp. tahini*
- *4 tsp. curry powder*
- *1 tsp. ground cinnamon*

Direction: Preparation Time: 12 minutes Cooking Time: 13 minutes Servings: 3

✓ *In a big mixing cup, add the milk, tahini, curry powder, and cinnamon.*

✓ *Add the chicken, apple, celery, cashews, and green onions. Stir to blend.*

✓ *To offer it ever something of a tropical feel, this salad can be eaten on its own, as a snack, or in plucked-out papaya.*

Nutrition: Calories: 139 Fat: 8g Carbohydrate: 19g

28) *Homemade Chicken Nuggets*

Ingredients:

- ½ cup almond flour
- 1tbsp. Italian seasoning
- 2tbsp. extra virgin olive oil
- ½ tsp. salt
- ½ tsp. pepper

Direction: Preparation Time: 15 minutes Cooking Time: 23 minutes Servings: 2

✓ *Preheat the oven to 200°C (400°F), Use parchment paper to arrange a large baking dish.*

✓ *Whisk the Italian seasoning, almond flour, pepper, and salt together in a dish.*

✓ *Start cutting and remove any fat from the chicken breasts, after which slice into 1-inch-thick bits. Sprinkle the extra virgin olive oil to the chicken.*

✓ *Place each chicken piece in the flour bowl and toss until thoroughly covered, then move the chicken to the baking sheet that has been prepared.*

✓ *Roast for 20 minutes.*

✓ *To get exterior crispy, toggle the broiler and put the chicken nuggets underneath the broiler for 3–4 minutes.*

Nutrition: Calories: 149 Fat: 9gCarbohydrate: 29g

29) *Beef Fajitas*

Ingredients:

- 1 lb. beef stir-fry strips
- 1 medium red onion
- 1 red bell pepper
- 1 yellow bell pepper
- ½ tsp. cumin
- ½ tsp. chili powder
- Splash oil
- Salt Pepper
- ½ lime, juiced
- Freshly chopped cilantro (also called coriander)
- 1 avocado

Direction: Preparation Time: 6 minutes Cooking Time: 19 minutes Servings: 4

✓ *Over medium fire, steam a cast-iron pan.*

✓ *Clean and dress bell peppers, cut them into long strips of 0.5cm thick and then Set aside.*

✓ *Clean and cut the red onion into strips. Set aside.*

✓ *Add a little bit of oil once the skillet is heated. Add 2–3 packets of stir-fry strips while the oil is hot. Please ensure the strips wouldn't hit 1 another.*

✓ *Inside the pan, stir-fry each beef batch thoroughly with salt and pepper. Cook on each side for around 1 minute, set aside on a plate, and cover to stay warm.*
Introduce chopped onion as well as ringer peppers to the residual meat juice when all the beef is finished cooking and set aside. Sweetened with chili powder and cumin, then simmer-fry till the preferred consistency is achieved.

✓ *Move the stir-fry strips of vegetables and beef to just a plate and eat alongside a chopped avocado, a sprinkling of lemon juice, and a spray of fresh cilantro.*

✓ *Serve.*

Nutrition: Calories: 151 Fat: 6g Carbohydrate: 27g

30) *Keto Salad*

Ingredients:

- 4 cherry tomatoes
- Half avocado
- 1 hard-boiled egg
- 2 cups mixed green salad
- 2 oz. chicken breast, shredded
- 1 oz. feta cheese, crumbled
- ¼ cup cooked bacon, crumbled

Direction: Preparation Time: 11 minutes Cooking Time: 0 minutes Servings: 2

✓ *Slice the avocado and tomatoes. Slice the hard-boiled egg.*

✓ *On a large plate, put the mixed greens. Quantify the pulverized chicken breast, crushed bacon, and feta cheese.*

✓ *Position the tomatoes, egg, chicken, avocado, feta, and bacon on top of the greens in horizontal rows.*

Nutrition: Calories: 152 Fat: 9g Carbohydrate: 24g

31) *Instant Pot Chicken Chili*

Ingredients:

- 1 tbsp. vegetable oil
- 1 yellow diced onion
- 4 minced garlic cloves
- 1 tsp. ground cumin

- *1tsp. oregano*
- *2½ lb. chicken breasts, boneless and skinless*
- *16 oz. salsa Verde*

For Toppings

- *2 packages of queso fresco (crumbled) or sour cream*
- *2 diced avocados*
- *Finely chopped radishes*
- *Eight springs cilantro (optional)*

Direction: (Cooking Time:) Preparation Time: 6 minutes Cooking Time: 21 minutes Servings: 2

✓ *Set the Instant Pot to a medium sauté setting.*

✓ *Add the oil to the vegetables.*

✓ *Attach the onion and simmer for 3 mins till the onion starts to melt, stirring regularly.*

✓ *Apply the garlic, then stir for a minute.*

✓ *Add the oregano and cumin and simmer for the next minute.*

✓ *Through the pot, add ½ of the salsa Verde. Finish only with the breasts of the chicken and spill over the chicken mostly with leftover salsa Verde. Position the cover on the Instant Pot, switch the nozzle to "seal," and choose "manual." set the timer to 10 minutes.*

✓ *Then let the pressure release naturally when the timer is up.*

✓ *Lift the cover, move the chicken to a small bowl just after pressure has dropped, and slice it with a fork.*

✓ *To mix mainly with remaining ingredients, transfer the meat to the pot and stir.*

Nutrition: Calories: 144 Fat: 7g Carbohydrate: 20g

32)   *Smoked Cheese Wraps with Salmon and Cream*

Ingredients:

- *18-inch low carb flour tortilla*
- *2 oz. smoked salmon*
- *2tsp. low-fat cream cheese*
- *1 ½ oz. red onion*
- *Handful arugulas*
- *½ tsp. fresh or dried basil*
- *A pinch pepper*

Direction: Preparation Time: 12 minutes Cooking Time: 15 minutes Servings: 2

✓ *In the oven or microwave, warm the tortilla (pro tip: to prevent it from drying out, warm it between 2 pieces of moist paper towel).*

✓ *The cream cheese, basil, and pepper are mixed and then scattered over the tortilla.*
With the salmon, arugula, and finely sliced onion,

finish it off. Roll it up and enjoy the wrap!

Nutrition: Calories: 138 Fat: 6g Carbohydrate: 19g

33)   *Cheese Yogurt*

Ingredients:

- *1 thick and Creamy Yogurt or store-bought yogurt*
- *½ tsp. kosher salt*

Direction: Preparation Time: 12 minutes Cooking Time: 15 minutes Servings: 2

✓ *Line a strainer of twice the normal or plastic cheesecloth thickness.*

✓ *Place the strainer on top of a bowl and apply the yogurt.*
Cover and refrigerate for 2 hours. Stir in the salt and continue to drip for another 2 hours until the yogurt cheese is ready to spread.

Nutrition: Calories: 83 Protein: 5g Fat: 5.4g

34)   *Muffins of Savory Egg*

Ingredients:

- *1½ cups water*
- *2tbsp. unsalted butter*
- *1 (6 oz.) package Stove, Top lower-sodium Stuffing Mix for chicken*
- *3 oz. bulk pork sausage*
- *Cooking spray*
- *6 eggs, beaten*
- *½ cup (1.5 oz.) Monterey Jack cheese, shredded*
- *½ cup finely chopped red bell pepper*
- *¼ cup sliced green onions*

Direction: Preparation Time: 12 minutes Cooking Time: 33 minutes Servings: 6

✓ *Preheat oven to 400°F.*

✓ *In a medium saucepan, put 1 ½ cups water and butter to a boil. Stir in the blend of stuffing. Cover, and leave to stand for 5 minutes; use a fork to fluff. Let stand 10 minutes or before cool enough to hold, uncovered.*

✓ *Cook the sausage in a small skillet over medium-high heat until browned while the stuffing is cooling; stir to crumble. Coat the fingers with a mist for frying.*
Press approximately ¼ cup stuffing into the bottom and sides of each of the 12 deeply coated muffin cups with cooking oil. Pour the egg uniformly into the cups stuffing. Layer cheese, ham, bell pepper, and green onions equally over the egg if desired.

✓ *Bake for 18 to 20 minutes at 400°F or until the centers are centered. Let it stand before serving for 5 minutes. Run a thin, sharp knife along the edges* to loosen the muffin cups. Delete from the casseroles. Immediately serve.

Nutrition: Calories: 292 Fat: 16.7g Protein: 14.6g

35) *Parfaits of Yogurt, Honey, and Walnut*

Ingredients:

- cups Greek-style plain yogurt (don't use nonfat)
- ½ tsp. vanilla extract
  ½ cup honey

Direction: Preparation Time: 25 minutes Cooking Time: 15 minutes Servings: 6

✓ Preheat the oven to 375°F. Brush with the molten butter on a rimmed baking dish. Lay a tray of pastry on top.

✓ Sprinkle with more honey, then add sugar and nuts. Repeat with the remaining sheets of pastry, butter, sugar, and nuts.
Bake 10 to 15 minutes until golden brown and crisp. Enable it to cool on a wire rack on a baking sheet. Break the pastry into chunks.

✓ Mix the yogurt and vanilla in a tub. There are alternating layers of yogurt, honey, and phyllo bits in 4 glasses. Immediately serve.

Nutrition: Calories: 420 Fat: 22g Protein: 14g

36) *Greek-Yogurt Style*

Ingredients:

- 1 thick and Creamy Yogurt
  or store-bought yogurt

Direction: Preparation Time: 12 minutes Cooking Time: 15 minutes Servings: 2

✓ Line a double thickness strainer with standard or synthetic cheesecloth
Place the strainer on top of a bowl and apply the yogurt. Chill and cover. Depending on how dense you want it, let it drain for 1 to 2 ½ hours.

Nutrition: Calories: 240 Protein: 14g Fat: 14g

37) *Shrimp and Grits Cajun-Style*

Ingredients:

- 1 tbsp. olive oil
- ½ cups (2 oz.) Tasso ham, minced
- 1 cup chopped onion 1 garlic clove, minced
- Thirty-6 medium shrimp, peeled (about 1 ¼ lb.)
- 1 tsp. Cajun seasoning
- 2½ cups water, divided
- 1 tbsp. unsalted butter
- 1 cup fat-free milk
- ¼ tsp. salt

- 1 cup uncooked quick-cooking grits
- 1 cup (4 oz.) of sharp cheddar cheese, shredded
- ½ cup sliced green onions

Direction: Preparation Time: 12 minutes Cooking Time: 20 minutes Servings: 6

✓ Heat the olive oil over medium-high heat in a large skillet. Add Tasso; sauté for 2 minutes or until golden on the edges. Stir in the onion; sauté for 2 minutes. Stir in garlic; sauté for 1 minute.

✓ Sprinkle with Cajun seasoning, add the shrimp to the grill, and cook for 3 minutes, rotating once. Apply ¼ cup water to loosen the browned pieces, scratching the pan. Remove from heat; mix with butter, stirring until melted. Cover yourself and stay warm.
On medium-high heat, put milk, salt, and 2 cups of water to a boil—heat elimination. Add the grits steadily, and cook until thick and sparkling (about 5 minutes), stirring continuously with a whisk. Drop the grits from the high temperatures; add the cheese and stir until the cheese melts, with a whisk.

✓ On 6 plates, the spoon grates evenly. Using seafood, ham combination, and green onions to finish uniformly.

Nutrition: Calories: 346 Fat: 14g Protein: 24g

38) *Scramble for Lox, Eggs, and Onion*

Ingredients:

- 6 eggs
- 4 egg whites
- 1 tsp. canola oil
- 1/3 cup sliced green onions
- 4 oz. smoked salmon, cut into ½-inch pieces
- ¼ cup reduced-fat cream
- cheese, cut into 12 pieces
- ¼ tsp. freshly ground black pepper
- 4 slices pumpernickel bread, toasted

Direction: Preparation Time: 12 minutes Cooking Time: 15 minutes Servings: 4

✓ Place the eggs and egg whites in a bowl; stir until mixed with a whisk.

✓ Over medium-high prepare, heat a medium nonstick skillet. In a bath, apply oil; swirl to coat. In the pan, add the green onions; sauté for 2 minutes or until tender. Attach a tray of the egg mixture. Until the mixture settles on the rim, cook without stirring.
Draw a spatula to form curds over the bottom of the tub. Add the cream cheese and salmon. Continue to draw the spatula across the bottom of the pan until the egg mixture is somewhat thick but still moist; do not continuously stir.

✓ Remove directly from the pan. Sprinkle the pepper with the egg mixture. Serve the toast of *pumpernickel.*

Nutrition: Calories: 297 Fat: 14.5g Protein: 22.8g

39) *Peach and Pancakes with Blueberry*

Ingredients:

- *1½ cups all-purpose flour 2 tbsp. sugar*
- *2tbsp. flaxseed (optional)*
- *1 tbsp. Baking powder*
- *½ tsp. kosher salt*
- *1½ cups nonfat buttermilk*
- *1 tsp. grated lemon rind*
- *2eggs*
- *1 cup fresh or frozen blueberries, thawed*
- *1 cup chopped fresh or frozen peaches, thawed*
- *2 tbsp. unsalted butter*
- *Fresh blueberries (optional)*

Direction: Preparation Time: 12 minutes Cooking Time: 16 minutes Servings: 6

✓ *Weigh or spoon the flour gently into dry measuring cups; level it with a knife. In a large cup, mix the flour, sugar, flaxseed, baking powder, and salt if necessary, and stir with a fork.*

✓ *In a medium cup, mix the buttermilk, lemon rind, and eggs and stir with a fork. To the flour mixture, apply the buttermilk mixture, stirring only, so it is moist. Fold in the blueberries and peaches kindly. Heat a nonstick griddle or nonstick skillet over medium heat. Pour ⅓ of a cup flour into the pan per pancake. Cook for 2 to 3 minutes over medium heat or until bubbles cover the tops and the edges appear fried. Switch the cakes over gently; cook for 2–3 mins or until the bottoms become golden brown.*

Nutrition: Calories: 238 Fat 2.8g Protein: 8.1g

40) *Omelet with Turmeric, Tomato, and Onions*

Ingredients:

- *4 large eggs*
- *Kosher salt*
- *1 tbsp. olive oil*
- *¼ tsp. brown mustard seeds Turmeric powder*
- *2 green onions, finely chopped*
- *¼ cup diced plum tomato*
- *Dash black pepper*

Direction: Preparation Time: 8 minutes Cooking Time: 15 minutes Servings: 2

✓ *Whisk the eggs and salt together.*

✓ *Heat oil over medium-high heat in a large cast-iron skillet. Apply the mustard and turmeric seeds; simmer for 30 seconds or until the seeds pop up, stirring regularly. Add onions; simmer for 30 seconds or until tender, stirring regularly. Add the tomato; simmer for 1 minute or until very tender, stirring regularly.*
Pour the plate with the egg mixture; scatter uniformly. Cook until the edges are set (about 2 minutes). Slide the spatula's front edge between the omelet edge and the plate. Raise the omelet edge softly, tilting the pan to allow the pan to come into contact with any uncooked egg mixture.

✓ *Procedure to replicate on the opposite edge. Continue to cook till the center is really just set (about 2 minutes). Loosen the omelet and fold it in half with a spatula. Slide the omelet carefully onto a platter. Halve the omelet and dust it with black pepper.*

Nutrition: Calories: 216 Fat: 16.9g Protein: 13.3g

41) *Breakfast Bowl of Yogurt*

Ingredients:

- *1 tsp. tandoori spice or curry powder*
- *¼ cup honey*
- *2 cups 2% plain Greek yogurt*
- *½ cup all-natural granola*
- *1 cup fresh berries*
- *1 cup freeze-dried mango, pineapple, and/or berries*
- *Small sprigs of fresh cilantro*

Direction: Preparation Time: 8 minutes Cooking Time: 15 minutes Servings: 4

✓ *Toast the spices on low in a small skillet, stirring, until very fragrant, for about 2 minutes. Take it out of the oven, add honey and, stir.*
Break the yogurt into 4 cups. Drizzle with spiced honey; finish with cilantro, granola, and mango. Just serve.

Nutrition: Calories: 227 Fat: 3.1g Protein: 11g

42) *Tex-Mex Migas*

Ingredients:

- *3 large eggs*
- *3 egg whites*
- *1 tbsp. canola oil*
- *4 corn tortillas, cut into ½-inch-wide strips*
- *½ cup chopped onion*
- *2 large seeded jalapeño peppers*
- *2-third cup lower-sodium salsa*
- *½ cup Monterey Jack cheese, shredded*
- *½ cup sliced green onions*

- *Hot sauce (optional)*
- *Lower-sodium red salsa (optional)*
- *Lower-sodium green salsa (optional)*

Direction: Preparation Time: 9 minutes Cooking Time: 15 minutes Servings: 4

✓ *Place the eggs and egg whites in a bowl; stir until mixed with a whisk.*

✓ *Over medium-high prepare, heat a medium nonstick skillet. In a bath, apply oil; swirl to coat. Apply tortilla strips to the skillet and cook, stirring constantly, for 3 minutes or until brown.*
In a sauce, add the onion and jalapeño peppers; sauté for 2 minutes or until tender. Stir in 2/3 of a cup salsa, and simmer for 1 minute, stirring continuously.

✓ *Add the mixture of eggs; simmer for 2 minutes or until the eggs are tender, stirring periodically. Sprinkle the cheese with the egg mixture. Cook for thirty seconds or until the cheese is molten. Cover with the green onions, then serve right away. If preferred, serve with hot sauce, red salsa, or green salsa.*

Nutrition: Calories: 193 Fat: 10.4g Protein: 10.2g

43) *Barley Breakfast with Banana &Sunflower Breakfast Bowl of Yogurt Seeds*

Ingredients:

- *-third cup water*
- *1 third cup uncooked quick- Cooking pearl barley*
- *1 banana, sliced*
- *1 tsp. honey*
- *1 tbsp. unsalted sunflower seeds*

Direction: Preparation Time: 5 minutes Cooking Time: 11 minutes Servings: 1

✓ *In a shallow microwave-safe cup, mix water and barley a high 6-minute microwave.*

✓ *Delete and leave to stand for 2 minutes.*

✓ *Cover with slices of banana, sunflower seeds, and honey.*

Nutrition: Calories: 410 Fat: 6g Protein: 10g

44) *Banana Smoothie for Breakfast*

Ingredients:

- *½ cup 1% low-fat milk*
- *½ cup crushed ice*
- *1 tbsp. honey*
- *½ tsp. ground nutmeg*
- *1 frozen sliced ripe large banana*
- *1 cup plain 2% reduced-fat Greek yogurt*

Direction: Preparation Time: 12 minutes Cooking Time: 0 minute Servings: 2

✓ *In a blender, combine the first 5 ingredients; mix for 2 minutes or until smooth. Add the yogurt; just process until it's blended. Immediately serve.*

Nutrition: Calories: 212 Fat: 3.6g Protein: 14.2g

45) *Blackberry-Mango Shake*

Ingredients:

- *1 cup orange juice*
- *1 cup refrigerated bottled mango slices*
- *¼ cup light firm silken tofu 3 tbsp. honey*
- *1 ½ cups frozen blackberries*

Direction: Preparation Time: 12 minutes Cooking Time: 0 minutes Servings: 4

✓ *In a blender, place all ingredients in the order given; process until smooth*

Nutrition: Calories: 162 Fat: 0.6g Protein: 3.7g

46) *Bulgur Porridge Breakfast*

Ingredients:

- *4 cups 1% low-fat milk*
- *1 cup bulgur*
- *1/3 cup dried cherries*
- *¼ tbsp. salt*
- *1/3 cup dried apricots, coarsely chopped*
- *½ cup sliced almonds*

Direction: Preparation Time: 5 minutes Cooking Time: 15 minutes Servings: 4

✓ *Combine the milk, bulgur, dried cherries, and salt in a medium saucepan; bring it to a boil. Reduce heat to low and simmer, stirring regularly, until tender and the oatmeal consistency of the bulgur is tender (10–15 minutes).*
Divide into 4 bowls of hot porridge; top with the apricots and almonds.

Nutrition: Calories: 340 Fat: 6.7g Protein: 15g

47) *Turkey Meatballs*

Ingredients:

- *20 oz. ground turkey*
- *4 oz. fresh or frozen spinach ¼ cup oats*
- *2 egg whites*
- *2 celery sticks*
- *3 garlic cloves*
- *Half green bell peppers Half red onion*
- *½ cup parsley*
- *½ tsp. cumin*
- *1 tsp. mustard powder 1*
- *tsp. Thyme*

- ½ tbsp. Turmeric
- ½ tsp. chipotle pepper
- 1 tsp. salt
- Pinch pepper

Direction: Preparation Time: 16 minutes Cooking Time: 25 minutes Servings: 5

✓ Preheat the oven to 350ºF (175ºC).

✓ Chop very finely (or use a food processor) the onion, garlic, and celery, and add to a large mixing cup.

✓ In the dish, add the ham, egg whites, oats, and spices and combine well. Make sure the blend has no pockets of spices or oats.

✓ Spinach, green peppers (stalked and seeded), and parsley are chopped. The bits need to be about a dime's size.
To the tub, add the vegetables and mix them until well-combined.

✓ Line the parchment paper with a baking sheet.

✓ Roll the turkey mixture (about the size of golf balls) into 15 balls and put them on the baking sheet.

✓ Bake for 25 minutes, until fully baked.

Nutrition: Calories: 349 Fat: 7g Protein: 19g

48)   *Berry Avocado Smoothie*

Ingredients:

- Half an avocado
- 1 cup strawberries
- ¼ cup blueberries
- ½ cup low-fat milk
- ½ cup 2% Greek yogurt
- 1 tsp. raw honey, optional

Direction: Preparation Time: 7 minutes Cooking Time: 20 minutes Servings: 2

✓ Fill the blender with avocado, strawberries, blueberries, and milk.

✓ Blend until perfectly smooth.

✓ Taste, then, if using honey, you can add.

✓ Serve or put in a refrigerator for up to 2 days.

Nutrition: Calories: 350 Fat: 17g Protein: 24g

49)   *Bagel Hummus Toast*

Ingredients:

- soft boiled egg halved
- 6 tbsp. plain hummus
- 2 pieces' gluten-free bread, toasted
- Pinch paprika
- 2 tsp. Everything Bagel Spice
- Drizzle olive oil

Direction: Preparation Time: 30 minutes Cooking Time: 4 hours Servings: 2

✓ Spread each bread piece with 3 tbsp. Hummus.

✓ Attach a slice of halved egg and finish with 1 tsp. of 'Bagel' spice each.

✓ Sprinkle a small amount of paprika, muzzle with olive oil, and serve at once.

Nutrition: Calories: 213 Fat 11.6g Protein: 6.5g

50)   *Cinnamon Apple Chips*

Ingredients:

- 1 medium apple, sliced thin
- ¼ tsp. cinnamon
- ¼ tsp. nutmeg Nonstick cooking spray

Direction: Preparation Time: 6 minutes Cooking Time: 11 minutes Servings: 2

✓ Heat oven to 375°F. Spray a baking sheet with cooking spray.

✓ Place apples in a mixing bowl and add spices. Toss to coat.
Arrange apples, in a single layer, on the prepared pan. Bake 4 minutes, turn apples over and bake 4 minutes more.

✓ Serve immediately or store in an airtight container.

Nutrition: Calories: 58 Protein: 0.1g Fat 0.3g

51)   *Whole-Grain Breakfast Cookies*

Ingredients:

- cups rolled oats
- 1/2 cup whole-wheat flour
- ¼ cup ground flaxseed
- 1 teaspoon baking powder
- 1 cup unsweetened applesauce
- 2 large eggs
- 2 tablespoons vegetable oil
- 2 teaspoons vanilla extract
- 1 teaspoon ground cinnamon
- 1/2 cup dried cherries
- ¼ cup unsweetened shredded coconut
- 2 ounces dark chocolate, chopped

Direction: Preparation time: 20 minutesCooking time: 10 minutes Servings: 18 cookies

✓ Preheat the oven to 350F.

✓ In a large bowl, combine the oats, flour, flaxseed, and baking powder. Stir well to mix.

✓ In a medium bowl, whisk the applesauce, eggs, vegetable oil, vanilla, and cinnamon. Pour the wet mixture into the dry mixture, and stir until just combined.

✓ Fold in cherries, coconut, and chocolate. Drop tablespoon-size balls of dough onto a baking sheet. Bake for 10 to 12 minutes, until browned and cooked through.

✓ Let cool for about 3 minutes, remove from the baking sheet, and cool completely before serving. Store in an airtight container for up to 1 week.

Nutrition: Calories: 136; Total fat: 7g; Protein: 4g; Carbs: 14g;

52)   Blueberry Breakfast Cake

Ingredients:

FOR THE TOPPING

* ¼ cup finely chopped walnuts
* 1/2 teaspoon ground cinnamon
* 2 tablespoons butter, chopped into small pieces
* 2 tablespoons sugar
* or frozen blueberries

FOR THE CAKE

* Nonstick cooking spray
* 1 cup whole-wheat pastry flour
* 1 cup oat flour
* ¼ cup sugar
* 2 teaspoons baking powder
* 1 large egg, beaten
* 1/2 cup skim milk
* 2 tablespoons butter, melted
* 1 teaspoon grated lemon peel
* 2 cups fresh

Direction: Preparation time: 15 minutesCooking time: 45 minutes Servings: 12

✓ TO MAKE THE TOPPING

✓ In a small bowl, stir together the walnuts, cinnamon, butter, and sugar. Set aside.

✓ TO MAKE THE CAKE

✓ Preheat the oven to 350F. Spray a 9-inch square pan with cooking spray. Set aside.

✓ In a large bowl, stir together the pastry flour, oat flour, sugar, and baking powder. Add the egg, milk, butter, and lemon peel, and stir until there are no dry spots.

✓ Stir in the blueberries, and gently mix until incorporated. Press the batter into the prepared pan, using a spoon to flatten it into the dish.

✓ Sprinkle the topping over the cake.

✓ Bake for 40 to 45 minutes, until a toothpick inserted into the cake, comes out clean, and serve.

Nutrition: Calories: 177; Total fat: 7g; Saturated fat: 3g; Protein: 4g; Carbs: 26g; Sugar: 9g; Fiber: 3g;

53)   Whole-Grain Pancakes

Ingredients:

* 2 cups whole-wheat pastry flour
* 4 teaspoons baking powder
* 2 teaspoons ground cinnamon
* 1/2 teaspoon salt
* 2 cups skim milk, plus more as needed
* 2 large eggs
* 1 tablespoon honey
* Nonstick cooking spray
* Maple syrup, for serving
* Fresh fruit, for serving

Direction: Preparation time: 10 minutesCooking time: 15 minutes Servings: 4 to 6

✓ In a large bowl, stir together the flour, baking powder, cinnamon, and salt.

✓ Add the milk, eggs, and honey, and stir well to combine. If needed, add more milk, 1 tablespoon at a time, until there are no dry spots and you have a pourable batter.

✓ Heat a large skillet over medium-high heat, and spray it with cooking spray.
Using a ¼-cup measuring cup, scoop 2 or 3 pancakes into the skillet at a time. Cook for a couple of minutes, until bubbles form on the surface of the pancakes, flip, and cook for 1 to 2 minutes more, until golden brown and cooked through. Repeat with the remaining batter.

✓ Serve topped with maple syrup or fresh fruit.

Nutrition: Calories: 392; Total fat: 4g; Saturated fat: 1g; Protein: 15g; Carbs: 71g; Sugar: 11g; Fiber: 9g; Cholesterol: 95mg; Sodium: 396mg

54)   Buckwheat Grouts Breakfast Bowl

Ingredients:

* 3 cups skim milk
* 1 cup buckwheat grouts
* ¼ cup chia seeds
* 2 teaspoons vanilla extract
* 1/2 teaspoon ground cinnamon
* Pinch salt
* 1 cup water
* 1/2 cup unsalted pistachios
* 2 cups sliced fresh strawberries
* ¼ cup cacao nibs (optional)

Direction: Preparation time: 5 minutes, plus overnight to soak Cooking time: 10 to 12 minutes Servings: 4

✓ In a large bowl, stir together the milk, groats, chia seeds, vanilla, cinnamon, and salt. Cover and refrigerate overnight.

✓ *The next morning, transfer the soaked mixture to a medium pot and add the water. Bring to a boil over medium-high heat, reduce the heat to maintain a simmer, and cook for 10 to 12 minutes, until the buckwheat is tender and thickened.*
Transfer to bowls and serve, topped with the pistachios, strawberries, and cacao nibs (if using).

Nutrition: Calories: 340; Total fat: 8g; Saturated fat: 1g; Protein: 15g; Carbs: 52g; Sugar: 14g; Fiber: 10g;

55) *Peach Muesli Bake*

Ingredients:

- *Nonstick cooking spray*
- *2 cups skim milk*
- *11/2 cups rolled oats*
- *1/2 cup chopped walnuts*
- *1 large egg*
- *2 tablespoons maple syrup*
- *1 teaspoon ground cinnamon*
- *1 teaspoon baking powder*
- *1/2 teaspoon salt*
- *2 to 3 peaches, sliced*

Direction: Preparation time: 10 minutes Cooking time: 40 minutes Servings: 8

✓ *Preheat the oven to 375F. Spray a 9-inch square baking dish with cooking spray. Set aside.*

✓ *In a large bowl, stir together the milk, oats, walnuts, egg, maple syrup, cinnamon, baking powder, and salt. Spread half the mixture in the prepared baking dish.*

✓ *Place half the peaches in a single layer across the oat mixture.*
Spread the remaining oat mixture over the top. Add the remaining peaches in a thin layer over the oats. Bake for 35 to 40 minutes, uncovered until thickened and browned.

✓ *Cut into 8 squares and serve warm.*

Nutrition: Calories: 138; Total fat: 3g; Saturated fat: 1g; Protein: 6g; Carbs: 22g; Sugar: 10g; Fiber: 3g;

56) *Steel-Cut Oatmeal Bowl with Fruit and Nuts*

Ingredients:

- *1 cup steel-cut oats*
- *2 cups almond milk*
- *¾ cup water*
- *1 teaspoon ground cinnamon*
- *¼ teaspoon salt*
- *2 cups chopped fresh fruit, such as blueberries, strawberries, raspberries, or peaches*
- *1/2 cup chopped walnuts*

- *¼ cup chia seeds*

Direction: Preparation time: 5 minutes

Cooking time: 20 minutes Servings: 4

✓ *In a medium saucepan over medium-high heat, combine the oats, almond milk, water, cinnamon, and salt.*

✓ *Bring to a boil, reduce the heat to low, and simmer for 15 to 20 minutes, until the oats are softened and thickened*

✓ *Top each bowl with 1/2 cup of fresh fruit, 2 tablespoons of walnuts, and 1 tablespoon of chia seeds before serving.*

Nutrition: Calories: 288; Total fat: 11g; Saturated fat: 1g; Protein: 10g; Carbs: 38g; Sugar: 7g; Fiber: 10g; Cholesterol: 0mg; Sodium: 329mg

57) *Whole-Grain Dutch Baby Pancake*

Ingredients:

- *2 tablespoons coconut oil*
- *1/2 cup whole-wheat flour*
- *¼ cup skim milk*
- *3 large eggs*
- *1 teaspoon vanilla extract*
- *1/2 teaspoon baking powder*
- *¼ teaspoon salt*
- *¼ teaspoon ground cinnamon*
- *Powdered sugar, for dusting*

Direction: Preparation time: 5 minutes Cooking time: 25 minutes Servings: 4

✓ *Preheat the oven to 400F.*

✓ *Put the coconut oil in a medium oven-safe skillet, and place the skillet in the oven to melt the oil while it preheats.*

✓ *In a blender, combine the flour, milk, eggs, vanilla, baking powder, salt, and cinnamon. Process until smooth.*
Carefully remove the skillet from the oven and tilt it to spread the oil around evenly.

✓ *Pour the batter into the skillet and return it to the oven for 23 to 25 minutes, until the pancake puffs and lightly browns.*

✓ *Remove, dust lightly with powdered sugar, cut into 4 wedges, and serve.*

Nutrition: Calories: 195; Total fat: 11g; Saturated fat: 7g; Protein: 8g; Carbs: 16g; Sugar: 1g; Fiber: 2g;

58) *Mushroom, Zucchini, and Onion Frittata*

Ingredients:

- *1 tablespoon extra-virgin olive oil*

- *1/2 onion, chopped*
- *1 medium zucchini, chopped*
- *11/2 cups sliced mushrooms*
- *6 large eggs, beaten*
- *2 tablespoons skim milk*
- *Salt*
- *Freshly ground black pepper*
- *1 ounce feta cheese, crumbled*

Direction: Preparation time: 10 minutes Cooking time: 20 minutes Servings: 4

- ✓ *Preheat the oven to 400F.*
- ✓ *In a medium oven-safe skillet over medium-high heat, heat the olive oil.*
- ✓ *Add the onion and sauté for 3 to 5 minutes, until translucent.*
- ✓ *Add the zucchini and mushrooms, and cook for 3 to 5 more minutes, until the vegetables are tender. Meanwhile, in a small bowl, whisk the eggs, milk, salt, and pepper. Pour the mixture into the skillet, stirring to combine, and transfer the skillet to the oven. Cook for 7 to 9 minutes, until set.*
- ✓ *Sprinkle with the feta cheese, and cook for 1 to 2 minutes more, until heated through.*
- ✓ *Remove, cut into 4 wedges, and serve.*

Nutrition: Calories: 178; Total fat: 13g; Protein: 12g; Carbs: 5g; Sugar: 3g; Fiber: 1g;

59)   *Spinach and Cheese Quiche*

Ingredients:

- *Nonstick cooking spray*
- *8 ounces Yukon Gold potatoes, shredded*
- *1 tablespoon plus 2 teaspoons extra-virgin olive oil, divided*
- *1 teaspoon salt, divided*
- *Freshly ground black pepper*
- *1 onion, finely chopped*
- *1 (10-ounce) bag fresh spinach*
- *4 large eggs*
- *1/2 cup skim milk*
- *1 ounce Gruyere cheese, shredded*

Direction: Preparation time: 10 minutes, plus 10 minutes to rest Cooking time: 50 minutes Servings: 4 to 6

- ✓ *Preheat the oven to 350F. Spray a 9-inch pie dish with cooking spray. Set aside.*
- ✓ *In a small bowl, toss the potatoes with 2 teaspoons of olive oil, 1/2 teaspoon of salt, and season with pepper. Press the potatoes into the bottom and sides of the pie dish to form a thin, even layer. Bake for 20 minutes, until golden brown. Remove from the oven and set aside to cool.*
- ✓ *In a large skillet over medium-high heat, heat the*

remaining 1 tablespoon of olive oil.
- ✓ *Add the onion and sauté for 3 to 5 minutes, until softened.*
  By handfuls, add the spinach, stirring between each addition, until it just starts to wilt before adding more. Cook for about 1 minute, until it cooks down.
- ✓ *In a medium bowl, whisk the eggs and milk. Add the Gruyère, and season with the remaining 1/2 teaspoon of salt and some pepper. Fold the eggs into the spinach. Pour the mixture into the pie dish and bake for 25 minutes, until the eggs are set.*
- ✓ *Let rest for 10 minutes before serving.*

Nutrition: Calories: 445; Total fat: 14g; Saturated fat: 4g; Protein: 19g; Carbs: 68g; Sugar: 6g; Fiber: 7g; Cholesterol: 193mg; Sodium: 773mg

60)   *Spicy Jalapeno Popper Deviled Eggs*

Ingredients:

- *4 large whole eggs, hardboiled*
- *2 tablespoons Keto-Friendly mayonnaise*
- *¼ cup cheddar cheese, grated*
- *2 slices bacon, cooked and crumbled*
- *1 jalapeno, sliced*

Direction: Preparation Time: 5 minutes Cooking Time: 5 minutes Servings: 4

- ✓ *Cut eggs in half, remove the yolk and put them in a bowl*
- ✓ *Lay egg whites on a platter*
- ✓ *Mix in remaining ingredients and mash them with the egg yolks*
  Transfer yolk mix back to the egg whites
- ✓ *Serve and enjoy!*

Nutrition: Calories: 176; Fat: 14g; Carbohydrates: 0.7g; Protein: 10g

61)   *Lovely Porridge*

Ingredients:

- *2 tablespoons coconut flour*
- *2 tablespoons vanilla protein powder*
- *3 tablespoons Golden Flaxseed meal*
- *1 and 1/2 cups almond milk, unsweetened*
- *Powdered erythritol*

Direction: Preparation Time: 15 minutes

Cooking Time: Nil Servings: 2

- ✓ *Take a bowl and mix in flaxseed meal, protein powder, coconut flour and mix well*
- ✓ *Add mix to the saucepan (placed over medium heat)*
- ✓ *Add almond milk and stir, let the mixture thicken*

✓ *Add your desired amount of sweetener and serve*

Nutrition: Calories: 259; Fat: 13g; Carbohydrates: 5g;
Protein: 16g

62) *Salty Macadamia Chocolate Smoothie*

Ingredients:

- *2 tablespoons macadamia nuts, salted*
- *1/3 cup chocolate whey protein powder, low carb*
- *1 cup almond milk, unsweetened*

Direction: Preparation Time: 5 minutes

Cooking Time: Nil Servings: 1

✓ *Add the listed ingredients to your blender and blend until you have a smooth mixture*
Chill and enjoy it!

Nutrition: Cal: 165; Fat: 2g; Carbs: 1g; Protein: 12g

63) *Chocolate Chip Blondies*

Ingredients:

- *1 egg*
- *½ cup semi-sweet chocolate chips*
- *¹/3 cup flour*
- *¹/3 cup whole wheat flour*
- *¼ cup Splenda brown sugar*
- *1 egg*
- *½ cup semi-sweet chocolate chips*
- *¹/3 cup flour*
- *¹/3 cup whole wheat flour*
- *¼ cup Splenda brown sugar*

Direction: Preparation Time: 6 minutes Cooking Time: 21 minutes Servings: 12

✓ *Heat oven to 350°F. Spray an 8-inch square baking dish with cooking spray.*

✓ *In a small bowl, combine dry ingredients.*

✓ *In a large bowl, whisk together egg, oil, honey, and vanilla. Stir in the dry ingredients until combined. Stir in chocolate chips.*

✓ *Spread batter in prepared dish. Bake 20–22 minutes or until they pass the toothpick test. Cool on a wire rack then cut into bars.*

Nutrition: Calories: 136 Protein: 2g Fat: 6g

64) *Cinnamon and Coconut Porridge*

Ingredients:

- *2 cups of water*
- *1 cup 36% heavy cream*

- *1/2 cup unsweetened dried coconut, shredded*
- *2 tablespoons flaxseed meal*
- *1 tablespoon butter*
- *1 and 1/2 teaspoon stevia*
- *1 teaspoon cinnamon*
- *Salt to taste*
- *Toppings as blueberries*

Direction: Preparation Time: 5 minutes Cooking Time: 5 minutes Servings: 4

✓ *Add the listed ingredients to a small pot, mix well*

✓ *Transfer pot to stove and place it over medium-low heat*

✓ *Bring to mix to a slow boil*
Stir well and remove the heat

✓ *Divide the mix into equal servings and let them sit for 10 minutes*

✓ *Top with your desired toppings and enjoy!*

Nutrition: Calories: 171; Fat: 16g; Carbohydrates: 6g; Protein: 2g

65) *An Omelet of Swiss chard*

Ingredients:

- *4 eggs, lightly beaten*
- *4 cups Swiss chard, sliced*
- *2 tablespoons butter*
- *1/2 teaspoon garlic salt*
- *Fresh pepper*

Direction: Preparation Time: 5 minutes

Cooking Time: 5 minutes Servings: 4

✓ *Take a non-stick frying pan and place it over medium-low heat*

✓ *Once the butter melts, add Swiss chard and stir cook for 2 minutes*

✓ *Pour egg into the pan and gently stir them into Swiss chard*
Season with garlic salt and pepper

✓ *Cook for 2 minutes*

✓ *Serve and enjoy!*

Nutrition: Calories: 260; Fat: 21g; Carbohydrates: 4g; Protein: 14g

66) *Cheesy Low-Carb Omelet*

Ingredients:

- *2 whole eggs*
- *1 tablespoon water*
- *1 tablespoon butter*
- *3 thin slices of salami*
- *5 fresh basil leaves*
- *5 thin slices, fresh ripe tomatoes*

- *2 ounces fresh mozzarella cheese*
- *Salt and pepper as needed*

Direction: Preparation Time: 5 minutes Cooking Time: 5 minutes Servings: 5

✓ *Take a small bowl and whisk in eggs and water*

✓ *Take a non-stick Sauté pan and place it over medium heat, add butter and let it melt*

✓ *Pour egg mixture and cook for 30 seconds Spread salami slices on half of egg mix and top with cheese, tomatoes, basil slices*

✓ *Season with salt and pepper according to your taste*

✓ *Cook for 2 minutes and fold the egg with the empty half*

✓ *Cover and cook on LOW for 1 minute*

✓ *Serve and enjoy!*

Nutrition: Calories: 451; Fat: 36g; Carbohydrates: 3g; Protein:33g

67) *Yogurt And Kale Smoothie*

Ingredients:

- *1 cup whole milk yogurt*
- *1 cup baby kale greens*
- *1 pack stevia*
- *1 tablespoon MCT oil*
- *1 tablespoon sunflower seeds*
- *1 cup of water*

Direction: Servings: 1 Preparation Time: 10 minutes

✓ *Add listed ingredients to the blender*

✓ *Blend until you have a smooth and creamy texture Serve chilled and enjoy!*

Nutrition: Calories: 329; Fat: 26g; Carbohydrates: 15g; protein: 11g

68) *Chili Lime Tortilla Chips*

Ingredients:

- *12 6-inch corn tortillas, cut into 8 triangles*
- *3 tbsp. lime juice*
- *1 tsp. cumin*
- *1 tsp. chili powder*

Direction: Preparation Time: 6 minutes Cooking Time: 15 minutes Servings: 10

✓ *Heat oven to 350°F.*

✓ *Place tortilla triangles in a single layer on a large baking sheet.*

✓ *In a small bowl stir together spices.*

✓ *Sprinkle half the lime juice over tortillas, followed by ½ the spice mixture. Bake 7 minutes.*

✓ *Remove from oven and turn tortillas over. Sprinkle with remaining lime juice and spices. Bake another 8 minutes or until crisp, but not brown. Serve with your favorite salsa, the serving size is 10 chips.*

Nutrition: Calories: 65 Protein: 2g Fat 1g

69) *Grilled Chicken Platter*

Ingredients:

- *3 large chicken breast, sliced half lengthwise*
- *10-ounce spinach, frozen and drained*
- *3-ounce mozzarella cheese, part-skim*
- *1/2 a cup of roasted red peppers, cut in long strips*
- *1 teaspoon of olive oil*
- *2 garlic cloves, minced*
- *Salt and pepper as needed*

Direction: Preparation Time: 5 minutes Cooking Time: 10 minutes Servings: 6

✓ *Preheat your oven to 400 degrees Fahrenheit*

✓ *Slice 3 chicken breast lengthwise*

✓ *Take a non-stick pan and grease with cooking spray*

✓ *Bake for 2-3 minutes each side Take another skillet and cook spinach and garlic in oil for 3 minutes*

✓ *Place chicken on an oven pan and top with spinach, roasted peppers, and mozzarella*

✓ *Bake until the cheese melted*

✓ *Enjoy!*

Nutrition: Calories: 195; Fat: 7g; Carbohydrates: 3g; Protein: 30g

70) *Parsley Chicken Breast*

Ingredients:

- *1 tablespoon dry parsley*
- *1 tablespoon dry basil*
- *4 chicken breast halves, boneless and skinless*
- *1/2 teaspoon salt*
- *1/2 teaspoon red pepper flakes, crushed*
- *2 tomatoes, sliced*

Direction: Preparation Time: 10 minutes

Cooking Time: 40 minutes Servings: 4

✓ *Preheat your oven to 350 degrees F*

✓ *Take a 9x13 inch baking dish and grease it up with cooking spray*

✓ *Sprinkle 1 tablespoon of parsley, 1 teaspoon of basil and spread the mixture over your baking dish*

✓ *Arrange the chicken breast halves over the dish and sprinkle garlic slices on top Take a small bowl and add 1 teaspoon parsley, 1* teaspoon of basil, salt, basil, red pepper and mix well. Pour the mixture over the chicken breast

✓ Top with tomato slices and cover, bake for 25 minutes

✓ Remove the cover and bake for 15 minutes more

✓ Serve and enjoy!

Nutrition: Calories: 150; Fat: 4g; Carbohydrates: 4g; Protein: 25g

71)   *Mustard Chicken*

Ingredients:

- 4 chicken breasts
- 1/2 cup chicken broth
- 3-4 tablespoons mustard
- 3 tablespoons olive oil
- 1 teaspoon paprika
- 1 teaspoon chili powder
- 1 teaspoon garlic powder

Direction: Preparation Time: 10 minutes

Cooking Time: 40 minutes Servings: 4

✓ Take a small bowl and mix mustard, olive oil, paprika, chicken broth, garlic powder, chicken broth, and chili

✓ Add chicken breast and marinate for 30 minutes Take a lined baking sheet and arrange the chicken

✓ Bake for 35 minutes at 375 degrees Fahrenheit

✓ Serve and enjoy!

Nutrition: Calories: 531; Fat: 23g; Carbohydrates: 10g; Protein: 64g

72)   *Balsamic Chicken*

Ingredients:

- 6 chicken breast halves, skinless and boneless
- 1 teaspoon garlic salt
- Ground black pepper
- 2 tablespoons olive oil
- 1 onion, thinly sliced
- 14 and 1/2 ounces tomatoes, diced
- 1/2 cup balsamic vinegar
- 1 teaspoon dried basil
- 1 teaspoon dried oregano
- 1 teaspoon dried rosemary
- 1/2 teaspoon dried thyme

Direction: Preparation Time: 10 minutes Cooking Time: 25 minutes Servings: 6

✓ Season both sides of your chicken breasts thoroughly with pepper and garlic salt

✓ Take a skillet and place it over medium heat

✓ Add some oil and cook your seasoned chicken for 3-4 minutes per side until the breasts are nicely browned

✓ Add some onion and cook for another 3-4 minutes until the onions are browned
Pour the diced up tomatoes and balsamic vinegar over your chicken and season with some rosemary, basil, thyme, and rosemary

✓ Simmer the chicken for about 15 minutes until they are no longer pink

✓ Take an instant-read thermometer and check if the internal temperature gives a reading of 165 degrees Fahrenheit

✓ If yes, then you are good to go!

Nutrition: Calories: 196; Fat: 7g; Carbohydrates: 7g; Protein: 23g

73)   *Greek Chicken Breast*

Ingredients:

- 4 chicken breast halves, skinless and boneless
- 1 cup extra virgin olive oil
- 1 lemon, juiced
- 2 teaspoons garlic, crushed
- 1 and 1/2 teaspoons black pepper
- 1/3 teaspoon paprika

Direction: Preparation Time: 10 minutes Cooking Time: 25 minutes Servings: 4

✓ Cut 3 slits in the chicken breast

✓ Take a small bowl and whisk in olive oil, salt, lemon juice, garlic, paprika, pepper and whisk for 30 seconds

✓ Place chicken in a large bowl and pour marinade

✓ Rub the marinade all over using your hand Refrigerate overnight

✓ Pre-heat grill to medium heat and oil the grate

✓ Cook chicken in the grill until the center is no longer pink

✓ Serve and enjoy!

Nutrition: Calories: 644; Fat: 57g; Carbohydrates: 2g; Protein: 27g

74)   *Chipotle Lettuce Chicken*

Ingredients:

- 1 pound chicken breast, cut into strips
- Splash of olive oil
- 1 red onion, finely sliced
- 14 ounces tomatoes
- 1 teaspoon chipotle, chopped
- 1/2 teaspoon cumin
- Pinch of sugar

- *Lettuce as needed*
- *Fresh coriander leaves*
- *Jalapeno chilies, sliced*
- *Fresh tomato slices for garnish*
- *Lime wedges*

Direction: Preparation Time: 10 minutes Cooking Time: 25 minutes Servings: 6

✓ *Take a non-stick frying pan and place it over medium heat*
✓ *Add oil and heat it up*
✓ *Add chicken and cook until brown*
✓ *Keep the chicken on the side*
✓ *Add tomatoes, sugar, chipotle, cumin to the same pan and simmer for 25 minutes until you have a nice sauce*
  Add chicken into the sauce and cook for 5 minutes
✓ *Transfer the mix to another place*
✓ *Use lettuce wraps to take a portion of the mixture and serve with a squeeze of lemon*
✓ *Enjoy!*

Nutrition: Calories: 332; Fat: 15g; Carbohydrates: 13g; Protein: 34g

75) *Stylish Chicken-Bacon Wrap*

Ingredients:

- *8 ounces lean chicken breast*
- *6 bacon slices*
- *3 ounces shredded cheese*
- *4 slices ham*

Direction: Preparation Time: 5 minutes Cooking Time: 50 minutes Servings: 3

✓ *Cut chicken breast into bite-sized portions*
✓ *Transfer shredded cheese onto ham slices*
✓ *Roll up chicken breast and ham slices in bacon slices*
✓ *Take a skillet and place it over medium heat*
  Add olive oil and brown bacon for a while
✓ *Remove rolls and transfer to your oven*
✓ *Bake for 45 minutes at 325 degrees F*
✓ *Serve and enjoy!*

Nutrition: Calories: 275; Fat: 11g; Carbohydrates: 0.5g; Protein: 40g

76) *Healthy Cottage Cheese Pancakes*

Ingredients:

- *1/2 cup of Cottage cheese (low-fat)*
- *1/3 cup (approx. 2 egg whites) Egg whites*
- *¼ cup of Oats*
- *1 teaspoon of Vanilla extract*

- *Olive oil cooking spray*
- *1 tablespoon of Stevia (raw)*
- *Berries or sugar-free jam (optional)*

Direction: Preparation Time: 10 minutes

Cooking Time: 15 Servings: 1

✓ *Begin by taking a food blender and adding in the egg whites and cottage cheese. Also, add in the vanilla extract, a pinch of stevia, and oats. Palpitate until the consistency is well smooth.*
✓ *Get a nonstick pan and oil it nicely with the cooking spray. Position the pan on low heat.*
  After it has been heated, scoop out half of the batter and pour it on the pan—Cook for about 21/2 minutes on each side.
✓ *Position the cooked pancakes on a serving plate and cover them with sugar-free jam or berries.*

Nutrition: Calories: 205 calories per serving Fat – 1.5 g, Protein – 24.5 g, Carbs– 19 g

77) *Avocado Lemon Toast*

Ingredients:

- *Whole-grain bread – 2 slices*
- *Fresh cilantro (chopped) – 2 tablespoons*
- *Lemon zest – ¼ teaspoon*
- *Fine sea salt – 1 pinch*
- *Cayenne pepper – 1 pinch*
- *Chia seeds – ¼ teaspoon*
- *Avocado – 1/2*
- *Fresh lemon juice – 1 teaspoon*

Direction: Preparation Time: 10 minutesCooking Time: 13 minutes Servings: 2

✓ *Begin by getting a medium-sized mixing bowl and adding in the avocado. Make use of a fork to crush it properly.*
✓ *Then, add in the cilantro, lemon zest, lemon juice, sea salt, and cayenne pepper. Mix well until combined.*
  Toast the bread slices in a toaster until golden brown. It should take about 3 minutes.
✓ *Top the toasted bread slices with the avocado mixture and finalize by drizzling with chia seeds.*

Nutrition: Calories: 72 calories per serving; Protein – 3.6 g; Fat – 1.2 g; Carbs – 11.6 g

78) *Healthy Baked Eggs*

Ingredients:

- *Olive oil – 1 tablespoon*
- *Garlic – 2 cloves*
- *Eggs – 8 large*
- *Sea salt – 1/2 teaspoon*

- *Shredded mozzarella cheese (medium-fat) – 3 cups*
- *Olive oil spray*
- *Onion (chopped) – 1 medium*
- *Spinach leaves – 8 ounces*
- *Half-and-half – 1 cup*
- *Black pepper – 1 teaspoon*
- *Feta cheese – 1/2 cup*

Direction: Preparation Time: 10 minutesCooking Time: 1 hour Servings: 6

✓ *Begin by heating the oven to 375F.*

✓ *Get a glass baking dish and grease it with olive oil spray. Arrange aside.*

✓ *Now take a nonstick pan and pour in the olive oil. Position the pan on allows heat and allows it heat.*

✓ *Immediately you are done, toss in the garlic, spinach, and onion. Prepare for about 5 minutes. Arrange aside.*

✓ *You can now Get a large mixing bowl and add in half eggs, pepper, and salt. Whisk thoroughly to combine.*
Put in the feta cheese and chopped mozzarella cheese (reserve 1/2 cup of mozzarella cheese for later).

✓ *Put the egg mixture and prepared spinach into the prepared glass baking dish. Blend well to combine. Drizzle the reserved cheese over the top.*

✓ *Bake the egg mix for about 45 minutes.*

✓ *Extract the baking dish from the oven and allow it to stand for 10 minutes.*

✓ *Dice and serve!*

Nutrition: Calories: 323 calories per serving; Fat 22.3 g; Protein 22.6 g; Carbs 7.9 g

79)   *Quick Low-Carb Oatmeal*

Ingredients:

- *Almond flour – 1/2 cup*
- *Flax meal – 2 tablespoons*
- *Cinnamon (ground) – 1 teaspoon*
- *Almond milk (unsweetened) – 11/2 cups*
- *Salt – as per taste*
- *Chia seeds – 2 tablespoons*
- *Liquid stevia – 10 – 15 drops*
- *Vanilla extract – 1 teaspoon*

Direction: Preparation Time: 10 minutes Cooking Time: 15 minutes Servings: 2

✓ *Begin by taking a large mixing bowl and adding in the coconut flour, almond flour, ground cinnamon, flax seed powder, and chia seeds. Mix properly to combine.*

✓ *Position a stockpot on low heat and add in the dry ingredients. Also, add in the liquid stevia, vanilla*

extract, and almond milk. Mix well to combine. Prepare the flour and almond milk for about 4 minutes. Add salt if needed.

✓ *Move the oatmeal to a serving bowl and top with nuts, seeds, and pure and neat berries.*

Nutrition: Calories: calories per serving; Protein – 11.7 g; Fat – 24.3 g; Carbs – 16.7 g

80)   *Cranberry & Almond Granola Bars*

Ingredients:

- *1 egg*
- *egg white*
- *cup low-fat granola*
- *¼ cup dried cranberries, sweetened*
- *¼ cup almonds, chopped*
- *2 tbsp. Splenda*
- *tsp. Almond extract*
- *½ tsp. cinnamon*

Direction: Preparation Time: 14 minutes Cooking Time: 21 minutes Servings: 12

✓ *Heat oven to 350°F. Line the bottom and sides of an 8-inch baking dish with parchment paper.*

✓ *In a large bowl, combine dry ingredients, including the cranberries.*

✓ *In a small bowl, whisk together egg, egg white, and extract. Pour over dry ingredients and mix until combined.*

✓ *Press mixture into the prepared pan. Bake 20 minutes or until light brown.*

✓ *Cool in the pan for 5 minutes. Then carefully lift the bars from the pan onto a cutting board. Use a sharp knife to cut into 12 bars. Cool completely and store in an airtight container.*

Nutrition: Calories: 85 Protein: 3g Fat: 3g

81)   *Cinnamon Apple Popcorn*

Ingredients:

- *4 tbsp. margarine, melted*
- *10 cup plain popcorn*
- *2 cup dried apple rings, unsweetened and chopped*
- *½ cup walnuts, chopped*
- *2 tbsp. Splenda brown sugar 1 tsp. Cinnamon*
- *½ tsp. vanilla*

Direction: Preparation Time: 31 minutes Cooking Time: 50 minutes Servings: 11

✓ *Heat oven to 250°F.*

✓ *Place chopped apples in a 9x13-inch baking dish and bake for 20 minutes. Remove from oven and stir in popcorn and nuts.*

✓ In a small bowl, whisk together margarine, vanilla, Splenda, and cinnamon. Drizzle evenly over popcorn and toss to coat.
Bake 30 minutes, stirring quickly every 10 minutes. If apples start to turn a dark brown, remove them immediately.

✓ Pout onto waxed paper to cool for at least 30 minutes. Store in an airtight container.

Nutrition: Calories: 133 Protein: 3g Fat 8g

82)   Crab & Spinach Dip

Ingredients:

- 1 pkg. frozen chopped spinach, thawed and squeezed nearly dry
- 8 oz. reduced-fat cream cheese
- 6 ½ oz. can crab meat, drained and shredded
- 6 oz. jar marinated artichoke hearts, drained and diced fine
- ¼ tsp. hot pepper sauce
- Melba toast or whole-grain crackers (optional)

Direction: Preparation Time: 9 minutes Cooking Time: 2 hours Servings: 10

✓ Remove any shells or cartilage from the crab.

✓ Place all the ingredients in a small crockpot. Cover and cook on high for 1

✓ ½–2 hours, or until heated through and cream cheese is melted. Stir after 1 hour.
Serve with Melba toast or whole-grain crackers. The serving size is ¼ cup.

Nutrition: Calories: 106 Protein: 5g Fat 8g

83)   Tomato and Zucchini Sauté

Ingredients:

- Vegetable oil – 1 tablespoon
- Tomatoes (chopped) – 2
- Green bell pepper (chopped)
- Black pepper (freshly ground) – as per taste
  Onion (sliced)
- 1 Zucchini (peeled) – 2 pounds and cut into 1-inch-thick slices
- Salt – as per taste
- Uncooked white rice – ¼ cup

Direction: Preparation Time: 10 minutes Cooking Time: 43 minutes Servings: 6

✓ Begin by getting a nonstick pan and putting it over low heat. Stream in the oil and allow it to heat through.

✓ Put in the onions and sauté for about 3 minutes.

✓ Then pour in the zucchini and green peppers. Mix well and spice with black pepper and salt.
Reduce the heat and cover the pan with a lid. Allow the veggies to cook on low for 5 minutes.

✓ While you're done, put in the water and rice. Place the lid back on and cook on low for 20 minutes.

Nutrition: Calories: 94 calories per serving; Fat – 2.8 g; Protein – 3.2 g; Carbs – 16.1 g

84)   Steamed Kale with Mediterranean Dressing

Ingredients:

- Kale (chopped) – 12 cups
- Olive oil – 1 tablespoon
- Soy sauce – 1 teaspoon
- Pepper (freshly ground) – as per taste
- Lemon juice – 2 tablespoons
- Garlic (minced) – 1 tablespoon
- Salt – as per taste

Direction: Preparation Time: 10 minutes Cooking Time: 25 minutes Servings: 6

✓ Get a gas steamer or an electric steamer and fill the bottom pan with water. If making use of a gas steamer, position it on high heat. Making use of an electric steamer, place it on the highest setting.

✓ Immediately the water comes to a boil, put in the shredded kale and cover with a lid. Boil for about 8 minutes. The kale should be tender by now. During the kale is boiling, take a big mixing bowl and put in the olive oil, lemon juice, soy sauce, garlic, pepper, and salt. Whisk well to mix.

✓ Now toss in the steamed kale and carefully enclose it into the dressing. Be assured the kale is well-coated.

✓ Serve while it's hot!

Nutrition: Calories: 91 calories per serving; Fat – 3.5 g; Protein – 4.6 g; Carbs – 14.5 g

85)   Vegetable Noodles Stir-Fry

Ingredients:

- White sweet potato – 1 pound
- Zucchini – 8 ounces
- Garlic cloves (finely chopped) – 2 large
- Vegetable broth – 2 tablespoons
- Salt – as per taste
- Carrots – 8 ounces
- Shallot (finely chopped) – 1
- Red chili (finely chopped) – 1
- Olive oil – 1 tablespoon
- Pepper – as per taste

Direction: Preparation Time: 10 minutes

Cooking Time: 40 minutes Servings: 4

✓ Begin by scrapping the carrots and sweet potato.

Make Use a spiralizer to make noodles out of the sweet potato and carrots.

✓ *Rinse the zucchini thoroughly and spiralize it as well.*

✓ *Get a large skillet and position it on a high flame. Stream in the vegetable broth and allow it to come to a boil.*
Toss in the spiralized sweet potato and carrots. Then put in the chili, garlic, and shallots. Stir everything using tongs and cook for some minutes.

✓ *Transfer the vegetable noodles into a serving platter and generously spice with pepper and salt.*

✓ *Finalize by sprinkling olive oil over the noodles. Serve while hot!*

Nutrition: Calories: 169 calories per serving; Fat 3.7 g; Protein 3.6 g; Carbs – 31.2 g

86) Millet Porridge

Ingredients:

- *1 cup millet, rinsed and drained*
- *Pinch of salt*
- *3 cups water*
- *2 tablespoons almonds, chopped finely*
- *6-8 drops liquid stevia*
- *1 cup unsweetened almond milk*
- *2 tablespoons fresh blueberries*

Direction: Preparation Time: 10 minutes Cooking Time: 25 minutes Servings: 4

✓ *In a nonstick pan, add the millet over medium-low heat and cook for about 3 minutes, stirring continuously.*

✓ *Add the salt and water and stir to combine. Increase the heat to medium and bring to a boil.*

✓ *Cook for about 15 minutes.*

✓ *Stir in the almonds, stevia and almond milk and cook for 5 minutes.*
Top with the blueberries and serve. **Meal Prep Tip:**

✓ *Transfer the cooled porridge to an airtight container and preserve it in the refrigerator for up to 2 days.*

✓ *Just before serving, reheat in the microwave.*

✓ *Serve with the topping of berries.*

Nutrition: Calories 219 Total Fat 4.5 g Saturated Fat 0.6 g Cholesterol 0 mg Total Carbs 38.2 g Sugar 0.6 g Fiber 5 g Sodium 92 mg Potassium 1721 mg Protein 6.4 g

87) Sweet Potato Waffles

Ingredients:

- *1 medium sweet potato, peeled, grated and squeezed*
- *1 teaspoon fresh thyme, minced*

- *1 teaspoon fresh rosemary, minced*
- *1/8 teaspoon red pepper flakes, crushed*
- *Salt and ground black pepper, as required*

Direction: Preparation Time: 10 minutes Cooking Time: 20 minutes Servings: 2

✓ *Preheat the waffle iron and then grease it.*

✓ *In a large bowl, add all ingredients and mix till well combined.*

✓ *Place half of the sweet potato mixture into preheated waffle iron and cook for about 8-10 minutes or until golden brown.*

✓ *Repeat with the remaining mixture.*

✓ *Serve warm.*
Meal Prep Tip:

✓ *Store these cooled waffles into an airtight container by placing a piece of wax paper between each waffle.*

✓ *Refrigerate for up to 5 days. Reheat in the microwave for about 1-2 minutes.*

Nutrition: Calories 72 Total Fat 0.3 g Saturated Fat 0.1 g Cholesterol 0 mg Total Carbs 16.3 g Sugar 4.9 g Fiber 3 g Sodium 28 mg Potassium 369 mg Protein 1.6 g

88) Quinoa Bread

Ingredients:

- *1 ¾ cups uncooked quinoa, rinsed, soaked overnight and drained*
- *¼ cup chia seeds, soaked in ½ cup of water overnight*
- *½ teaspoon bicarbonate soda*
- *Pinch of sea salt*
- *½ cup filtered water*
- *¼ cup olive oil, melted*
- *1 tablespoon fresh lemon juice*

Direction: Preparation Time: 10 minutes Cooking Time: 1½ hours Servings: 12

✓ *Preheat the oven to 320 degrees F. Line a loaf pan with parchment paper.*

✓ *In a food processor, add all the ingredients and pulse for about 3 minutes.*

✓ *Transfer the mixture into the prepared loaf pan evenly.*

✓ *Bake for about 1½ hours or until a wooden skewer inserted in the center of the loaf comes out clean.*

✓ *Remove the pan from the oven and place it onto a wire rack to cool for about 10-15 minutes.*

✓ *Carefully remove the bread from the loaf pan and place it onto the wire rack to cool completely before slicing.*
With a sharp knife, cut the bread loaf into desired-sized slices and serve.

Meal Prep Tip:

✓ In a resealable plastic bag, place the bread and seal the bag after squeezing out the excess air.

✓ Set the bread away from direct sunlight and preserve it in a cool and dry place for about 1-2 days.

Nutrition: Calories 137 Total Fat 6.5 g Saturated Fat 0.9 g Cholesterol 0 mg Total Carbs 16.9 g Sugar 0 g Fiber 2.6 g Protein 4 g

89) *Veggie Frittata*

Ingredients:

- 1 tablespoon olive oil
- 1 large sweet potato, peeled and cut into thin slices
- 1 yellow squash, sliced
- 1 zucchini, sliced
- ½ of red bell pepper, seeded and sliced
- ½ of yellow bell pepper, seeded and sliced
- 8 eggs
- Salt and ground black pepper, as required
- 2 tablespoons fresh cilantro, chopped finely

Direction: Preparation Time: 15 minutes Cooking Time: 25 minutes Servings: 6

✓ Preheat the oven to the broiler.

✓ In a large oven-proof skillet, heat the oil over medium-low heat and cook the sweet potato for about 6-7 minutes.

✓ Add the yellow squash, zucchini and bell peppers and cook for about 3-4 minutes.

✓ Meanwhile, in a bowl, add the eggs, salt and black pepper and beat until well combined.

✓ Pour egg mixture over vegetable mixture evenly.

✓ Immediately, reduce the heat to low and cook for about 8-10 minutes or until just done.
Transfer the skillet in the oven and broil for about 3-4 minutes or until the top becomes golden brown.

✓ With a sharp knife, cut the frittata in desired size slices and serve with the garnishing of cilantro.

Meal Prep Tip:

✓ In a resealable plastic bag, place the cooled frittata slices and seal the bag.

✓ Refrigerate for about 2-4 days.

✓ Reheat in the microwave on High for about 1 minute before serving.

Nutrition: Calories 143 Total Fat 8.4 g Saturated Fat 2.2 g Cholesterol 218 mg Total Carbs 9.3 g Sugar 4.2

90) *Chicken & Sweet Potato Hash*

Ingredients:

- 2 tablespoons olive oil, divided
- 1½ pounds boneless, skinless chicken breasts, cubed

- Salt and ground black pepper, as required
- 2 celery stalks, chopped
- 1 medium white onion, chopped
- 4 garlic cloves, minced
- 1 tablespoon fresh oregano, chopped
- 1 tablespoon fresh thyme, chopped
- 2 large sweet potatoes, peeled and cubed
- 1 cup low-sodium chicken broth
- 1 cup scallion, chopped
- 2 tablespoons fresh lime juice

Direction: Preparation Time: 15 minutes Cooking Time: 35 minutes Servings: 8

✓ In a large skillet, heat 1 tablespoon of oil over medium heat and cook the chicken with a little salt and black pepper for about 4-5 minutes.

✓ Transfer the chicken into a bowl. In the same skillet, heat the remaining oil over medium heat and sauté celery and onion for about 3-4 minutes.

✓ Add the garlic and herbs and sauté for about 1 minute. Add the sweet potato and cook for about 8-10 minutes.
Add the broth and cook for about 8-10 minutes.

✓ Add the cooked chicken and scallion and cook for about 5 minutes.

✓ Stir in lemon juice, salt and serve. **Meal Prep Tip:** Transfer the cooled hash in an airtight container and preserve it in the refrigerator for up to 2 days. Just before serving, reheat in the microwave.

Nutrition: Calories 253 Total Fat 10 g Saturated Fat 2.3 g Cholesterol 76 mg Total Carbs 14 g Sugar 1.2 g Fiber 2.6 g Sodium 92 mg Protein 26 g

91) *Strawberry & Spinach Smoothie*

Ingredients:

- 1½ cups fresh strawberries, hulled and sliced
- 2 cups fresh baby spinach
- ½ cup fat-free plain Greek yogurt
- 1 cup unsweetened almond milk
- ¼ cup ice cubes

Direction: Preparation Time: 10 minutes Servings: 2

✓ In a high-speed blender, add all the ingredients and pulse until smooth. Pour into serving glasses and serve immediately.

Meal Prep Tip:

✓ In 2 zip lock bags, divide the strawberries and spinach. Seal the bags and store them in the freezer for about 2-3 days.

✓ Just before serving, remove from the freezer and transfer into a blender with yogurt, almond milk and ice cubes and pulse until smooth.

Nutrition: Calories 96 Total Fat 2.3 g Saturated Fat 0.2 g Cholesterol 1 mg Total Carbs 12.3 g Sugar 7.7 g Fiber 3.9 g Sodium 144 mg Potassium 428 mg Protein 8.1 g

92)   *Quinoa Porridge Recipe 1*

Ingredients:

- 2 cups water 1 cup dry quinoa, rinsed
- ½ teaspoon organic vanilla extract
- ½ cup unsweetened almond milk
- 10-12 drops liquid stevia
- ¼ teaspoon lemon peel, grated freshly
- ½ teaspoon ground cinnamon
- ½ teaspoon ground nutmeg
- Pinch of ground cloves
- 1 cup fresh mixed berries

Direction: Preparation Time: 10 minutes Cooking Time: 15 minutes Servings: 4

✓ In a pan, mix together the water, quinoa and vanilla essence over low heat and cook for about 15 minutes, stirring occasionally.

✓ Stir in the almond milk, stevia, lemon peel and spices and immediately remove from the heat.

✓ Top with the berries and serve warm.

✓ **Meal Prep Tip:**

✓ Transfer the cooled porridge to an airtight container and preserve it in the refrigerator for up to 2 days.

✓ Just before serving, reheat in the microwave. Serve with the topping of berries.

Nutrition: Calories 186 Total Fat 3.3 g Saturated Fat 0.4 g Cholesterol 0 mg Total Carbs 32.3 g Sugar 2.7 g Fiber 4.6 g Sodium 25 mg Protein 6.4 g

93)   *Millet Porridge 2*

Ingredients:

- 1 cup millet, rinsed and drained
- Pinch of salt
- 3 cups water
- 2 tablespoons almonds, and Nuts chopped finely
- 8-10 drops liquid stevia
- 1 cup unsweetened almond milk or Coconut Milk
- 2 tablespoons fresh blueberries or Strawberries

Direction: Preparation Time: 12 minutes Cooking Time: 25 minutes Servings: 4

✓ In a nonstick pan, add the millet over medium-low heat and cook for about 3 minutes, stirring continuously.

✓ Add the salt and water and stir to combine. Increase the heat to medium and bring to a boil.

✓ Cook for about 15 minutes.

✓ Stir in the almonds, stevia, and almond milk and cook for 5 minutes.
Top with the blueberries and serve.

✓ **Meal Prep Tip:**

✓ Transfer the cooled porridge to an airtight container and preserve it in the refrigerator for up to 2 days.

✓ Just before serving, reheat in the microwave.

✓ Serve with the topping of berries.

Nutrition: Calories 219 Total Fat 4.5 g Saturated Fat 0.6 g Cholesterol 0 mg Total Carbs 38.2 g Protein 6.4 g

94)   *Bell Pepper Pancakes*

Ingredients:

- ½ cup chickpea flour
- ¼ teaspoon baking powder
- Pinch of sea salt Pinch of red pepper flakes, crushed
- ½ cup plus
- 2 tablespoons filtered water
- ¼ cup green bell peppers, seeded and chopped finely
- ¼ cup scallion, chopped finely
- 2 teaspoons olive oil

Direction: Preparation Time: 15 minutes Cooking Time: 8 minutes Servings: 2

✓ In a bowl, mix together flour, baking powder, salt and red pepper flakes.

✓ Add the water and mix until well combined.

✓ Fold in bell pepper and scallion. In a large frying pan, heat the oil over low heat.

✓ Add half of the mixture and cook for about 1-2 minutes per side.
Repeat with the remaining mixture.

✓ Serve warm.

Meal Prep Tip:

✓ Store these cooled pancakes into an airtight container by placing a piece of wax paper between each pancake.

✓ Refrigerate for up to 4 days.

✓ Reheat in the microwave for about 1½-2 minutes.

Nutrition: Calories 232 Total Fat 7.8 g Saturated Fat 1 g Cholesterol 0 mg Total Carbs 32.7 g Sugar 6.4 g Fiber 9.3 g Sodium 132 mg Potassium 566 mg Protein 10 g

95)   *Red Pepper, Goat Cheese, and Arugula Open-Faced Grilled Sandwich*

Ingredients:

- 1 red bell pepper, seeded
- Nonstick cooking spray
- 2 slice whole-wheat thin-sliced bread
- 4 tbsp. crumbled goat cheese
- Pinch dried thyme

- *1 cup arugula*

Direction: Preparation Time: 5 minutes Cooking Time: 15 minutes Servings: 2

✓ *Preheat the broiler to high heat. Line a baking sheet with parchment paper.*

✓ *Cut the ½ bell pepper lengthwise into 2 pieces and arrange the prepared baking sheet with the skin facing up.*

✓ *Broil until the skin is blackened for about 5 to 10 minutes. Transfer to a covered container to steam for 5 minutes, then remove the skin from the pepper using your fingers. Cut the pepper into strips. Heat a small skillet over medium-high heat. Spray it with nonstick cooking spray and place the bread in the skillet. Top with the goat cheese and sprinkle with the thyme. Pile the arugula on top, followed by the roasted red pepper strips. Press down with a spatula to hold in place.*

✓ *Cook for 2 to 3 minutes until the bread is crisp and browned and the cheese is warmed through.*

Nutrition: Calories: 109 Fat: 2g Protein: 4g

96)   *Tofu Scramble*

Ingredients:

- *½ tablespoon olive oil*
- *1 small onion, chopped finely*
- *1 small red bell pepper, seeded and chopped finely*
- *1 cup cherry tomatoes, chopped finely*
- *1½ cups firm tofu pressed and crumbled*
- *Pinch of ground turmeric*
- *Pinch of cayenne pepper*
- *1 tablespoon fresh parsley, chopped*

Direction: Preparation Time: 15 minutes Cooking Time: 15 minutes Servings: 2

✓ *In a skillet, heat the oil over medium heat and sauté the onion and bell pepper for about 4-5 minutes.*

✓ *Add the tomatoes and cook for about 1-2 minutes.*

✓ *Add the tofu, turmeric and cayenne pepper and cook for about 6-8 minutes.*

✓ *Garnish with parsley and serve.* **Meal Prep Tip:**

✓ *Transfer the cooled scrambled into an airtight container and refrigerate for up to 3 days.*

✓ *Reheat in microwave before serving.*

Nutrition: Calories 213 Total Fat 11.8 g Saturated Fat 2.2 g Cholesterol 0 mg Total Carbs 14.7 g Sugar 8 g Fiber 4.5 g Sodium 31 mg Protein 17.3 g

97)   *Apple Omelet*

Ingredients:

- *4 teaspoons olive oil, divided*

- *2 small green apples, cored and sliced thinly*
- *¼ teaspoon ground cinnamon*
- *Pinch of ground cloves*
- *Pinch of ground nutmeg*
- *4 large eggs*
- *¼ teaspoon organic vanilla extract*
- *Pinch of salt*

Direction: Preparation Time: 10 minutes Cooking Time: 10 minutes Servings: 3

✓ *In a large nonstick frying pan, heat 1 teaspoon of oil over medium-low heat. Place the apple slices and sprinkle with spices.*

✓ *Cook for about 4-5 minutes, flipping once halfway through.*

✓ *Meanwhile, in a bowl, add the eggs, vanilla extract and salt and beat until fluffy.*

✓ *Add the remaining oil to the pan and let it heat completely.*
Place the egg mixture over apple slices evenly and cook for about 3-5 minutes or until desired doneness.

✓ *Carefully turn the pan over a serving plate and immediately fold the omelet.*

✓ *Serve immediately.*

✓ **Meal Prep Tip:**

✓ *In a resealable plastic bag, place the cooled omelet slices and seal the bag.*

✓ *Refrigerate for about 2-4 days.*

✓ *Reheat in the microwave on High for about 1 minute before serving.*

Nutrition: Calories 228 Total Fat 13.2 g Saturated Fat 3 g Total Carbs 21.3 g Sugar 16.1 g Protein 8.8 g

98)   *Spiced Overnight Oats*

Ingredients:

- *2 cups old-fashioned oats*
- *1 cup fat-free milk*
- *1 tablespoon vanilla extract*
- *1 teaspoon liquid stevia extract*
- *1 teaspoon ground cinnamon*
- *¼ teaspoon ground nutmeg*
- *½ cup toasted walnuts, chopped*

Direction: Servings: 6 Cooking Time: None

✓ *Stir together the oats, milk, vanilla extract, liquid stevia extract, cinnamon, and nutmeg in a large bowl. Cover and chill overnight until thick.*
Stir in the yogurt just before serving and spoon into cups.

✓ *Top with chopped walnuts and fresh fruit to serve.*

Nutrition: Calories 140, Total Fat 7.1g, Total Carbs 12.7g, Net Carbs 10.4g, Protein 5.6g, Sugar 2.6g,

99)   *Almond & Berry Smoothie*

Ingredients:

- ⅔ cup frozen raspberries
- ½ cup frozen banana, sliced
- ½ cup almond milk (unsweetened)
- 3 tablespoons almonds, sliced flakes (unsweetened)
- ¼ teaspoon ground cinnamon
- ⅛ teaspoon vanilla extract
- ¼ cup blueberries
- 1 tablespoon coconut

Direction: Cooking Time: 0 Minute Servings: 1

✓ Put the ingredients in a blender except for coconut flakes. Pulse until smooth.
   Top with the coconut flakes before serving.

Nutrition: Calories 360 Total Fat 19 g Carbohydrate 46 g Dietary Total Sugars 21 g Protein 9 g

100)   *Keto Low Carb Crepe*

Ingredients:

- 2 eggs
- 1 egg white
- 1 tbsp unsalted butter
- 1 1/3 tbsp cream cheese
- 2/3 tbsp psyllium husk

Direction: Servings: 2 Cooking Time: 4 Minutes

✓ Put all the ingredients in a bowl, except for butter, and then whisk using a stick blender until smooth and very liquid.

✓ Bring out a skillet pan, put it over medium heat, add ½ tbsp butter and when it melts, pour in half of the batter, spread evenly, and cook until the top has firmed.
   Carefully flip the crepe, continue cooking for 2 minutes until cooked and then move it to a plate.

✓ Add remaining butter and when it melts, cook another crepe in the same manner and then serve.

Nutrition: 118 Cal 9.4 g Fats 6.5 g Protein 1 g Net Carb 0.9 g Fiber

101)   *Cinnamon Oat Pancakes*

Ingredients:

- 1 cup old-fashioned oats
- 1 cup whole-wheat flour
- 2 teaspoons baking powder
- 1 teaspoon salt
- 1 ½ cups fat-free milk

- ¼ cup canola oil
- 2 large eggs, whisked
- 1 teaspoon lemon juice
- ½ to 1 teaspoon liquid stevia extract

Direction: Servings: 6 Cooking Time: 15 Minutes

✓ Combine the oats, flour, baking powder, and salt in a medium mixing bowl. In a separate bowl, stir together the milk, canola oil, eggs, lemon juice, and stevia extract.

✓ Stir the wet ingredients into the dry until just combined.

✓ Heat a large skillet or griddle to medium-high heat and grease with cooking spray.
   Spoon the batter in ¼ cups into the skillet and cook until bubbles form on the surface.

✓ Flip the pancakes and cook to brown on the other side. Slide onto a plate and repeat with the remaining batter.

✓ Store the extra pancakes in an airtight container and reheat in the microwave or oven.

Nutrition: Calories 230, Total Fat 11.4g, Saturated Fat 1.3g, Total Carbs 24.3g, Protein 7.1g, Sugar 3.3g,

102)   *Keto Creamy Bacon Dish*

Ingredients:

- ½ tsp dried basil
- ½ tsp minced garlic
- ½ tsp tomato paste
- 2 oz unsalted butter, softened
- 3 slices of bacon, chopped

Direction: Servings: 2 Cooking Time: 5 Minutes

✓ Bring out a skillet pan, put it over medium heat, add 1 tbsp butter and when it starts to melts, add chopped bacon and cook for 5 minutes.
   Then remove the pan from heat, add remaining butter, along with basil and tomato paste, season with salt and black pepper and stir until well mixed.

✓ Move bacon butter into an airtight container, cover with the lid, and refrigerate for 1 hour until solid.

Nutrition: 150 Cal 16 g Fats 1 g Protein 0.5 g Net Carb 1 g Fiber

103)   *Egg "dough" In A Pan*

Ingredients:

- ¼ tsp salt
- ½ of medium red bell pepper, chopped
- 1/8 tsp ground black pepper
- 2 eggs
- 2 tbsp chopped chives

Direction: Servings: 2 Cooking Time: 4 Minutes

✓ Turn on the oven, then set it to 350 degrees F and let it preheat. In the meantime, crack eggs in a bowl, add remaining ingredients and whisk until combined.
Bring out a small heatproof dish, pour in egg mixture, and bake for 5 to 8 minutes until set. When done, cut it into two squares and then serve.

Nutrition: 87 Cal 5.4 g Fats 7.2 g Protein 1.7 g Net Carb 0.7 g Fiber

104)   *Healthy Carrot Muffins*

Ingredients:

- *Dry ingredients*
- *Tapioca starch ¼ cup*
- *Baking soda – 1 teaspoon*
- *Cinnamon – 1 tablespoon*
- *Cloves – ¼ teaspoon*
- *Wet ingredients*
- *Vanilla extract – 1 teaspoon*
- *Water – 11/2 cups*
- *Carrots (shredded) – 11/2*
- *Almond flour – 1¾ cups*
- *Granulated sweetener of choice – 1/2 cup*
- *Baking powder – 1 teaspoon*
- *Nutmeg – 1 teaspoon*
- *Salt – 1 teaspoon*
- *Coconut oil – 1/3 cup*
- *Flax meal – 4 tablespoons*
- *Banana (mashed) – 1 medium*

Direction: Servings: 8 Cooking Time: 40 Minutes

✓ Begin by heating the oven to 350F. Get a muffin tray and position paper cups in all the molds.
✓ Arrange aside. Get a small glass bowl and put half a cup of water and a flax meal.
✓ Allow this rest for about 5 minutes. Your flax egg is prepared.
✓ Get a large mixing bowl and put in the almond flour, tapioca starch, granulated sugar, baking soda, baking powder, cinnamon, nutmeg, cloves, and salt.
✓ Mix well to combine. Conform a well in the middle of the flour mixture and stream in the coconut oil, vanilla extract, and flax egg.
Mix well to conform to a mushy dough. Then put in the chopped carrots and mashed banana.
✓ Mix until well-combined. Make use of a spoon to scoop out an equal amount of mixture into 8 muffin cups.
✓ Position the muffin tray in the oven and allow it to bake for about 40 minutes.

✓ Extract the tray from the microwave and allow the muffins to stand for about 10 minutes.
✓ Extract the muffin cups from the tray and chill until they reach the room degree of hotness and coldness.
✓ Serve and enjoy!

Nutrition: Calories: 189 calories per serving; Fat 13.9 g; Protein 3.8 g; Carbs 17.3 g

105)   *Breakfast Smoothie Bowl With Fresh Berries*

Ingredients:

- *Almond milk (unsweetened) – 1/2 cup*
- *Psyllium husk powder – 1/2 teaspoon*
- *Strawberries (chopped) –2 ounces*
- *Coconut oil – 1 tablespoon*
- *Crushed ice – 3 cups*
- *Liquid stevia – 5 to 10 drops*
- *Pea protein powder – 1/3 cup*

Direction: Servings: 2 Cooking Time: 5 Minutes

✓ Begin by taking a blender and adding in the mashed ice cubes. Allow them to rest for about 30 seconds.
✓ Then put in the almond milk, shredded strawberries, pea protein powder, psyllium husk powder, coconut oil, and liquid stevia.
Blend well until it turns into a smooth and creamy puree.
✓ Vacant the prepared smoothie into 2 glasses.
✓ Cover with coconut flakes and pure and neat strawberries.

Nutrition: Calories: 166 calories per serving; Fat – 9.2 g; Carbs – 4.1 g; Protein – 17.6 g

106)   *Egg "dough" In A Pan*

Ingredients:

- *¼ tsp salt*
- *½ of medium red bell pepper, chopped*
- *1/8 tsp ground black pepper*
- *2 eggs*
- *2 tbsp chopped chives*

Direction: Servings: 2 Cooking Time: 4 Minutes

✓ Turn on the oven, then set it to 350 degrees F and let it preheat. In the meantime, crack eggs in a bowl, add remaining ingredients and whisk until combined.
Bring out a small heatproof dish, pour in egg mixture, and bake for 5 to 8 minutes until set. When done, cut it into two squares and then serve.

Nutrition: 87 Cal 5.4 g Fats 7.2 g Protein 1.7 g Net Carb 0.7 g Fiber

107) Eggs Florentine

Ingredients:

- 1 cup washed, fresh spinach leaves
- 2 tbsp freshly grated parmesan cheese
- Sea salt and pepper
- 1 tbsp white vinegar
- 2 eggs

Direction: Servings: 2 Cooking Time: 10 Minutes

✓ Cook the spinach in the microwave or steam until wilted.

✓ Sprinkle with parmesan cheese and seasoning.

✓ Slice into bite-size pieces

✓ Simmer a pan of water and add the vinegar. Stir quickly with a spoon.
Break an egg into the center.

✓ Turn off the heat and cover until set.

✓ Repeat with the second egg. Place the eggs on top of the spinach and serve.

Nutrition: 180 cal.10g fat 7g protein 5g carbs.

108) Quick Low-carb Oatmeal

Ingredients:

- Almond flour – 1/2 cup
- Flax meal – 2 tablespoons
- Cinnamon (ground) – 1 teaspoon
- Almond milk (unsweetened) – 11/2 cups
- Salt – as per taste
- Chia seeds – 2 tablespoons
- Liquid stevia – 10 – 15 drops
- Vanilla extract – 1 teaspoon

Direction: Servings: 2 Cooking Time: 15 Minutes

✓ Begin by taking a large mixing bowl and adding coconut flour, almond flour, ground cinnamon, flax seed powder, and chia seeds.

✓ Mix properly to combine. Position a stockpot on low heat and add in the dry ingredients.
Also, add in the liquid stevia, vanilla extract, and almond milk. Mix well to combine. Prepare the flour and almond milk for about 4 minutes. Add salt if needed.

✓ Move the oatmeal to a serving bowl and top with nuts, seeds, and pure and neat berries.

Nutrition: Calories: calories per serving; Protein – 11.7 g; Fat – 24.3 g; Carbs – 16.7 g

109) Cucumber & Yogurt

Ingredients:

- 1 cup low-fat yogurt
- ½ cup cucumber, diced
- ¼ teaspoon lemon zest
- ¼ teaspoon lemon juice
- ¼ teaspoon fresh mint, chopped Salt to taste

Direction: Servings: 1 Cooking Time: 0 Minute

✓ Mix all the ingredients in a jar.
Refrigerate and serve.

Nutrition: Calories 164 Total Fat 4 g Saturated Fat 2 g Cholesterol 15 mg Total Carbohydrate 19 g Dietary Fiber 1 g Total Sugars 18 g Protein 13 g

110) Eggs Baked In Peppers

Ingredients:

- 4 medium bell peppers, assorted
- 1 cup shredded low-fat cheddar cheese
- 8 large eggs Salt and pepper
- Fresh chopped parsley, to serve

Direction: Servings: 4 Cooking Time: 25 Minutes

✓ Preheat the oven to 400°F and slice the peppers in half.

✓ Remove the seeds and pith from each pepper and place them cut-side up in a baking dish large enough to fit them all.
Divide the shredded cheese among the pepper halves and crack an egg into each.

✓ Season with salt and pepper then bake for 20 to 25 minutes until done to your liking.

✓ Garnish with fresh chopped parsley to serve.

Nutrition: Calories 260, Total Fat 16.3g, Saturated Fat 6.6g, Total Carbs 10.9g, Net Carbs 9.3g, Protein 20.8g, Sugar 6.8g, Fiber 1.6g, Sodium 374mg

111) Easy Egg Scramble

Ingredients:

- 2 large eggs
- 1 tablespoon fat-free milk Salt and pepper
- ¼ cup diced green pepper
- 2 tablespoons diced onion
- ¼ cup diced tomatoes

Direction: Servings: 1 Cooking Time: 10 Minutes

✓ Whisk together the eggs, milk, salt, and pepper in a small bowl. Heat a medium skillet over medium-high heat and grease with cooking spray.

✓ Add the green pepper and onion then cook for 2 to 3 minutes.
Spoon the veggies into a bowl then reheat the skillet. Pour in the egg mixture and cook until the eggs start to thicken.

✓ Spoon in the cooked veggies and diced tomatoes.

Stir the mixture and cook until the egg is set and scrambled. Serve hot.

Nutrition: Calories 170, Total Fat 10.1g, Saturated Fat 3.1g, Total Carbs 6.3g, Net Carbs 4.9g, Protein 13.9g, Sugar 4.1g, Fiber 1.4g, Sodium 152mg

112) Bacon And Chicken Garlic Wrap

Ingredients:

- *1 chicken fillet, cut into small cubes*
- *8-9 thin slices bacon, cut to fit cubes*
- *6 garlic cloves, minced*

Direction: Servings: 4 Cooking Time: 10 Minutes

- ✓ *Preheat your oven to 400 degrees F Line a baking tray with aluminum foil*
- ✓ *Add minced garlic to a bowl and rub each chicken piece with it. Wrap bacon piece around each garlic chicken bite*
  Secure with toothpick Transfer bites to the baking sheet, keeping a little bit of space between them
- ✓ *Bake for about 15-20 minutes until crispy Serve and enjoy!*

Nutrition: Calories: 260; Fat: 19g; Carbohydrates: 5g; Protein: 22g

113) Strawberry Puff Pancake

Ingredients:

- *3 eggs, large*
- *1/8 teaspoon cinnamon, ground*
- *1 cup strawberry, sliced*
- *3/4 cup milk, fat-free*
- *What you will need from the store cupboard:*
- *1 teaspoon vanilla extract*
- *¾ cup of all-purpose flour*
- *2 tablespoons of butter*
- *1 tablespoon cornstarch*
- *½ cup of water*
- *1/8 teaspoon salt*

Direction: Servings: 4 Cooking Time: 20 Minutes

- ✓ *Keep the butter on a pie plate and keep in an oven for 4 to 5 minutes. In the meantime, whisk the vanilla, milk, and eggs in a bowl.*
- ✓ *Take another bowl and bring together the cinnamon, salt, and flour in it. Whisk this into the egg mix until it blends well. Pour this into the plate. Bake for 15 minutes. The sides should be golden brown and crisp. Add the cornstarch to your saucepan.*
- ✓ *Stir the water in until it turns smooth. Now add the strawberries.*
- ✓ *Cook while stirring till it thickens. Mash the strawberries coarsely and serve with the pancake.*

Nutrition: Calories 277, Carbohydrates 38g, Fiber 2g, Cholesterol 175mg, Total Fat 10g, Protein 9g, Sodium 187mg

114) Egg Porridge

Ingredients:

- *2 organic free-range eggs*
- *1/3 cup organic heavy cream without food additives*
- *2 packages of your preferred sweetener*
- *2 tbsp grass-fed butter ground organic cinnamon to taste*

Direction: Servings: 1 Cooking Time: 10 Minutes

- ✓ *In a bowl add the eggs, cream and sweetener, and mix. Melt the butter in a saucepan over medium heat.*
- ✓ *Lower the heat once the butter is melted. Combine with the egg and cream mixture.*
  While Cooking, mix until it thickens and curdles.
- ✓ *When you see the first signs of curdling, remove the saucepan immediately from the heat.*
- ✓ *Pour the porridge into a bowl. Sprinkle cinnamon on top and serve immediately.*

Nutrition: 604 cal 45g fat 8g protein 2.8g carbs.

115) Breakfast Parfait

Ingredients:

- *4 oz. unsweetened applesauce*
- *6 oz. non-fat and sugar-free vanilla yogurt*
- *¼ teaspoon pumpkin pie spice*
- *¼ teaspoon honey*
- *1 cup low-fat granola*

Direction: Servings: 2 Cooking Time: 0 Minute

- ✓ *Mix the ingredients except for the granola in a bowl.*
  Layer the mixture with the granola in a cup.
  Refrigerate before serving

Nutrition: Calories 287 Total Fat 3 g Saturated Fat 1 g Cholesterol 28 mg Sodium 186 mg Total Carbohydrate 57 g Dietary Fiber 4 g Total Sugars2 g Protein 8 g

116) Oatmeal Blueberry Pancakes

Ingredients:

- *½ cup rolled oats*
- *½ cup unsweetened almond milk*
- *¼ cup unsweetened applesauce*
- *¼ cup unsweetened vegan protein powder*
- *½ tablespoon flax meal*

- *1 teaspoon baking powder*
- *½ teaspoon vanilla extract*
- *¼ teaspoon baking soda*
- *¼ teaspoon ground cinnamon*
- *1/8 teaspoon salt*
- *½ cup fresh blueberries*

Direction: Servings: 4 Cooking Time: 40 Minutes

✓ *Place all ingredients (except for blueberries) in a food processor and pulse until smooth.*

✓ *Transfer the mixture into a bowl and set aside for 5 minutes. Gently, fold in blueberries.*
Place a lightly greased medium skillet over medium heat until heated.

✓ *Place the desired amount of the mixture and cook for about 3–5 minutes per side.*

✓ *Repeat with the remaining mixture. Serve warm.*

Nutrition: Calories 105 Total Fat 1.8 g Saturated Fat 0.2 g Cholesterol 0 mg Sodium 204 mg Total Carbs 15.4 g Fiber 2.2 g Sugar 5.2 g Protein 8 g

117) *Bulgur Porridge*

Ingredients:

- *2/3 cup unsweetened soy milk*
- *1/3 cup bulgur, rinsed*
Pinch of salt
- *1 ripe banana, peeled and mashed*
- *2 kiwis, peeled and sliced*

Direction: Servings: 2 Cooking Time: 15 Minutes

✓ *In a pan, add the soy milk, bulgur, and salt over medium-high heat and bring to a boil.*

✓ *Adjust the heat to low and simmer for about 10 minutes.*
Remove the pan of bulgur from heat and immediately stir in the mashed banana.

✓ *Serve warm with the topping of kiwi slices.*

Nutrition: Calories 223 Total Fat 2.3 g Saturated Fat 0.3 g Cholesterol 0 mg Sodium 126 mg Total Carbs 47.5 g Fiber 8.6 g Sugar 17.4 g Protein 7.1 g

118) *Turkey-broccoli Brunch Casserole*

Ingredients:

- *2-1/2 cups turkey breast, cubed and cooked*
- *16 oz. broccoli, chopped and drained*
- *1-1/2 cups of milk, fat-free*
- *1 cup cheddar cheese, low-fat, shredded*
- *10 oz. Cream of chicken soup. low sodium and low fat*

What you will need from the store cupboard:

- *8 oz. egg substitute*
- *¼ teaspoon of poultry seasoning*

- *¼ cup of sour cream, low fat*
- *½ teaspoon pepper*
- *1/8 teaspoon salt 2 cups of seasoned stuffing cubes*
- *Cooking spray*

Direction: Servings: 6 Cooking Time: 20 Minutes

✓ *Bring together the egg substitute, soup, milk, pepper, sour cream, salt, and poultry seasoning in a big bowl.*

✓ *Now stir in the broccoli, turkey, ¾ cup of cheese and stuffing cubes.*
Transfer to a baking dish. Apply cooking spray.

✓ *Bake for 10 minutes. Sprinkle the remaining cheese.*

✓ *Bake for another 5 minutes.*

✓ *Keep it aside for 5 minutes. Serve.*

Nutrition: Calories 303, Carbohydrates 26g, Fiber 3g, Sugar 0.8g, Cholesterol 72mg, Total Fat 7g, Protein 33g Cheesy

119) *Low-carb Omelet*

Ingredients:

- *2 whole eggs*
- *1 tablespoon water*
- *1 tablespoon butter*
- *3 thin slices of salami*
- *5 fresh basil leaves*
- *5 thin slices, fresh ripe tomatoes*
- *2 ounces fresh mozzarella cheese*
- *Salt and pepper as needed*

Direction: Servings: 5 Cooking Time: 5 Minutes

✓ *Take a small bowl and whisk in eggs and water*

✓ *Take a non-stick Sauté pan and place it over medium heat, add butter and let it melt*

✓ *Pour egg mixture and cook for 30 seconds. Spread salami slices on half of egg mix and top with cheese, tomatoes, basil slices*
Season with salt and pepper according to your taste

✓ *Cook for 2 minutes and fold the egg with the empty half*

✓ *Cover and cook on LOW for 1 minute. Serve and enjoy!*

Nutrition: Calories: 451; Fat: 36g; Carbohydrates: 3g; Protein:33g

120) *Apple & Cinnamon Pancake*

Ingredients:

- *¼ teaspoon ground cinnamon*
- *1 ¾ cups Better Baking Mix*

- *1 tablespoon oil*
- *1 cup water*
- *2 egg whites*
- *½ cup sugar-free applesauce*
- *Cooking spray*
- *1 cup plain yogurt*
- *Sugar substitute*

Direction: Servings: 4 Cooking Time: 10 Minutes

✓ *Blend the cinnamon and the baking mix in a bowl.*

✓ *Create a hole in the middle and add the oil, water, egg and applesauce.*

✓ *Mix well. Spray your pan with oil.*
  Place it on medium heat. Pour ¼ cup of the batter.

✓ *Flip the pancake and cook until golden.*

✓ *Serve with yogurt and sugar substitute.*

Nutrition: Calories 231 Total Fat 6 g Saturated Fat 1 g Total Carbohydrate 37 g Dietary Fiber 4 g Total Sugars 1 g Protein 8 g

121)   *Guacamole Turkey Burgers*

Ingredients:

- *12 oz. turkey, ground*
- *1-1/2 avocados*
- *2 teaspoons of juice from a lime*
- *½ teaspoon cumin*
- *1 red chili, chopped*

What you will need from the store cupboard:

- *½ teaspoon garlic powder*
- *½ teaspoon onion powder*
- *3 teaspoons of olive oil*
- *½ teaspoon salt*

Direction: Servings: 3 Cooking Time: 15 Minutes

✓ *Mix the turkey with the cumin, chili, salt, garlic powder, and onion powder in a medium-sized bowl.*

✓ *Create 3 patties. Pour 3 teaspoons olive oil in a skillet and heat over medium heat.*
  Now cook your patties. Make sure that both sides are brown. Make the guacamole in the meantime.

✓ *Mash together the garlic powder, juice from lime and avocados in a bowl.*

✓ *Add salt for seasoning. Serve the burgers with guacamole on the patties.*

Nutrition: Calories 316, Carbohydrates 9g, Fiber 8g, Sugar 0g, Cholesterol 80mg, Total Fat 21g, Protein 24g

122)   *Ham And Goat Cheese Omelet*

Ingredients:

- *1 slice of ham, chopped*
- *4 egg whites*

- *2 teaspoons of water*
- *2 tablespoons onion, chopped*
- *1 tablespoon parsley, minced*

What you will need from the store cupboard:

- *2 tablespoons green pepper, chopped*
- *1/8 teaspoon pepper*
- *2 tablespoons goat cheese, crumbled Cooking spray*

Direction: Servings: 1 Cooking Time: 10 Minutes

✓ *Whisk together the water, pepper and egg whites in a bowl till everything blends well. Stir in the green pepper, ham, and onion.*

✓ *Now heat your skillet over medium heat after applying the cooking spray. Pour in the egg white mix towards the edge.*
  As it sets, it pushes the cooked parts to the center. Allow the uncooked portions to flow underneath.

✓ *Sprinkle the goat cheese to one side when there is no liquid egg. Now fold your omelet into half.*

✓ *Sprinkle the parsley.*

Nutrition: Calories 143, Carbohydrates 5g, Fiber 1g, Sugar 0.3g, Cholesterol 27mg, Total Fat 4g, Protein 21g

123)   *Banana Matcha Breakfast Smoothie*

Ingredients:

- *1 cup fat-free milk*
- *1 medium banana, sliced*
- *¼ cup frozen chopped pineapple*
- *½ cup ice cubes*
- *1 tablespoon matcha powder*
- *¼ teaspoon ground cinnamon*
- *Liquid stevia extract, to taste*

Direction: Servings: 1 Cooking Time: None

✓ *Combine the ingredients in a blender.*

✓ *Pulse the mixture several times to chop the ingredients.*
  Blend for 30 to 60 seconds until smooth and well combined. Sweeten to taste with liquid stevia extract, if desired.

✓ *Pour into a glass and serve immediately.*

Nutrition: Calories 230, Total Fat 0.4g, Saturated Fat 0.1g, Total Carbs 44.9g, Net Carbs 38g, Protein 12.6g, Sugar 30.9g, Fiber 6.9g, Sodium 135mg

124)   *Tofu And Vegetable Scramble*

Ingredients:

- *Firm tofu (drained) – 16 ounces*

- Sea salt – 1/2 teaspoon
- Garlic powder – 1 teaspoon
- Fresh coriander – for garnishing
- Red onion – 1/2 medium
- Cumin powder – 1 teaspoon
- Lemon juice – for topping
- Green bell pepper – 1 medium
- Garlic powder – 1 teaspoon
- Fresh coriander – for garnishing
- Red onion – 1/2 medium
- Cumin powder – 1 teaspoon
- Lemon juice – for topping

Direction: Servings: 2 Cooking Time: 15 Minutes

✓ Begin by preparing the ingredients. For this, you are to extract the seeds of the tomato and green bell pepper. Shred the onion, bell pepper, and tomato into small cubes. Get a small mixing bowl and position the fairly hard tofu inside it.

✓ Make use of your hands to break the fairly hard tofu. Arrange aside. Get a nonstick pan and add in the onion, tomato, and bell pepper.

✓ Mix and cook for about 3 minutes. Put the somewhat hard crumbled tofu to the pan and combine well.
Get a small bowl and put in the water, turmeric, garlic powder, cumin powder, and chili powder.

✓ Combine well and stream it over the tofu and vegetable mixture. Allow the tofu and vegetable crumble to cook with seasoning for 5 minutes.

✓ Continuously stir so that the pan is not holding the ingredients. Drizzle the tofu scramble with chili flakes and salt.

✓ Combine well. Transfer the prepared scramble to a serving bowl and give it a proper spray of lemon juice.

✓ Finalize by garnishing with pure and neat coriander. Serve while hot!

Nutrition: Calories: 238 calories per serving; Carbohydrates – 16.6 g; Fat – 11 g

125)   Basil And Tomato Baked Eggs

Ingredients:

- 1 garlic clove, minced
- 1 cup canned tomatoes
- ¼ cup fresh basil leaves, roughly chopped
- 1/2 teaspoon chili powder
- 1 tablespoon olive oil
- 4 whole eggs
- Salt and pepper to taste

Direction: Servings: 4 Cooking Time: 15 Minutes

✓ Preheat your oven to 375 degrees F. Take a small

baking dish and grease with olive oil

✓ Add garlic, basil, tomatoes chili, olive oil into a dish and stir

✓ Crackdown eggs into a dish, keeping space between the two
Sprinkle the whole dish with salt and pepper

✓ Place in oven and cook for 12 minutes until eggs are set and tomatoes are bubbling Serve with basil on top Enjoy!

Nutrition: Calories: 235; Fat: 16g; Carbohydrates: 7g; Protein: 14g

126)   Cream Cheese Pancakes

Ingredients:

- 2 oz cream cheese 2 eggs
- ½ tsp cinnamon
- 1 tbsp keto coconut flour
- ½ to 1 packet of Stevia

Direction: Servings: 1 Cooking Time: 5 Minutes

✓ Skillet with butter in the pan or coconut oil on medium-high. Make them as you would normal pancakes.
Cook and flip one side to cook the other side! Top with some butter and/or sugar-free syrup.

Nutrition: 340 cal.30g fat 7g protein 3g carbs

127)   Chia And Coconut Pudding

Ingredients:

- Light coconut milk – 7 ounces
- Liquid stevia – 3 to 4 drops
- Kiwi – 1
- Chia seeds – ¼ cup
- Clementine – 1
- Shredded coconut (unsweetened)

Direction: Servings: 2 Cooking Time: 5 Minutes

✓ Begin by getting a mixing bowl and putting in the light coconut milk. Set in the liquid stevia to sweeten the milk. Combine well. Put the chia seeds to the milk and whisk until well-combined.

✓ Arrange aside. Scrape the clementine and carefully extract the skin from the wedges.

✓ Leave aside. Also, scrape the kiwi and dice it into small pieces.
Get a glass vessel and gather the pudding.

✓ For this, position the fruits at the bottom of the jar; then put a dollop of chia pudding.

✓ Then spray the fruits and then put another layer of chia pudding.

✓ Finalize by garnishing with the rest of the fruits

and chopped coconut.

Nutrition: Calories: 201 calories per serving; Protein – 5.4 g; Fat – 10 g; Carbs – 22.8 g

128) *Mashed Cauliflower*

Ingredients:

- *1 cauliflower head*
- *1/8 cup plain yogurt, skim milk or butter*
- *1 red chili, diced*
- *1 tomato, sliced ½ chopped onion*

What you will need from the store cupboard:

- *1 garlic clove, optional Salt and pepper Paprika to taste*

Direction: Servings: 6 Cooking Time: 10 Minutes

✓ *Steam the cauliflower till it becomes tender. You can steam with a garlic clove as well. Now cut your cauliflower into small pieces.*

✓ *Keep in your blender with yogurt, butter or milk. Season with pepper and salt. Whip until it gets smooth. Pour the cauliflower into a small baking dish.*

✓ *Sprinkle the paprika. Bake in the oven till it becomes bubbly.*

Nutrition: Calories 57, Carbohydrates 12g, Total Fat 0g, Protein 4g, Fiber 5g, Sodium 91mg, Sugars 5g

129) *Quinoa Porridge Recipe 2*

Ingredients:

- *1 cup dry quinoa, rinsed*
- *1½ cups unsweetened almond milk*
- *1 teaspoon vanilla extract*
- *1 teaspoon ground cinnamon blueberries*
- *2 tablespoons maple syrup*
- *4 tablespoons peanut butter*
- *¼ cup fresh strawberries, hulled and chopped*
- *¼ cup fresh*

Direction: Servings: 2 Cooking Time: 20 Minutes

✓ *In a small pan, place quinoa, almond milk, vanilla extract, and cinnamon over medium heat and bring to a boil.*

✓ *Now, adjust the heat to low and simmer, covered for about 15 minutes or until all the liquid is absorbed.*

✓ *Remove the pan of quinoa from heat and stir in maple syrup and peanut butter.*

✓ *Serve warm with the topping of berries.*

Nutrition: Calories 608 Total Fat 24 g Saturated Fat 4.2 g Cholesterol 0 mg Sodium 289 mg Total Carbs 81 g Fiber 10 g Sugar 17.9 g Protein 21.1 g

130) *Vanilla Mixed Berry Smoothie*

Ingredients:

- *1 cup fat-free milk*
- *½ cup nonfat Greek yogurt, plain*
- *½ cup frozen blueberries*
- *¼ cup frozen strawberries*
- *3 to 4 ice cubes*
- *1 teaspoon fresh lemon juice*
- *Liquid stevia extract, to taste*

Direction: Servings: 1 Cooking Time: None

✓ *Combine the ingredients in a blender.*

✓ *Pulse the mixture several times to chop the ingredients.*

✓ *Blend for 30 to 60 seconds until smooth and well combined.*
Sweeten to taste with liquid stevia extract, if desired.

✓ *Pour into a glass and serve immediately.*

Nutrition: Calories 220, Total Fat 0.3g, Saturated Fat 0g, Total Carbs 31.6g, Net Carbs 28.3g, Protein 21.6g, Sugar 27.3g, Fiber 3.3g, S

131) *Granola With Fruits*

Ingredients:

- *3 cups quick-cooking oats*
- *1 cup almonds, sliced*
- *½ cup wheat germ*
- *3 tablespoons butter*
- *1 teaspoon ground cinnamon*
- *1 cup honey*
- *3 cups whole-grain cereal flakes*
- *½ cup raisins*
- *½ cup dried cranberries*
- *½ cup dates, pitted and chopped*

Direction: Servings: 6 Cooking Time: 35 Minutes

✓ *Preheat your oven to 325 degrees F.*

✓ *Place the almonds on a baking sheet.*

✓ *Bake for 15 minutes.*

✓ *Mix the wheat germ, butter, cinnamon, and honey in a bowl.*
Add the toasted almonds and oats. Mix well.

✓ *Spread on the baking sheet.*

✓ *Bake for 20 minutes.*

✓ *Mix with the rest of the ingredients. Let cool and serve.*

Nutrition: Calories 210 Total Fat 7 g Saturated Fat 2 g Cholesterol 5 mg Sodium 58 mg Total Carbohydrate 36 g Dietary Fiber 4 g Total Sugars 2 g Protein 5 g Potassium 250 mg

132) Egg Muffins

Ingredients:

- *1 tbsp green pesto*
- *3 oz/75g shredded cheese*
- *5 oz/150g cooked bacon*
- *1 scallion, chopped*
- *6 eggs*

Direction: Servings: 6 Cooking Time: 20 Minutes

✓ *You should set your oven to 350°F/175°C.*
✓ *Place liners in a regular cupcake tin.*
✓ *This will help with easy removal and storage. Beat the eggs with pepper, salt, and pesto.*
✓ *Mix in the cheese.*
✓ *Pour the eggs into the cupcake tin and top with the bacon and scallion.*
✓ *Cook for 15-20 minutes*

Nutrition: 190 cal.15g fat 7g protein 4g carbs.

133) Eggs On The Go

Ingredients:

- *4 oz/110g bacon, cooked*
- *Pepper Salt*
  12 eggs

Direction: Servings: 4 Cooking Time: 5 Minutes

✓ *You should set your oven to 200°C.*
✓ *Place liners in a regular cupcake tin.*
✓ *This will help with easy removal and storage. Crack an egg into each of the cups and sprinkle some bacon onto each of them.*
✓ *Season with some pepper and salt.*
✓ *Bake for 15 minutes, or until the eggs are set.*

Nutrition: 75 cal. 6g fat 8g protein 1g carbs.

134) Breakfast Mix

Ingredients:

- *5 tbsp coconut flakes, unsweetened*
- *7 tbsp hemp seeds*
- *5 tbsp flaxseed, ground*
- *2 tbsp sesame, ground*
- *2 tbsp cocoa, dark, unsweetened*

Direction: Servings: 1 Cooking Time: 5 Minutes

✓ *Grind the sesame and flaxseed. only grind the sesame seeds for a small period.*
✓ *Mix all ingredients in a jar and shake it well. Keep refrigerated until ready to eat.*
Serve softened with black coffee or even with still

water and add coconut oil if you want to increase the fat content.
✓ *It also blends well with cream or with mascarpone cheese.*

Nutrition: 150 cal.9g fat 8g protein 4g carbs.

135) Lovely Porridge

Ingredients:

- *2 tablespoons coconut flour*
- *2 tbsp vanilla protein powder*
- *3 tablespoons golden flaxseed meal*
  1 and 1/2 cups almond milk, unsweetened
- *Powdered erythritol*

Direction: Servings: 2 Cooking Time: Nil

✓ *Take a bowl and mix in flaxseed meal, protein powder, coconut flour and mix well*
✓ *Add mix to the saucepan (placed over medium heat)*
Add almond milk and stir, let the mixture thicken
✓ *Add your desired amount of sweetener and serve*
✓ *Enjoy!*

Nutrition: Calories: 259; Fat: 13g; Carbohydrates: 5g; Protein: 16g

136) Vegetable Omelet

Ingredients:

- *½ cup yellow summer squash, chopped*
- *½ cup canned diced tomatoes with herbs, drained*
- *½ ripe avocado, pitted and chopped*
- *½ cup cucumber, chopped*
- *2 eggs*
- *2 tablespoons water*
- *Salt and pepper to taste*
- *1 teaspoon dried basil, crushed*
- *Cooking spray ¼ cup low-fat*
- *Monterey Jack cheese, shredded*
- *Chives, chopped*

Direction: Servings: 4 Cooking Time: 25 Minutes

✓ *In a bowl, mix the squash, tomatoes, avocado and cucumber.*
✓ *In another bowl, mix the eggs, water, salt, pepper and basil.*
✓ *Spray oil on a pan over medium heat.*
Pour egg mixture on the pan. Put the vegetable mixture on top of the egg.
✓ *Lift and fold.*
✓ *Cook until the egg has set.*

✓ Sprinkle cheese and chives on top.

Nutrition: Calories 128 Total Fat 6 g Saturated Fat 2 g Cholesterol 97 mg Sodium 357 mg Total Carbohydrate 7 g Dietary Fiber 3 g Total Sugars 4 g Protein 12 g Potassium 341 mg

137) *Vegetable Frittata*

Ingredients:

- 1 cup mushrooms, sliced
- 4 eggs, beaten lightly
- 2 tablespoons onion, chopped
- ½ cup broccoli, chopped
- ¼ cup cheddar cheese, shredded, low-fat

What you will need from the store cupboard:

- 2 tablespoons green pepper, chopped
- Dash of pepper
- 1/8 teaspoon of salt
- Cooking spray

Direction: Servings: 2 Cooking Time: 20 Minutes

✓ Bring together all the ingredients in your bowl. Coat your baking dish with cooking spray and pour everything into it.

✓ Bake for 20 minutes and serve immediately.

Nutrition: Calories 230, Carbohydrates 6g, Fiber 1g, Sugar 0.2g, Cholesterol 386mg, Total Fat 14g, Protein 20g

138) *Egg-veggie Scramble*

Ingredients:

- ¼ tsp salt
- 1 tbsp unsalted butter
- 1/8 tsp ground black pepper
- 3 eggs, beaten
- 4 oz spinach

Direction: Servings: 2 Cooking Time: 3 Minutes

✓ Bring out a frying pan, put it over medium heat, add butter and when it melts, add spinach and cook for 5 minutes until leaves have wilted.
Then pour in eggs, season with salt and black pepper, and cook for 3 minutes until eggs have scramble to the desired level.

Nutrition: 90 Cal 7 g Fats 5.6 g Protein; 0.7 g Net Carb 0.6 g Fiber

139) *Apple Omelet*

Ingredients:

- 4 teaspoons olive oil, divided
- 2 small green apples, cored and sliced thinly
- ¼ teaspoon ground cinnamon Pinch of salt

- Pinch of ground cloves
- Pinch of ground nutmeg
- 4 large eggs
- ¼ teaspoon organic vanilla extract

Direction: Servings: 3 Cooking Time: 10 Minutes

✓ Over medium-low heat in a frying pan, heat 1 teaspoon. Place the apple slices and sprinkle with spices.

✓ Cook for about 4-5 minutes, flipping once halfway through.

✓ Meanwhile, in a bowl, add the eggs, vanilla extract and salt and beat until fluffy.

✓ Add the remaining oil in the pan and let it heat completely.
Place the egg mixture over apple slices evenly and cook for about 3-5 minutes or until desired doneness.

✓ Carefully turn the pan over a serving plate and immediately fold the omelet.

✓ Serve immediately.

Nutrition: Calories 228 Total Fat 13.2 g Saturated Fat 3 g Cholesterol 248 mg Total Carbs 21.3 g Sugar 16.1 g Fiber 3.8 g Sodium 145 mg Potassium 251 mg Protein 8.8 g Mix

140) *Veggie Fritters*

Ingredients:

- ½ tsp nutritional yeast
- 1 oz chopped broccoli
  1 zucchini, grated, squeezed
- 2 eggs
- 2 tbsp almond flour

Direction: Servings: 2 Cooking Time: 3 Minutes

✓ Wrap grated zucchini in a cheesecloth, twist it well to remove excess moisture, and then

✓ Put zucchini in a bowl.

✓ Add remaining ingredients, except for oil, and then whisk well until combined.
Bring out a skillet pan, put it over medium heat, add oil, and when hot, drop zucchini mixture in four portions, shape them into flat patties and cook for 4 minutes per side until thoroughly cooked.

Nutrition: 191 Cal 16.6 g Fats 9.6 g Protein 0.8 g Net Carb 0.2 g Fiber

141) *Yummy...Millet Porridge*

Ingredients:

- 1 and ½ cup millet, rinsed and drained
- Pinch of salt
- 3 cups water

- *2 tablespoons Chia seeds ,*
- *3 drops liquid stevia*
- *1 cup unsweetened Coconut Milk*
- *1 tablespoons fresh berries*

Direction: Servings: 4 Cooking Time: 25 Minutes

✓ *In a nonstick pan, add the millet over medium-low heat and cook for about 3 minutes, stirring continuously.*

✓ *Add the salt and water and stir to combine Increase the heat to medium and bring to a boil— Cook for about 15 minutes.*

✓ *Stir in the almonds, stevia and almond milk and cook for 5 minutes.*

✓ *Top with the blueberries and serve.*

Nutrition: Calories 219 Total Fat 4.5 g Saturated Fat 0.6 g Cholesterol 0 mg Total Carbs 38.2 g Sugar 0.6 g Fiber 5 g Sodium 92 mg Protein 6.4 g

142) *Steel-cut Oatmeal Bowl With Fruit And Nuts*

Ingredients:

- *1 cup steel-cut oats*
- *2 cups almond milk*
- *¾ cup water*
- *1 teaspoon ground cinnamon*
- *¼ teaspoon salt*
- *2 cups chopped fresh fruit, such as blueberries, strawberries, raspberries, or peaches*
- *1/2 cup chopped walnuts*
- *¼ cup chia seeds*

Direction: Servings: 4 Cooking Time: 20 Minutes

✓ *In a medium saucepan over medium-high heat, combine the oats, almond milk, water, cinnamon, and salt.*
Bring to a boil, reduce the heat to low, and simmer for 15 to 20 minutes, until the oats are softened and thickened.

✓ *Top each bowl with 1/2 cup of fresh fruit, 2 tablespoons of walnuts, and 1 tablespoon of chia seeds before serving.*

Nutrition: Calories: 288; Total fat: 11g; Saturated fat: 1g; Protein: 10g; Carbs: 38g; Sugar: 7g;

143) *Tofu & Zucchini Muffins*

Ingredients:

- *12 ounces extra-firm silken tofu, drained and pressed*
- *¾ cup unsweetened soy milk*
- *2 tablespoons canola oil*

- *1 tablespoon apple cider vinegar*
- *1 cup whole-wheat pastry flour*
- *½ cup chickpea flour*
- *1 teaspoon baking powder*
- *½ teaspoon baking soda*
- *1 teaspoon smoked paprika*
- *1 teaspoon onion powder*
- *1 teaspoon salt*
- *½ cup zucchini, chopped*
- *¼ cup fresh chives, minced*

Direction: Servings: 6 Cooking Time: 40 Minutes

✓ *Preheat your oven to 400ºF. Line a 12-cup muffin tin with paper liners.*

✓ *In a bowl, place tofu and with a fork, mash until smooth. Add almond milk, oil, vinegar, and mix until slightly smooth in the bowl of tofu.*

✓ *In a separate large bowl, add flours, baking powder, baking soda, spices, salt, and mix well. Transfer the mixture into muffin cups evenly.*

✓ *Bake for approximately 35–40 minutes or until a toothpick inserted in the center comes out clean.*

✓ *Remove the muffin tin from the oven and place it onto a wire rack to cool for about 10 minutes.*

✓ *Carefully invert the muffins onto a platter and serve warm.*

Nutrition: Calories 237 Total Fat 9 g Saturated Fat 1 g Cholesterol 0 mg Sodium 520 mg Total Carbs 2293.3 g Fiber 5.9 g Sugar 3.7 g Protein 11.1 g

144) *Savory Keto Pancake*

Ingredients:

- *¼ cup almond flour*
- *1 ½ tbsp unsalted butter*
- *2 eggs*
- *2 oz cream cheese, softened*

Direction: Servings: 2 Cooking Time: 2 Minutes

✓ *Bring out a bowl, crack eggs in it, whisk well until fluffy, and then whisk in flour and cream cheese until well combined.*
Bring out a skillet pan, put it over medium heat, add butter and when it melts, drop pancake batter in four sections, spread it evenly, and cook for 2 minutes per side until brown.

Nutrition: 166.8 Cal 15 g Fats 5.8 g Protein 1.8 g Net Car 0.8 g Fiber

145) *Buckwheat Porridge*

Ingredients:

- *1½ cups water*

- *1 cup buckwheat groats, rinsed*
- *¾ teaspoon vanilla extract*
- *½ teaspoon ground cinnamon*
- *¼ teaspoon salt*
- *2 tablespoons maple syrup*
- *1 ripe banana, peeled and mashed*
- *1½ cups unsweetened soy milk*
- *1 tablespoon peanut butter*
- *1/3 cup fresh strawberries, hulled and chopped*

Direction: Servings: 2 Cooking Time: 15 Minutes

✓ *Place the water, buckwheat, vanilla extract, cinnamon, and salt in a pan and bring to a boil.*

✓ *Now, adjust the heat to medium-low and simmer for about 6 minutes, stirring occasionally. Stir in maple syrup, banana, soy milk, and simmer, covered for about 6 minutes.*

✓ *Remove the pan of porridge from heat and stir in peanut butter. Serve warm with the topping of strawberry pieces.*

Nutrition: Calories 453 Total Fat 9.4 g Saturated Fat 1.7 g Cholesterol 0 mg Sodium 374 mg Total Carbs 82.8 g Fiber 9.4 g Sugar 28.8 g Protein 16.

146) *Breakfast Sandwich*

Ingredients:

- *2 oz/60g cheddar cheese*
- *1/6 oz/30g smoked ham*
- *2 tbsp butter 4 eggs*

Direction: Servings: 2 Cooking Time: 0 Minutes

✓ *Fry all the eggs and sprinkle the pepper and salt on them.*

✓ *Place an egg down as the sandwich base. Top with the ham and cheese and a drop or two of Tabasco.*

✓ *Place the other egg on top and enjoy.*

Nutrition: 600 cal.50g fat 12g protein 7g carbs.

147) *Berry-oat Breakfast Bars*

Ingredients:

- *2 cups fresh raspberries or blueberries*
- *2 tablespoons sugar*
- *2 tablespoons freshly squeezed lemon juice*
- *1 tablespoon cornstarch*
- *11/2 cups rolled oats*
- *1/2 cup whole-wheat flour*
- *1/2 cup walnuts*
- *¼ cup chia seeds*
- *¼ cup extra-virgin olive oil*

- *¼ cup honey*
- *1 large egg*

Direction: Servings: 12 Cooking Time: 25 Minutes

✓ *Preheat the oven to 350F. In a small saucepan over medium heat, stir together the berries, sugar, lemon juice, and cornstarch.*

✓ *Bring to a simmer. Reduce the heat and simmer for 2 to 3 minutes, until the mixture thickens.*

✓ *In a food processor or high-speed blender, combine the oats, flour, walnuts, and chia seeds. Process until powdered. Add the olive oil, honey, and egg.*

✓ *Pulse a few more times, until well combined. Press half of the mixture into a 9-inch square baking dish. Spread the berry filling over the oat mixture. Add the remaining oat mixture on top of the berries.*

✓ *Bake for 25 minutes, until browned. Let cool completely, cut into 12 pieces, and serve. Store in a covered container for up to 5 days.*

Nutrition: Calories: 201; Total fat: 10g; Saturated fat: 1g; Protein: 5g; Carbs: 26g; Sugar: 9g; Fiber: 5g; Cholesterol: 16mg; Sod

148) *Eggplant Omelet*

Ingredients:

- *1 large eggplant*
- *1 tbsp coconut oil, melted*
- *1 tsp unsalted butter*
- *2 eggs*
- *2 tbsp chopped green onions*

Direction: Servings: 2 Cooking Time: 5 Minutes

✓ *Set the grill and let it preheat at the high setting.*

✓ *In the meantime, prepare the eggplant, and for this, cut two slices from eggplant, about 1-inch thick, and reserve the remaining eggplant for later use.*

✓ *Brush slices of eggplant with oil, season with salt on both sides, put the slices on the grill and cook for 3 to 4 minutes per side. Move grilled eggplant to a cutting board, let it cool for 5 minutes, and then make a home in the center of each slice by using a cookie cutter.*

✓ *Bring out a frying pan, put it over medium heat, add butter and when it melts, add eggplant slices in it and crack an egg into each hole.*

✓ *Let the eggs cook, carefully flip the eggplant slice,*

✓ *and continue cooking for 3 minutes until the egg is thoroughly cooked. Season egg with salt and black pepper, move them to a plate, then garnish with green onions and serve.*

Nutrition: 184 Cal 14.1 g Fats 7.8 g Protein 3 g Net Carb 3.5 g Fiber

LUNCH

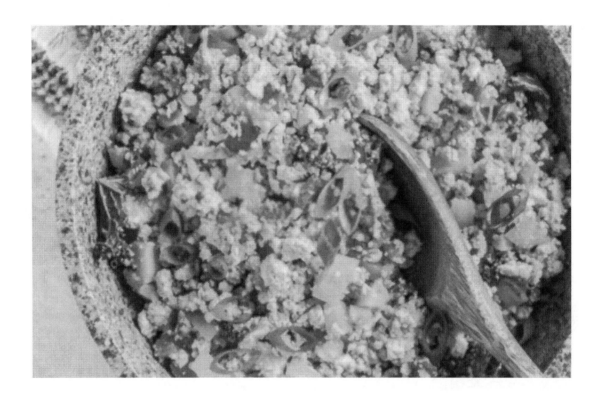

149) *Gazpacho*

Ingredients:

- *3 pounds ripe tomatoes*
- *1 cup low-sodium tomato juice*
- *½ red onion, chopped 1 cucumber*
- *red bell pepper 2 celery stalks*
- *2 tbsp. parsley*
- *2 garlic cloves*
- *2 tbsp. Extra-virgin olive oil*
- *2 tbsp. red wine vinegar*
- *1 tsp. Honey*
- *½ tsp. salt*
- *¼ tsp. freshly ground black pepper*

Direction: Preparation Time: 15 minutes Cooking Time: 0 minute Servings: 4

✓ *In a blender jar, combine the tomatoes, tomato juice, onion, cucumber, bell pepper, celery, parsley, garlic, olive oil, vinegar, honey, salt, and pepper. Pulse until blended but still slightly chunky.*

✓ *Adjust the seasonings as needed and serve.*

Nutrition: Calories: 170 Carbohydrates: 24g Sugar: 16g

150) *Tomato and Kale Soup*

Ingredients:

- *tbsp. extra-virgin olive oil*
- *1 medium onion*
- *2 carrots*
- *3 garlic cloves*
- *4 cups low-sodium vegetable broth*
- *1 (28 oz.) can crushed tomatoes*
- *½ tsp. dried oregano*
- *¼ tsp. dried basil*
- *4 cups chopped baby kale leaves*
- *¼ tsp. salt*

Direction: Preparation Time: 10 minutes Cooking Time: 15 minutes Servings: 4

✓ *In a huge pot, heat up oil over medium heat. Sauté onion and carrots for 3 to 5 minutes. Add the garlic and sauté for 30 seconds more, until fragrant.*

✓ *Add the vegetable broth, tomatoes, oregano, and basil to the pot and boil. Decrease the heat to low and simmer for 5 minutes. Using an immersion blender, purée the soup.*

✓ *Add the kale and simmer for 3 more minutes— season with salt. Serve immediately.*

Nutrition: Calories: 170 Carbohydrates: 31g Sugar: 13g

151) *Comforting Summer Squash Soup with Crispy Chickpeas*

Ingredients:

- *1 (15 oz.) can low-sodium chickpeas*
- *1 tsp. extra-virgin olive oil*
- *¼ tsp. smoked paprika Pinch salt, plus ½ tsp.*
- *3 medium zucchinis*
- *3 cups low-sodium vegetable broth*
- *½ onion*
- *3 garlic cloves*
- *2 tbsp. plain low-fat Greek yogurt*
- *Freshly ground black pepper*

Direction: Preparation Time: 10 minutes Cooking Time: 20 minutes Servings: 4

✓ *Preheat the oven to 425°F. Line a baking sheet with parchment paper.*

✓ *In a medium mixing bowl, toss the chickpeas with 1 tsp. of olive oil, the smoked paprika, and a pinch of salt. Transfer to the prepared baking sheet and roast until crispy, about 20 minutes, stirring once. Set aside.*

✓ *Meanwhile, in a medium pot, heat the remaining 1 tbsp—oil over medium heat. Add the zucchini, broth, onion, and garlic to the pot, and boil. Simmer, and cook for 20 minutes.*

✓ *In a blender jar, purée the soup. Return to the pot.*

✓ *Add the yogurt, remaining ½ tsp. of salt, and pepper, and*

✓ *stir well. Serve topped with roasted chickpeas.*

Nutrition: Calories: 188 Carbs: 24g Sugar: 7g

152) *Curried Carrot Soup*

Ingredients:

- *tbsp. extra-virgin olive oil*
- *1 small onion*
- *2 celery stalks*
- *1½ tsp. curry powder*
- *1 tsp. ground cumin*
- *1 tsp. minced fresh ginger*
- *6 medium carrots*
- *4 cups low-sodium vegetable broth*
- *¼ tsp. salt*
- *1 cup canned coconut milk*
- *¼ tsp. freshly ground black pepper*
- *1 tbsp. chopped fresh cilantro*

Direction: Preparation Time: 10 minutes Cooking Time: 5 minutes Servings: 6

✓ *Heat an Instant Pot to high and add the olive oil.*

✓ *Sauté the onion and celery for 2 to 3 minutes. Add*

the curry powder, cumin, and ginger to the pot and cook until fragrant, about 30 seconds.

✓ Add the carrots, vegetable broth, and salt to the pot. Close and seal, and set for 5

✓ minutes on high. Allow the pressure to release naturally.

✓ In a blender jar, carefully purée the soup in batches and transfer it back to the pot.

✓ Stir in the coconut milk and pepper, and heat through. Top with cilantro and serve.

Nutrition: Calories: 145 Carbs: 13g Sugar: 4g

153) *Thai Peanut, Carrot, and Shrimp Soup*

Ingredients:

- *1 tbsp. coconut oil*
- *1 tbsp. Thai red curry paste*
- *½ onion*
- *3 garlic cloves*
- *2 cups chopped carrots*
- *½ cup whole unsalted peanuts*
- *4 cups low-sodium vegetable broth*
- *½ cup unsweetened plain almond milk*
- *½ pound shrimp*
- *Minced fresh cilantro, for garnish*

Direction: Preparation Time: 10 minutes Cooking Time: 10 minutes Servings: 4

✓ In a big pan, heat oil over medium-high heat until shimmering.

✓ Cook curry paste, stirring continuously, for 1 minute. Add the onion, garlic, carrots, and peanuts to the pan, and continue to cook for 2 to 3 minutes. Boil broth. Reduce the heat to low and simmer for 5 to 6 minutes.

✓ Purée the soup until smooth and return it to the pot. Over low heat, pour almond milk and stir to combine—Cook shrimp in the pot for 2 to 3 minutes.

✓ Garnish with cilantro and serve.

Nutrition: Calories: 237 Carbs: 17g Sugar: 6g

154) *Chicken Tortilla Soup*

Ingredients:

- *1 tbsp. extra-virgin olive oil*
- *1 onion, thinly sliced*
- *1 garlic clove, minced*
- *jalapeño pepper, diced*
- *boneless, skinless chicken breasts*
- *4 cups low-sodium chicken broth*
- *Roma tomato, diced*
- *½ tsp. salt*

- *(6-inch) corn tortillas 1 lime, juiced*
- *Minced fresh cilantro for garnish*
- *¼ cup shredded cheddar cheese, for garnish*

Direction: Preparation Time: 10 minutes Cooking Time: 35 minutes Servings: 4

✓ In a medium pot, cook oil over medium-high heat. Add the onion and cook for 3 to 5 minutes until it begins to soften.

✓ Add the garlic and jalapeño, and cook until fragrant, about 1 minute more.

✓ Add the chicken, chicken broth, tomato, and salt to the pot and boil. Lower heat to medium and simmer mildly for 20 to 25 minutes.

✓ Remove the chicken from the pot and set it aside.

✓ Preheat a broiler too high.

✓ Spray the tortilla strips with nonstick cooking spray and toss to coat. Spread in a single layer on a baking sheet and broil for 3 to 5 minutes, flipping once, until crisp.

✓ Once the chicken is cooked, shred it with 2 forks and return to the pot.

✓ Season the soup with lime juice. Serve hot, garnished with cilantro, cheese, and tortilla strips.

Nutrition: Calories: 191 Carbs: 13g Sugar: 2g

155) *Beef and Mushroom Barley Soup*

Ingredients:

- *1 lb. beef stew meat, cubed*
- *¼ tsp. Salt*
- *¼ tsp. freshly ground black pepper*
- *1 tbsp. extra-virgin olive oil*
- *8 oz. sliced mushrooms*
- *1 onion, chopped*
- *2 carrots, chopped*
- *3 celery stalks, chopped*
- *6 garlic cloves, minced*
- *½ tsp. dried thyme*
- *4 cups low-sodium beef broth*
- *1 cup water*
- *½ cup pearl barley*

Direction: Preparation Time: 10 minutes Cooking Time: 80 minutes Servings: 6

✓ Season the meat well.

✓ In an Instant Pot, heat the oil over high heat—Cook meat on all sides. Remove from the pot and set aside.

✓ Add the mushrooms to the pot and cook for 1 to 2 minutes. Remove the mushrooms and set them aside with the meat.

✓ Sauté onion, carrots, and celery for 3 to 4 minutes. Add the garlic and continue to cook until fragrant, about 30 seconds longer.

✓ *Return the meat and mushrooms to the pot, then add the thyme, beef broth, and water. Adjust the pressure on high and cook for 15 minutes. Let the pressure release naturally.*

✓ *Open the Instant Pot and add the barley. Use the slow cooker function on the Instant Pot, affix the lid (vent open), and continue to cook for 1 hour. Serve.*

Nutrition: Calories: 245 Carbohydrates: 19g Sugar: 3g

156) *Tomato and Guaca Salad*

Ingredients:

- *1 cup cherry tomatoes*
- *1 large cucumber*
- *1 small red onion*
- *1 avocado*
- *2 tbsp. chopped fresh dill*
- *2 tbsp. extra-virgin olive oil*
- *1 lemon, juiced*
- *¼ tsp. Salt*
- *¼ tsp. freshly ground black pepper*

Direction: Preparation Time: 10 minutes Cooking Time: 0 minute Servings: 4

✓ *In a big mixing bowl, mix the tomatoes, cucumber, onion, avocado, and dill.*

✓ *In a small bowl, combine the oil, lemon juice, salt, and pepper, and mix well.*
Drizzle the dressing over the vegetables and toss to combine. Serve.

Nutrition: Calories: 151 Carbohydrates: 11g Sugar: 4g

157) *Coleslaw*

Ingredients:

- *2 cups green cabbage*
- *2 cups red cabbage*
- *2 cups grated carrots*
- *3 scallions*
- *2 tbsp. extra-virgin olive oil*
- *2 tbsp. rice vinegar*
- *1 tsp. honey*
- *1 garlic clove*
- *¼ tsp. salt*

Direction: Preparation Time: 15 minutes Cooking Time: 0 minute Servings: 4

✓ *Throw together the green and red cabbage, carrots, and scallions.*

✓ *In a small bowl, whisk together the oil, vinegar, honey, garlic, and salt.*
Pour the dressing over the veggies and mix to thoroughly combine.

✓ *Serve immediately, or cover and chill for several hours before serving.*

Nutrition: Calories: 80 Carbohydrates: 10g Sugar: 6g

158) *Green Salad with Berries and Sweet Potatoes*

Ingredients:

- *For the vinaigrette:*
- *1-pint blackberries*
- *2 tbsp. red wine vinegar*
- *1 tbsp. honey*
- *3 tbsp. extra-virgin olive oil*
- *¼ tsp. salt*
- *Freshly ground black pepper*

For The Salad:

- *1 sweet potato, cubed*
- *1 tsp. extra-virgin olive oil*
- *8 cups salad greens (baby spinach, spicy greens, romaine)*
- *½ red onion, sliced*
- *¼ cup crumbled goat cheese*

Direction: Preparation Time: 15 minutes Cooking Time: 20 minutes Servings: 4

✓ *For The Vinaigrette:*

✓ *In a blender jar, combine the blackberries, vinegar, honey, oil, salt, and pepper, and process until smooth. Set aside.*

✓ *For The Salad:*

✓ *Preheat the oven to 425°F. Line a baking sheet with parchment paper.*

✓ *Mix the sweet potato with olive oil. Transfer to the prepared baking sheet and roast for 20 minutes, stirring once halfway through, until tender. Remove and cool for a few minutes.*

✓ *In a large bowl, toss the greens with the red onion and cooled sweet potato, and drizzle with the vinaigrette. Serve topped with 1 tbsp—goat cheese per serving.*

Nutrition: Calories: 196 Carbohydrates: 21g Sugar: 10g

159) *Bean and Scallion Salad*

Ingredients:

- *1 (15 oz.) can low-sodium chickpeas*
- *1(15 oz.) can low-sodium kidney beans*
- *1 (15 oz.) can low-sodium white beans*
- *1 red bell pepper*
- *¼ cup chopped scallions*
- *¼ cup finely chopped fresh basil*

- 3 garlic cloves, minced
- 2 tbsp. extra-virgin olive oil
- 1 tbsp. red wine vinegar
- 1 tsp. Dijon mustard
- ¼ tsp. freshly ground black pepper

Direction: Preparation Time: 10 minutes Cooking Time: 0 minute Servings: 8

✓ Toss chickpeas, kidney beans, white beans, bell pepper, scallions, basil, and garlic gently.

✓ Blend together olive oil, vinegar, mustard, and pepper. Toss with the salad.

✓ Wrap and chill for 1 hour.

Nutrition: Calories: 193 Carbs: 29g Sugar: 3g

160) *Rainbow Bean Salad*

Ingredients:

- 1 (15 oz.) can low-sodium black beans
- 1 avocado, diced
- 1 cup cherry
- 3 tomatoes, halved
- 1 cup chopped baby spinach
- ½ cup red bell pepper
- ¼ cup jicama
- ½ cup scallions
- ¼ cup fresh cilantro
- 2 tbsp. lime juice
- 1 tbsp. extra-virgin olive oil
- 2 garlic cloves, minced
- 1 tsp. honey
- ¼ tsp. salt
- ¼ tsp. freshly ground black pepper

Direction: Preparation Time: 15 minutes Cooking Time: 0 minute Servings: 5

✓ Mix black beans, avocado, tomatoes, spinach, bell pepper, jicama, scallions, and cilantro.

✓ Blend lime juice, oil, garlic, honey, salt, and pepper. Add to the salad and toss.

✓ Chill for 1 hour before serving.

Nutrition: Calories: 169 Carbohydrates: 22g Sugar: 3g

161) *Warm Barley and Squash Salad*

Ingredients:

- 1 small butternut squash
- 3 tbsp. extra-virgin olive oil
- 2 cups broccoli florets
- 1 cup pearl barley

- cup toasted chopped walnuts
- 2 cups baby kale
- ½ red onion, sliced
- 2 tbsp. balsamic vinegar
- 2 garlic cloves, minced
- ½ tsp. salt
- ¼ tsp. black pepper

Direction: Preparation Time: 20 minutes Cooking Time: 40 minutes Servings: 8

✓ Preheat the oven to 400°F. Line a baking sheet with parchment paper.

✓ Peel off the squash and slice into dice. In a large bowl, toss the squash with 2 tsp. of olive oil. Transfer to the prepared baking sheet and roast for 20 minutes.

✓ While the squash is roasting, toss the broccoli in the same bowl with 1 tsp. of olive oil. After 20 minutes, flip the squash and push it to one side of the baking sheet. Add the broccoli to the other side and continue to roast for 20 more minutes until tender. While the veggies are roasting, in a medium pot, cover the barley with several inches of water. Boil, then adjust heat, cover, and simmer for 30 minutes until tender. Drain and rinse.

✓ Transfer the barley to a large bowl, and toss with the cooked squash and broccoli, walnuts, kale, and onion.

✓ In a small bowl, mix the remaining 2 tbsp. Olive oil, balsamic vinegar, garlic, salt, and pepper. Drizzle dressing over the salad and toss.

Nutrition: Calories: 274 Carbohydrates: 32g Sugar: 3g

162) *Citrus and Chicken Salad*

Ingredients:

- 4 cups baby spinach
- 2 tbsp. extra-virgin olive oil
- 1 tbsp. Lemon juice
- ⅛ tsp. salt
- 2 cups chopped cooked chicken
- 2 mandarin oranges
- ½ peeled grapefruit, sectioned
- ¼ cup sliced almonds

Direction: Preparation Time: 10 minutes Cooking Time: 0 minute Servings: 4

✓ Toss spinach with olive oil, lemon juice, salt, and pepper.

✓ Add the chicken, oranges, grapefruit, and almonds to the bowl. Toss gently.

✓ Arrange on 4 plates and serve.

Nutrition: Calories: 249 Carbs: 11g Sugar: 7g

163) Blueberry and Chicken Salad

Ingredients:

- 2 cups chopped cooked chicken
- 1 cup fresh blueberries
- ¼ cup almonds
- 1 celery stalk
- ¼ cup red onion
- 1 tbsp. fresh basil
- 1 tbsp. fresh cilantro
- ½ cup plain, vegan mayonnaise
- ¼ tsp. salt
- ¼ tsp. freshly ground black pepper
- 8 cups salad greens

Direction: Preparation Time: 10 minutes Cooking Time: 0 minute Servings: 4

✓ Toss chicken, blueberries, almonds, celery, onion, basil, and cilantro.

✓ Blend yogurt, salt, and pepper. Stir chicken salad to combine.

✓ Situate 2 cups of salad greens on each of 4 plates and divide the chicken salad among the plates to serve.

Nutrition: Calories: 207 Carbs: 11g Sugar: 6g

164) Crunchy Strawberry Salad

Ingredients:

- 0.6 lb. romaine lettuce leaves, roughly torn
- 0.6 lb. strawberries, sliced
- 0.2 lb. nuts of choice

Direction: Preparation Time: 10 minutes Cooking Time: 0 minutes Servings: 5

✓ In a large mixing bowl add strawberry slices, lettuce, and nuts; toss to combine.

✓ Add to a serving bowl.

Nutrition: Calories: 94 Fat: 0.3g Protein: 11g

165) Zucchini Noodle Salad with Almonds

Ingredients:

- 2–3 zucchini, noodled
- 2 tbsp. olive oil
- 1 carrot, peeled, noodled
- lb. red cabbage, thinly sliced
- 2 tbsp. lime juice
- Kosher salt and pepper, to taste
- lb. toasted almonds, chopped

- 3–4 tbsp. cilantro leaves

Direction: Preparation Time: 35 minutes Cooking Time: 10 minutes Servings: 4

✓ Combine zucchini, carrots, cabbage, and almonds. Season with salt, pepper, lemon juice, and olive oil then toss it well.

✓ Add to a serving platter.

Nutrition: Calories: 264 Fat: 2g Protein: 6g

166) Carrot and Spinach Salad

Ingredients:

- 0.8 lb. baby spinach leaves
- 2 carrots, peeled, grated
- 5 tbsp. olive oil
- 4 tbsp. lemon juice
- Salt and black pepper, to taste
- 1 tsp. thyme
- 1–2 garlic cloves, minced
- ¼ tsp. olive powder

Direction: Preparation Time: 60 minutes Cooking Time: 0 minutes Servings: 4

✓ Stir in lemon juice, olive oil, salt, pepper, onion powder, and garlic. Mix well.

✓ Add carrots and spinach leaves to the mixture. Toss to combine.
Cover the bowl with a plastic wrapper. Place it in the refrigerator for about 50 minutes before serving.

Nutrition: Calories: 215 Fat: 4.5g Protein: 14g

167) Red Cabbage Salad

Ingredients:

- lb. red cabbage, thinly sliced
- 2 carrots, peeled, thinly sliced
- 2 tbsp. olive oil
- Salt and black pepper, to taste
- 2 tbsp. lemon juice
- 2 tbsp. coriander leaves, chopped
- 1 tbsp. mint leaves, chopped

Direction: Preparation Time: 15 minutes Cooking Time: 0 minutes Servings: 4

✓ Combine cabbage, carrots, mint, and coriander. Mix in salt, pepper, lemon juice, and olive oil then toss it well. Transfer salad onto a serving platter

Nutrition: Calories: 226 Fat: 5g Protein: 12g

168) Quinoa Fruit Salad

Ingredients:

- *1 lb. cooked quinoa*
- *1 mango, peeled and diced*
- *½ lb. strawberries, quartered*
- *½ lb. blueberries*
- *2 tbsp. pine nuts*
- *Chopped mint leaves, for garnish*
- *4 tbsp. olive oil*
- *1 lemon zest, as required*
- *3 tbsp. freshly squeezed lemon juice*
- *1 tbsp. date sugar*

Direction: Preparation Time: 15 minutes Cooking Time: 0 minutes Servings: 3

✓ *For the vinaigrette, beat the olive oil, lemon zest, juice, and sugar in a small bowl. Set aside.*
✓ *Mix quinoa, mango, strawberries, blueberries, and pine nuts in a large bowl. Add the lemon vinaigrette.*

Nutrition: Calories: 490 Fat: 17.2g Protein: 9.8g

169)   *Beef and Red Bean Chili*

Ingredients:

- *1 cup dry red beans*
- *1 tbsp. olive oil*
- *pounds' boneless beef chuck*
- *large onion, coarsely chopped*
- *1 (14 ounces) can beef broth*
- *chipotle chili peppers in adobo sauce*
- *2 tsp. dried oregano, crushed*
- *1 tsp. ground cumin*
- *½ tsp. salt*
- *1 (14.5 ounces) can of tomatoes with mild green chilis*
- *1 (15 ounces) can tomato sauce*
- *¼ cup snipped fresh cilantro*
- *1 medium red sweet pepper*

Direction: Preparation Time: 10 minutes Cooking Time: 6 hours Servings: 4

✓ *Rinse out the beans, place them into a Dutch oven or big saucepan, and then add water enough to cover them. Allow the beans to boil then drop the heat down. Simmer the beans without a cover for 10 minutes. Take off the heat and keep covered for an hour.*
✓ *In a big fry pan, heat up the oil upon medium-high heat, then cook onion and half the beef until they brown a bit over medium-high heat. Move into a 3 ½ or 4-quart crockery cooker. Do this again with what's left of the beef.*
Add in tomato sauce, tomatoes (not drained), salt, cumin, oregano, adobo sauce, chipotle peppers, and broth, stirring to blend. Strain out and rinse beans

and stir in the cooker.
✓ *Cook while covered on a low setting for around 10–12 hours or on a*
✓ *high setting for 5–6 hours. Spoon the chili into bowls or mugs and top with sweet pepper and cilantro.*

Nutrition: Calories: 288 Carbs: 24g Sugar: 5g

170)   *Berry Apple Cider*

Ingredients:

- *4 cinnamon sticks, cut into 1-inch pieces*
- *1½ tsp. whole cloves*
- *4 cups apple cider*
- *4 cups low-calorie cranberry-raspberry juice drink*
- *1 medium apple*

Direction: Preparation Time: 15 minutes Cooking Time: 3 hours Servings: 3

✓ *To make the spice bag, cut out a 6-inch square from double-thick, pure cotton cheesecloth. Put in the cloves and cinnamon, then bring the corners up, tie it closed using a clean kitchen string that is pure cotton.*
✓ *In a 3 ½ 5-quart slow cooker, combine cranberry-raspberry juice, apple cider, and the spice bag. Cook while covered over a low heat setting for around 4–6 hours or on a high heat setting for 2-2 ½ hours.*
✓ *Throw out the spice bag. Serve right away or keep it warm while covered on warm or low-heat, setting up to 2 hours, occasionally stirring. Garnish each serving with apples (thinly sliced).*

Nutrition: Calories: 89 Carbohydrates: 22g Sugar: 19g

171)   *Brunswick Stew*

Ingredients:

- *4 oz. diced salt pork*
- *2 pounds chicken parts*
- *8 cups water*
- *3 potatoes, cubed*
- *3 onions, chopped*
- *1 (28 oz.) can whole peeled tomatoes*
- *2 cups canned whole kernel corn*
- *1 (10 oz.) package frozen lima beans*
- *1 tbsp. Worcestershire sauce*
- *½ tsp. salt*
- *¼ tsp. ground black pepper*

Direction: Preparation Time: 10 minutes Cooking Time: 45 minutes Servings: 3

✓ *Mix and boil water, chicken, and salt pork in a big*

pot on high heat. Lower heat to low. Cover then simmer until chicken is tender for 45 minutes.

✓ Take out chicken. Let cool until easily handled. Take the meat out. Throw out bones and skin. Chop meat into bite-sized pieces. Put back in the soup. Add ground black pepper, salt, Worcestershire sauce, lima beans, corn, tomatoes, onions, and potatoes. Mix well. Stir well and simmer for 1 hour, uncovered.

Nutrition: Calories: 368 Carbs: 25.9g Protein: 27.9g

172) *Buffalo Chicken Salads*

Ingredients:

- 1½ pounds chicken breast halves
- ½ cup Wing Time® Buffalo chicken sauce
- 4 tsp. cider vinegar
- 1 tsp. Worcestershire sauce
- 1 tsp. paprika
- 1/3 cup light mayonnaise
- 2 tbsp. fat-free milk
- 2 tbsp. crumbled blue cheese
- 2 romaine hearts, chopped
- cup whole-grain croutons
- ½ cup very thinly sliced red onion

Direction: Preparation Time: 7 minutes Cooking Time: 3 hours Servings: 5

✓ Place chicken in a 2/4 slow cooker. Mix together Worcestershire sauce, 2 tsp. of vinegar and Buffalo sauce in a small bowl; pour over chicken. Dust with paprika. Close and cook for 3 hours in a low-heat setting.

✓ Mix the leftover 2 tsp. of vinegar with milk and light mayonnaise together in a small bowl at serving time; mix in blue cheese. While chicken is still in the slow cooker, pull meat into bite-sized pieces using 2 forks.

✓ Split the romaine among 6 dishes. Spoon sauce and chicken over lettuce. Pour with blue cheese dressing then add red onion slices and croutons on top.

Nutrition: Calories: 274 Carbohydrates: 11g Fiber: 2g

173) *Cacciatore Style Chicken*

Ingredients:

- 2 cups sliced fresh mushrooms
- 1 cup sliced celery
- 1 cup chopped carrot
- 2 medium onions, cut into wedges
- 1 green, yellow, or red sweet peppers
- 4 garlic cloves, minced

- 12 chicken drumsticks
- ½ cup chicken broth
- ¼ cup dry white wine
- 2 tbsp. quick-cooking tapioca
- 2 bay leaves
- 1 tsp. dried oregano, crushed 1
- 1tsp. sugar
- ½ tsp. salt
- ¼ tsp. pepper
- 1 (14.5 ounces) can diced tomatoes
- 1/3 cup tomato paste
- Hot cooked pasta or rice

Direction: Preparation Time: 10 minutes Cooking Time: 4 hours Servings: 6

✓ Mix garlic, sweet pepper, onions, carrot, celery, and mushrooms in a 5 or 6-qt. slow cooker. Cover veggies with the chicken. Add pepper, salt, sugar, oregano, bay leaves, tapioca, wine, and broth.

✓ Cover. Cook for 3–3 ½ hours in a high-heat setting. Take chicken out; keep warm. Discard bay leaves. Turn to the high-heat setting if using the low-heat setting. Mix tomato paste and undrained tomatoes in. Cover. Cook on high-heat setting for 15 more minutes. Servings: Put the veggie mixture on top of pasta and chicken.

Nutrition: Calories: 324 Sugar: 7g Carbohydrates: 35g

174) *Carnitas Tacos*

Ingredients:

- 3 to 3½ lb. bone-in pork shoulder roast
- ½ cup chopped onion
- 1/3 cup orange juice 1 tbsp. ground cumin
- 1½ tsp. kosher salt
- 1 tsp. dried oregano, crushed
- ¼ tsp. cayenne pepper
- 1 lime
- 2 (5.3 ounces) containers of plain low-fat Greek yogurt
- 1 pinch kosher salt
- 16 (6 inches) soft yellow corn tortillas
- 4 leaves green cabbage, quartered
- 1 cup very thinly sliced red onion
- 1 cup salsa (optional)

Direction: Preparation Time: 10 minutes Cooking Time: 5 hours Servings: 4

✓ Take off meat from the bone; throw away bone— trim meat fat. Slice meat into 2 to 3-inch pieces; put in a slow cooker of 3 ½ or 4-quart in size. Mix in cayenne, oregano, salt, cumin, orange juice, and onion.

✓ Cover and cook for 4 to 5 hours on high. Take out the meat from the cooker—Shred meat with 2 forks. Mix in enough cooking liquid to moisten.
Take out 1 tsp. zest (put aside) for lime cream, then squeeze 2 tbsp. lime juice. Mix dash salt, yogurt, and lime juice in a small bowl.

✓ Serve lime cream, salsa (if wished), red onion, and cabbage with meat in tortillas. Scatter with lime zest.

Nutrition: Calories: 301 Carbs: 28g Sugar: 7g

175) *Chicken Vera Cruz*

Ingredients:

- 1 medium onion, cut into wedges
- 1 lb. yellow-skin potatoes
- 6 skinless, boneless chicken thighs
- 2 (14.5 oz.) cans of no-salt-added diced tomatoes
- 1 fresh jalapeño chili pepper
- 2 tbsp. Worcestershire sauce
- 1 tbsp. chopped garlic
- 1 tbsp. Dried oregano, crushed
- ¼ tsp. ground cinnamon
- ⅛ tsp. ground cloves
- ½ cup snipped fresh parsley
- ¼ cup chopped pimiento-stuffed green olives

Direction: Preparation Time: 7 minutes Cooking Time: 10 hours Servings: 5

✓ Put the onion in a 3 ½ or 4-quart slow cooker. Place chicken thighs and potatoes on top. Drain and discard juices from a can of tomatoes. Stir undrained and drained tomatoes, cloves, cinnamon, oregano, garlic, Worcestershire sauce, and jalapeño pepper together in a bowl. Pour over all in the cooker.
Cook with a cover for 10 hours in a low-heat setting.

✓ To make the topping: Stir chopped pimiento-stuffed green olives and snipped fresh parsley together in a small bowl. Drizzle the topping over each serving of chicken.

Nutrition: Calories: 228 Sugar: 9g Carbs: 25g

176) *Chicken and Cornmeal Dumplings*

Ingredients:

- Chicken and Vegetable Filling:
- 2 medium carrots, thinly sliced
- 1 stalk celery, thinly sliced
- 1/3 cup corn kernels
- ½ a medium onion, thinly sliced
- 2 garlic cloves, minced
- 1 tsp. snipped fresh rosemary

- ¼ tsp. ground black pepper
- 1 tbsp. all-purpose flour
Cornmeal Dumplings:
- ¼ cup flour
- ¼ cup cornmeal
- ½ tsp. baking powder
- 1 egg white
- 1 tbsp. fat-free milk
- 1 tbsp. canola oil
- 2 chicken thighs, skinned
- 1 cup reduced-sodium chicken broth
- ½ cup fat-free milk

Direction: Preparation Time: 8 minutes Cooking Time: 8 hours Servings: 4

✓ Mix ¼ tsp. pepper, carrots, garlic, celery, rosemary, corn, and onion in a 1 ½ or 2-quart slow cooker. Place chicken on top. Pour the broth atop the mixture into the cooker.

✓ Close and cook on low heat for 7 to 8 hours.

✓ If cooking with the low-heat setting, switch to a high-heat setting (or if the heat setting is not available, continue to cook). Place the chicken onto a cutting board and let cool slightly. Once cool enough to handle, chop off the chicken from bones and get rid of the bones. Chop the chicken and place it back into the mixture in the cooker. Mix flour and milk in a small bowl until smooth. Stir into the mixture in the cooker.

✓ Drop the Cornmeal Dumplings dough into 4 mounds atop hot chicken mixture using 2 spoons. Cover and cook for 20 to 25 minutes more or until a toothpick comes out clean when inserted into a dumpling. (Avoid lifting the lid when cooking.) Sprinkle each of the servings with coarse pepper if desired.

✓ Mix together ½ tsp. baking powder, ¼ cup flour, a dash of salt and, ¼ cup cornmeal in a medium bowl. Mix 1 tbsp. canola oil, 1 egg white, and 1 tbsp. fat-free milk in a small bowl. Pour the egg mixture into the flour mixture. Mix just until moistened.

Nutrition: Calories: 369 Sugar: 9g Carbohydrates: 47g

177) *Chicken and Pepperoni*

Ingredients:

- 3 ½ to 4 pounds' meaty chicken pieces
- ⅛ tsp. salt
- ⅛ tsp. black pepper
- 2 oz. sliced turkey pepperoni
- ¼ cup sliced pitted ripe olives
- ½ cup reduced-sodium chicken broth
- 1 tbsp. tomato paste
- 1 tsp. dried Italian seasoning, crushed

- *½ cup shredded part-skim mozzarella cheese (2 oz.)*

Direction: Preparation Time: 4 minutes Cooking Time: 4 hours Servings: 5

✓ *Put the chicken into a 3 ½ to 5-qt. slow cooker. Sprinkle pepper and salt on the chicken. Slice pepperoni slices in half. Put olives and pepperoni into the slow cooker. In a small bowl, blend Italian seasoning, tomato paste, and chicken broth together. Transfer the mixture into the slow cooker.*

✓ *Cook with a cover for 3–3 ½ hours on high.*

✓ *Transfer the olives, pepperoni, and chicken onto a serving platter with a slotted spoon. Discard the cooking liquid. Sprinkle cheese over the chicken. Use foil to loosely cover and allow to sit for 5 minutes to melt the cheese.*

Nutrition: Calories: 243 Carbohydrate: 1g Protein: 41g

178) <u>Chicken and Sausage Gumbo</u>

Ingredients:

- *¹/3 cup all-purpose flour*
- *1 (14 oz.) can reduced-sodium chicken broth*
- *2 cups chicken breast*
- *8 oz. smoked turkey sausage links*
- *2 cups sliced fresh okra*
- *1 cup water*
- *½ cup sliced celery*
- *4 garlic cloves, minced*
- *1 tsp. dried thyme*
- *½ tsp. ground black pepper*
- *¼ tsp. cayenne pepper*
- *3 cups hot cooked brown rice*
- *1 cup coarsely chopped onion*
- *1 cup sweet pepper*

Direction: Preparation Time: 6 minutes Cooking Time: 4 hours Servings: 5

✓ *To make the roux: Cook the flour upon medium heat in a heavy medium-sized saucepan, stirring periodically, for roughly 6 minutes or until the flour browns. Take off the heat and slightly cool, then slowly stir in the broth. Cook the roux until it bubbles and thickens up.*
Cook the soup covered on a high setting for 3–3 ½ hours. Take the fat off the top and serve atop hot cooked brown rice.

✓ *Pour the roux in a 3 ½ or 4/4 slow cooker, then add in cayenne pepper, black pepper, thyme, garlic, celery, sweet pepper, onion, water, okra, sausage, and chicken.*

Nutrition: Calories: 230 Sugar: 3g Protein: 19g

179) <u>Chicken, Barley, and Leek Stew</u>

Ingredients:

- *1 lb. chicken thighs*
- *1 tbsp. olive oil*
- *1 (49 ounces) can reduced-sodium chicken broth*
- *1 cup regular barley (not quick-cooking)*
- *2 medium leeks, halved lengthwise and sliced*
- *2 medium carrots, thinly sliced*
- *1½ tsp. dried basil or Italian seasoning, crushed*
- *¼ tsp. cracked black pepper*

Direction: Preparation Time: 10 minutes Cooking Time: 3 hours Servings: 2

✓ *In the big skillet, cook the chicken in hot oil till becoming brown on all sides. In the 4–5-qt. slow cooker, whisk the pepper, dried basil, carrots, leeks, barley, chicken broth, and chicken.*
Keep covered and cooked over a high heat setting for 2–2.5 hours or till the barley softens. As you wish, drizzle with the parsley or fresh basil prior to serving.

Nutrition: Calories: 248 Fiber: 6g Carbohydrate: 27g

180) <u>Cider Pork Stew</u>

Ingredients:

- *2 pounds' pork shoulder roast*
- *3 medium cubed potatoes*
- *3 medium carrots*
- *2 medium onions, sliced*
- *1 cup coarsely chopped apple*
- *½ cup coarsely chopped celery*
- *3 tbsp. quick-cooking tapioca*
- *2 cups apple juice*
- *1 tsp. salt*
- *1 tsp. caraway seeds*
- *¼ tsp. black pepper*

Direction: Preparation Time: 9 minutes Cooking Time: 12 hours Servings: 3

✓ *Chop the meat into 1-in. cubes. In the 3.5–5.5 qt. slow cooker, mix the tapioca, celery, apple, onions, carrots, potatoes, and meat. Whisk in pepper, caraway seeds, salt, and apple juice.*

✓ *Keep covered and cook over a low heat setting for 10–12 hours. If you want, use the celery leaves to decorate each of the servings.*

Nutrition: Calories: 244 Fiber: 5g Carbohydrate: 33g

181) <u>Creamy Chicken Noodle Soup</u>

Ingredients:

- *1 (32 fluid ounce) container reduced-sodium chicken broth*

- *3 cups water*
- *2½ cups chopped cooked chicken*
- *3 medium carrots, sliced*
- *3 stalks celery*
- *1½ cups sliced fresh mushrooms*
- *¼ cup chopped onion*
- *1½ tsp. dried thyme, crushed*
- *¾ tsp. garlic-pepper seasoning*
- *3 oz. reduced-fat cream cheese (Neufchatel), cut up*
- *2 cups dried egg noodles*

Direction: Preparation Time: 7 minutes Cooking Time: 8 hours Servings: 4

- ✓ *Mix together the garlic-pepper seasoning, thyme, onion, mushrooms, celery, carrots, chicken, water, and broth in a 5 to 6-quart slow cooker.*
- ✓ *Put the cover and let it cook for 6–8 hours on a low-heat setting.*
  Increase to the high-heat setting if you are using a low-heat setting. Mix in the cream cheese until blended. Mix in uncooked noodles. Put the cover and let it cook for an additional 20–30 minutes or just until the noodles become tender.

Nutrition: Calories: 170 Sugar: 3g Fiber: 2g

182)   *Cuban Pulled Pork Sandwich*

Ingredients:

- *1 tsp. Dried oregano, crushed*
- *¾ tsp. ground cumin*
- *½ tsp. ground coriander*
- *¼ tsp. salt*
- *¼ tsp. black pepper*
- *¼ tsp. ground allspice*
- *2 to 2½ lb. boneless pork shoulder roast*
- *1 tbsp. olive oil*
- *Nonstick cooking spray*
- *2 cups sliced onions*
- *2 sweet green peppers, cut into bite-size strips*
- *½ to 1 fresh jalapeño pepper*
- * 4 garlic cloves, minced*
- *¼ cup orange juice*
- *¼ cup lime juice*
- *6 heart-healthy wheat hamburger buns, toasted*
- *2 tbsp. jalapeño mustard*

Direction: Preparation Time: 6 minutes Cooking Time: 5 hours Servings: 5

- ✓ *Mix allspice, oregano, black pepper, cumin, salt, and coriander together in a small bowl. Press each side of the roast into the spice mixture. On medium-high heat, heat oil in a big non-stick pan; put in roast. Cook for 5mins until both sides of the roast*

are light brown. Turn the roast 1 time.

- ✓ *Using a cooking spray, grease a 3 ½ or 4qt slow cooker; arrange the garlic, onions, jalapeno, and green peppers in a layer. Pour in lime juice and orange juice. Slice the roast if needed to fit inside the cooker; put on top of the vegetables covered for 4 ½–5hrs on high heat setting.*
  Move roast to a cutting board using a slotted spoon. Drain the cooking liquid and keep the jalapeno, green peppers, and onions. Shred the roast with 2 forks then place it back in the cooker. Remove fat from the
- ✓ *liquid. Mix half cup cooking liquid and reserved vegetables into the cooker. Pour in more cooking liquid if desired. Discard the remaining cooking liquid.*
- ✓ *Slather mustard on rolls. Split the meat between the bottom roll halves. Add avocado on top if desired. Place the roll tops on sandwiches.*

Nutrition: Calories: 379 Carbohydrate: 32g Fiber: 4g

183)   *Lemon-Tarragon Soup*

Ingredients:

- *1 tbsp. avocado oil*
- *½ cup diced onion*
- *3 garlic cloves, crushed*
- *¼ plus ⅛ tsp. sea salt*
- *¼ plus ⅛ tsp. freshly ground black pepper*
- *1 (13.5 oz.) can full-fat coconut milk*
- *tbsp. freshly squeezed lemon juice*
- *½ cup raw cashews 1 celery stalk*
- *2 tbsp. chopped fresh tarragon*

Direction: Preparation Time: 10 minutes Cooking Time: 10 minutes Servings: 2

- ✓ *In a medium skillet over medium-high heat, heat up avocado oil. Sauté onion, garlic, salt, and pepper for 4 minutes.*
- ✓ *In a high-speed blender, blend together the coconut milk, lemon juice, cashews, celery, and tarragon with the onion mixture until smooth. Adjust seasonings, if necessary.*
- ✓ *Pour into 1 large or 2 small bowls and enjoy immediately, or transfer to a medium saucepan and warm on low heat for 3 to 5 minutes before serving.*

Nutrition: Calories: 264 Fiber: 11g Fats: 10g

184)   *Chilled Cucumber and Lime Soup*

Ingredients:

- *1 cucumber, peeled*
- *½ zucchini, peeled*
- *1 tbsp. freshly squeezed lime juice*
- *1 tbsp. fresh cilantro leaves*

- *garlic clove, crushed*
- *¼ tsp. sea salt*

Direction: Preparation Time: 25 minutes Cooking Time: 0 minute Servings: 2

✓ *In a blender, blend together the cucumber, zucchini, lime juice, cilantro, garlic, and salt until well combined. Add more salt, if necessary.*

✓ *Pour into 1 large or 2 small bowls and enjoy immediately, or refrigerate for 15 to 20 minutes to chill before serving.*

Nutrition: Calories: 254 Protein: 30g Fat: 8g

185) *Coconut, Cilantro, and Jalapeño Soup*

Ingredients:

- *2 tbsp. Avocado oil*
- *½ cup diced onions*
- *garlic cloves, crushed*
- *¼ tsp. sea salt*
- *1 (13.5 oz.) can full-fat coconut milk*
- *1 tbsp. freshly squeezed lime juice*
- *½ to 1 jalapeño*
- *tbsp. fresh cilantro leaves*

Direction: Preparation Time: 5 minutes Cooking Time: 5 minutes Servings: 2

✓ *Using a medium skillet over medium-high heat, heat up avocado oil. Sauté onion, garlic, and salt for 4 minutes.*

✓ *In a blender, blend together the coconut milk, lime juice, jalapeño, and cilantro with the onion mixture until creamy.*
Pour into 1 large or 2 small bowls and enjoy.

Nutrition: Calories: 159 Fat: 11g Protein: 37g

186) *Spicy Watermelon Gazpacho*

Ingredients:

- *2 cups cubed watermelon*
- *¼ cup diced onion*
- *¼ cup packed cilantro leaves*
- *½ to 1 jalapeño*
- *2 tbsp. freshly squeezed lime juice*

Direction: Preparation Time: 5 minutes Cooking Time: 0 minute Servings: 2

✓ *In a blender or food processor, pulse to combine the watermelon, onion, cilantro, jalapeño, and lime juice only long enough to break down the ingredients, leaving them very finely diced and taking care to not over process.*
Pour into 1 large or 2 small bowls and enjoy.

Nutrition: Calories: 207 Fat: 5g Protein: 36g

187) *Roasted Carrot and Leek Soup*

Ingredients:

- *6 carrots*
- *cup chopped onion*
- *1 fennel bulb, cubed*
- *2 garlic cloves, crushed*
- *2 tbsp. avocado oil*
- *1 tsp. sea salt*
- *1 tsp. freshly ground black pepper*
- *2 cups almond milk, plus more if desired*

Direction: Preparation Time: 10 minutes Cooking Time: 30 minutes Servings: 2 to 4

✓ *Preheat the oven to 400°F. Line a baking sheet with parchment paper. Cut the carrots into thirds, and then cut each third in half. Transfer to a medium bowl.*

✓ *Add the onion, fennel, garlic, and avocado oil, and toss to coat. Season with salt and pepper, and toss again.*

✓ *Transfer the vegetables to the prepared baking sheet and roast for 30 minutes. Remove from the oven and allow the vegetables to cool.*
In a high-speed blender, blend together the almond milk and roasted vegetables until creamy and smooth. Adjust the seasonings, if necessary, and add additional milk if you prefer a thinner consistency.

✓ *Pour into 2 large or 4 small bowls and enjoy.*

Nutrition: Calories: 220 Fiber: 15g Protein: 28g

188) *Lemon Cauliflower & Pine Nuts*

Ingredients:

- *1 tsp. lemon zest*
- *¼ tsp. sea salt*
- *(10 oz.) package cauliflower florets*
- *2 tbsp. extra virgin olive oil*
- *2 tbsp. pine nuts*
- *1 tbsp. parsley, fresh flat-leaf*
- *1 ½ tsp. lemon juice*
- *¼ tsp. fresh ground black pepper*

Direction: Preparation Time: 5 minutes Cooking Time: 20 minutes Servings: 4

✓ *Preheat your oven to 400°F.*

✓ *In a large bowl, combine all of your ingredients. Then set onto a baking sheet.*
Bake for 20 minutes, serve and enjoy!

Nutrition: Calories: 60 Protein: 4g Fat: 0.1g

189) Beef Tenderloin & Avocado Cream

Ingredients:

- 1 tsp. mustard
- (6 oz.) beef steaks
- ¼ cup sour cream
- 2 tsp. lemon juice, fresh
- ¹/3 avocado
- 1 tbsp. olive oil-slicked
- Sea salt along with fresh ground black pepper as needed

Direction: Preparation Time: 10 minutes Cooking Time: 8 minutes Servings: 2

✓ Preheat your oven to 450°F.

✓ Sprinkle the beef steaks with some salt and pepper.

✓ Mix the mustard and oil and spread the mixture over the meat.

✓ Place the steaks into a skillet over medium-high heat for 3 minutes.
Transfer the steaks to a baking sheet and place in the oven, then bake for 6 minutes.

✓ Blend the avocado with lemon juice and sour cream.

✓ Serve steaks with avocado cream and enjoy!

Nutrition: Calories: 205 Protein: 20g Fat: 15g

190) Salmon & Citrus Sauce

Ingredients:

- ¾ lb. salmon fillets
- ¹/3 cup fresh orange juice
- 1 tbsp. fresh lime juice
- 1 tbsp. fresh lemon juice
- 1 tbsp. honey
- 1 tbsp. olive oil
- 1 ½ tbsp. mustard
- Sea salt along with fresh ground black pepper as needed
- ¼ tsp. smoked paprika

Direction: Preparation Time: 10 minutes Cooking Time: 15 minutes Servings: 2

✓ Sprinkle fillets with paprika, salt, and pepper. Then, cook in a skillet over medium-high heat for 5 minutes per side.

✓ While fillets are cooking, mix the lemon, orange, lime juices, and honey, then add to a small saucepan. Add the mustard and stir to combine—
Cook over low heat for 10 minutes.
Add the salmon fillets to serving dishes, then pour the sauce over the fillets. Serve and enjoy!

Nutrition: Calories: 210 Protein: 20g Fat: 22g

191) Orange-Avocado Salad

Ingredients:

- ½ tsp. arugula
- 1 avocado
- 1 navel orange
- 1 tbsp. fresh lime juice
- 1 tbsp. extra-virgin olive oil

Direction: Preparation Time: 10 minutes Cooking Time: 0 minutes Servings: 2

✓ Mix your lime juice, arugula, and oil in a bowl.

✓ Add the peeled and sectioned pieces of orange, then toss.

✓ Add the diced avocado just before serving, then enjoy!

Nutrition: Calories: 30 Protein: 2g Fat: 2g

192) Avocados with Walnut-Herb

Ingredients:

- 1 avocado
- ¼ cup walnuts
- 1 ½ tsp. virgin olive oil
- 1 ½ tsp. lemon juice (fresh)
- 1 tbsp. fresh basil
- sea salt and black pepper to taste

Direction: Preparation Time: 7 minutes Cooking Time: 5 minutes Servings: 2

✓ Fry the chopped nuts for about 5 minutes over medium-low heat in a pan.

✓ In a small bowl, mix the chopped basil, lemon juice, oil, sea salt, and pepper.
Slice avocado in half, then top slices with the walnut mixture, serve, and enjoy!

Nutrition: Calories: 200 Protein: 2g Fat: 17g

193) Barbecue Brisket

Ingredients:

- 1 cup beef broth
- 2 lb. beef brisket
- 1 sweet onion, diced
- ½ cup barbecue sauce
- ½ tbsp. steak seasoning

Direction: Preparation Time: 15 minutes Cooking Time: 5 hours Servings: 4

✓ Add the prepared onion to your slow cooker. Rub the trimmed brisket with seasoning.

✓ Cut the brisket into pieces, and add to your slow cooker.

✓ Pour the beef broth and barbecue sauce over the brisket.

✓ Cook on low for 5 hours, slice brisket. Serve and enjoy!

Nutrition: Calories: 188 Protein: 13g Fat: 8g

194) Broccoli & Hot Sauce

Ingredients:

- 4 cups broccoli florets
- 1 tbsp. extra-virgin olive oil
- ½ tsp. hot sauce
- Sea salt along with black ground pepper as needed

Direction: Preparation Time: 5 minutes Cooking Time: 5 minutes Servings: 4

✓ Arrange your broccoli in a steamer basket. Steam your broccoli for about 5 minutes or until tender.

✓ Drizzle with the oil and sprinkle with hot sauce, sea salt, and black pepper. Serve and enjoy!

Nutrition: Calories: 30 Protein: 4g Fat: 0.1g

195) Chicken Thighs

Ingredients:

- 4 bone-in skinless chicken thighs
- ½ tsp. ginger
- 1 tbsp. olive oil
- 2 tbsp. soy sauce
- ¼ tsp. dry mustard
- 1 garlic clove
- ¼ tsp. red pepper
- ¼ tsp. all-spice

Direction: Preparation Time: 10 minutes Cooking Time: 40 minutes Servings: 4

✓ Preheat the oven to 400°F and sauté the minced garlic, ground allspice, ground ginger, crushed red pepper, and mustard in hot oil for 5 minutes. Remove from heat.

✓ Whisk in soy sauce, then place the chicken thighs on a baking sheet. Add the garlic mixture over the chicken, and toss.

Nutrition: Calories: 120 Protein: 8g Fat: 5g

196) Creamy Bell Pepper-Corn Salad & Seared Zucchini

Ingredients:

- 2 zucchinis
- ½ cup celery
- 1 green bell pepper, sliced and seeded
- 1 dozen cherry tomatoes
- 2 cups kernel corn
- 4 tbsp. sour cream
- ½ cup mayonnaise
- 2 tsp. sweetener
- sea salt along with ground black pepper as needed

Direction: Preparation Time: 10 minutes Cooking Time: 20 minutes Servings: 5

✓ Cook your corn by following package instructions.

✓ Mix the chopped celery, sliced bell pepper, whole cherry tomatoes, mayonnaise, sour cream, sweetener, salt, and pepper in a large salad bowl.

✓ Heat a skillet over medium-high heat. Cook the zucchini sliced lengthwise for about 10 minutes. Turn occasionally, then add salt to zucchini.

✓ Once zucchini is cooked, add it to the corn mixture.

✓ You can serve this dish alongside your favorite meat dish!

Nutrition: Calories: 100 Protein: 6g Fat: 3g

197) Sweet Potato, Kale, and White Bean Stew

Ingredients:

- 1 (15-ounce) can low-sodium cannellini beans, rinsed and drained, divided
- 1 tablespoon olive oil
- 1 medium onion, chopped
- 2 garlic cloves, minced
- 2 celery stalks, chopped
- 3 medium carrots, chopped
- 2 cups low-sodium vegetable broth
- 1 teaspoon apple cider vinegar
- 2 medium sweet potatoes (about 1¼ pounds)
- 2 cups chopped kale
- 1 cup shelled edamame
- ¼ cup quinoa
- 1 teaspoon dried thyme
- 1/2 teaspoon cayenne pepper
- 1/2 teaspoon salt
- ¼ teaspoon freshly ground black pepper

Direction: Preparation time: 15 minutes Cooking time: 25 minutes Servings: 4

✓ Put half the beans into a blender and blend until smooth. Set aside.

✓ In a large soup pot over medium heat, heat the oil. When the oil is shining, include the onion and garlic, and cook until the onion softens and the garlic is sweet about 3 minutes. Add the celery and carrots, and continue cooking until the vegetables soften, about 5 minutes.
Add the broth, vinegar, sweet potatoes, unblended beans, kale, edamame, and quinoa, and bring the

mixture to a boil. Reduce the heat and simmer until the vegetables soften, about 10 minutes.

✓ Add the blended beans, thyme, cayenne, salt, and black pepper, increase the heat to medium-high, and bring the mixture to a boil. Reduce the heat and simmer, uncovered, until the flavors combine, about 5 minutes.

✓ Into each of 4 containers, scoop 1¾ cups of stew.

Nutrition: calories: 373; total fat: 7g; saturated fat: 1g; protein: 15g; total carbs: 65g; fiber: 15g; sugar: 13g;

198)   *Slow Cooker Two-Bean Sloppy Joes*

Ingredients:

- 1 (15-ounce) can of low-sodium black beans
- 1 (15-ounce) can of low-sodium pinto beans
- 1 (15-ounce) can no-salt-added diced tomatoes
- 1 medium green bell pepper, cored, seeded, and chopped
- 1 medium yellow onion, chopped
- ¼ cup low-sodium vegetable broth
- 2 garlic cloves, minced
- 2 servings (¼ cup) meal prep barbecue sauce or bottled barbecue sauce
- ¼ teaspoon salt
- ¼ teaspoon freshly ground black pepper
- 4 whole-wheat buns

Direction: Preparation time: 10 minutes Cooking time: 6 hours Servings: 4

✓ In a slow cooker, combine the black beans, pinto beans, diced tomatoes, bell pepper, onion, broth, garlic, meal prep barbecue sauce, salt, and black pepper. Stir the ingredients, then cover and cook on low for 6 hours.

✓ Into each of 4 containers, spoon 1¼ cups of sloppy sloppy joe mix. Serve with 1 whole-wheat bun. Storage: place airtight containers in the refrigerator for up to 1 week. To freeze, place freezer-safe containers in the freezer for up to 2 months. To defrost, refrigerate overnight. To reheat individual portions, microwave uncovered on high for 2 to 2½ minutes. Alternatively, reheat the entire dish in a saucepan on the stovetop. Bring the sloppy joes to a boil, then reduce the heat and simmer until heated through, 10 to 15 minutes. Serve with a whole-wheat bun.

Nutrition: calories: 392; total fat: 3g; saturated fat: 0g; protein: 17g; total carbs: 79g; fiber: 19g; sugar: 15g;

199)   *Lighter Eggplant Parmesan*

Ingredients:

- Nonstick cooking spray
- 3 eggs, beaten, 1 tablespoon dried parsley
- 2 teaspoons ground oregano
- 1/8 teaspoon freshly ground black pepper
- 1 cup panko bread crumbs, preferably whole-wheat
- 1 large eggplant (about 2 pounds)
- 5 servings (2½ cups) chunky tomato sauce or jarred low-sodium tomato sauce
- 1 cup part-skim mozzarella cheese
- ¼ cup grated parmesan cheese

Direction: Preparation time: 15 minutes Cooking time: 35 minutes Servings: 4

✓ Preheat the oven to 450f. Coat a baking sheet with cooking spray.

✓ In a medium bowl, whisk together the eggs, parsley, oregano, and pepper.

✓ Pour the panko into a separate medium bowl.

✓ Slice the eggplant into ¼-inch-thick slices. Dip each slice of eggplant into the egg mixture, shaking off the excess. Then dredge both sides of the eggplant in the panko bread crumbs. Place the coated eggplant on the prepared baking sheet, leaving a 1/2-inch space between each slice.

✓ Bake for about 15 minutes until soft and golden brown. Remove from the oven and set aside to cool slightly.
Pour 1/2 cup of chunky tomato sauce on the bottom of an 8-by-15-inch baking dish. Using a spatula or the back of a spoon spread the tomato sauce evenly. Place half the slices of cooked eggplant, slightly overlapping, in the dish, and top with 1 cup of chunky tomato sauce, 1/2 cup of mozzarella and 2 tablespoons of grated parmesan. Repeat the layer, ending with the cheese.

✓ Bake uncovered for 20 minutes until the cheese is bubbling and slightly browned.

✓ Remove from the oven and allow cooling for 15 minutes before dividing the eggplant equally into 4 separate containers.

Nutrition: calories: 333; total fat: 14g; saturated fat: 6g; protein: 20g; total carbs: 35g; fiber: 11g; sugar: 15g

200)   *Lemony Salmon Burgers*

Ingredients:

- 2 (3-oz) cans boneless, skinless pink salmon
- 1/4 cup panko breadcrumbs
- 4 tsp. lemon juice
- 1/4 cup red bell pepper
- 1/4 cup sugar-free yogurt
- 1 egg
- 2 (1.5-oz) whole wheat hamburger toasted buns

Direction: Preparation Time: 10 Minutes Cooking

Time: 10 Minutes Servings: 4

✓ *Mix drained and flaked salmon, finely-chopped bell pepper, panko breadcrumbs.*

✓ *Combine 2 tbsp. cup sugar-free yogurt, 3 tsp. fresh lemon juice, and egg in a bowl. Shape mixture into 2 (3-inch) patties, bake on the skillet over medium heat 4 to 5 minutes per side.*
Stir together 2 tbsp. sugar-free yogurt and 1 tsp. lemon juice; spread over bottom halves of buns.

✓ *Top each with 1 patty, and cover with bun tops.*

✓ *This dish is very mouth-watering!*

Nutrition: Cal 131 / Protein 12 / Fat 1 g / Carbs 19 g

201) *Coconut-Lentil Curry*

Ingredients:

- *1 tablespoon olive oil*
- *1 medium yellow onion, chopped, 1 garlic clove, minced*
- *1 medium red bell pepper, diced*
- *1 (15-ounce) can green or brown lentils, rinsed and drained*
- *2 medium sweet potatoes, washed, peeled, and cut into bite-size chunks (about 1¼ pounds)*
- *1 (15-ounce) can no-salt-added diced tomatoes*
- *2 tablespoons tomato paste*
- *4 teaspoons curry powder*
- *1/8 teaspoon ground cloves*
- *1 (15-ounce) can light coconut milk*
- *¼ teaspoon salt*
- *2 pieces whole-wheat naan bread, halved, or 4 slices crusty bread*

Direction: Preparation time: 15 minutes Cooking time: 35 minutes Servings: 4

✓ *In a large saucepan over medium heat, heat the olive oil. When the oil is shimmering, add both the onion and garlic and cook until the onion softens and the garlic is sweet, for about 3 minutes.*

✓ *Add the bell pepper and continue cooking until it softens, about 5 minutes more. Add the lentils, sweet potatoes, tomatoes, tomato paste, curry powder, and cloves, and bring the mixture to a boil. are softened, about 20 minutes.*
Reduce the heat to medium-low, cover, and simmer until the potatoes

✓ *Add the coconut milk and salt, and return to a boil. Reduce the heat and simmer until the flavors combine, about 5 minutes.*

✓ *Into each of 4 containers, spoon 2 cups of curry.*

✓ *Enjoy each serving with half of a piece of naan bread or 1 slice of crusty bread.*

Nutrition: calories: 559; total fat: 16g; saturated fat: 7g; protein: 16g; total carbs: 86g; fiber: 16g; sugar: 18g; sodium: 819mg

202) *Maple-Mustard Salmon*

Ingredients:

- *Nonstick cooking spray*
- *1/2 cup 100% maple syrup*
- *2 tablespoons Dijon mustard*
- *¼ teaspoon salt*
- *4 (5-ounce) salmon fillets*
- *4 servings (4 cups) roasted broccoli with shallots*
- *4 servings (2 cups) parsleyed whole-wheat couscous*

Direction: Preparation time: 10 minutes, plus 30 minutes marinating time Cooking time: 20 minutes Servings: 4

✓ *Preheat the oven to 400f. Line a baking sheet with aluminum foil and coat with cooking spray.*

✓ *In a medium bowl, whisk together the maple syrup, mustard, and salt until smooth.*

✓ *Put the salmon fillets into the bowl and toss to coat. Cover and place in the refrigerator to marinate for at least 30 minutes and up to overnight.*
Shake off excess marinade from the salmon fillets and place them on the prepared baking sheet, leaving a 1-inch space between each fillet. Discard the extra marinade.

✓ *Bake for about 20 minutes until the salmon is opaque and a thermometer inserted in the thickest part of a fillet reads 145f.*

✓ *Into each of 4 resealable containers, place 1 salmon fillet, 1 cup of roasted broccoli with shallots, and 1/2 cup of parsleyed whole-wheat couscous.*

Nutrition: calories: 601; total fat: 29g; saturated fat: 4g; protein: 36g; total carbs: 51g; fiber: 3g; sugar: 23g; sodium: 610mg

203) *Stuffed Portobello with Cheese*

Ingredients:

- *4 Portobello mushroom caps*
- *1 tablespoon olive oil*
- *1/2 teaspoon salt, divided*
- *¼ teaspoon freshly ground black pepper, divided*
- *1 cup baby spinach, chopped*
- *11/2 cups part-skim ricotta cheese*
- *1/2 cup part-skim shredded mozzarella cheese*
- *¼ cup grated parmesan cheese*
- *1 garlic clove, minced*
- *1 tablespoon dried parsley*
- *2 teaspoons dried oregano*
- *4 teaspoons unseasoned bread crumbs, divided*
- *4 servings (4 cups) roasted broccoli with shallots*

Direction: Preparation time: 15 minutes Cooking

time: 25 minutes Servings: 4

✓ Preheat the oven to 375f. Line a baking sheet with aluminum foil.

✓ Brush the mushroom caps with olive oil, and sprinkle with ¼ teaspoon salt and 1/8 teaspoon pepper. Put the mushroom caps on the prepared baking sheet and bake until soft, about 12 minutes.

✓ In a medium bowl, mix together the spinach, ricotta, mozzarella, parmesan, garlic, parsley, oregano, and the remaining ¼ teaspoon of salt and 1/8 teaspoon of pepper.
Spoon 1/2 cup of cheese mixture into each mushroom cap, and sprinkle each with 1 teaspoon of bread crumbs. Return the mushrooms to the oven for an additional 8 to 10 minutes until warmed through.

✓ Remove from the oven and allow the mushrooms to cool for about 10 minutes before placing each in an individual container. Add 1 cup of roasted broccoli with shallots to each container.

Nutrition: calories: 419; total fat: 30g; saturated fat: 10g; protein: 23g; total carbs: 19g; fiber: 2g; sugar: 3g;

204) *Lighter Shrimp Scampi*

Ingredients:

- 11/2 pounds large peeled and deveined shrimp
- ¼ teaspoon salt
- 1/8 teaspoon freshly ground black pepper
- 2 tablespoons olive oil
- 1 shallot, chopped
- 2 garlic cloves, minced
- ¼ cup cooking white wine
- Juice of 1/2 lemon (1 tablespoon)
- 1/2 teaspoon sriracha
- 2 tablespoons unsalted butter, at room temperature
- ¼ cup chopped fresh parsley
- 4 servings (6 cups) zucchini noodles with lemon vinaigrette

Direction: Preparation time: 15 minutes

Cooking time: 15 minutes Servings: 4

✓ Season the shrimp with salt and pepper.

✓ In a medium saucepan over medium heat, heat the oil. Add the shallot and garlic, and cook until the shallot softens and the garlic is fragrant, about 3 minutes. Add the shrimp, cover, and cook until opaque, 2 to 3 minutes on each side. Using a slotted spoon, transfer the shrimp to a large plate.

✓ Bring the mixture to a boil, then reduce the heat and simmer until the liquid is reduced by about half, 3 minutes. Add the butter and stir until melted, about 3 minutes. Return the shrimp to the saucepan and toss to coat. Add the parsley and stir

to combine.

✓ Into each of 4 containers, place 11/2 cups of zucchini noodles with lemon vinaigrette, and top with ¾ cup of scampi.

Nutrition: calories: 364; total fat: 21g; saturated fat: 6g; protein: 37g; total carbs: 10g; fiber: 2g; sugar:6g;

205) *Chicken Salad with Grapes and Pecans*

Ingredients:

- 1/3 cup unsalted pecans, chopped
- 10 ounces cooked skinless, boneless chicken breast or rotisserie chicken, finely chopped
- 1/2 medium yellow onion, finely chopped
- 1 celery stalk, finely chopped
- ¾ cup red or green seedless grapes, halved
- ¼ cup light mayonnaise
- ¼ cup nonfat plain Greek yogurt
- 1 tablespoon Dijon mustard
- 1 tablespoon dried parsley
- ¼ teaspoon salt
- 1/8 teaspoon freshly ground black pepper
- 1 cup shredded romaine lettuce
- 4 (8-inch) whole-wheat pitas

Direction: Preparation Time: 15 Minutes Cooking Time: 5 Minutes Servings: 4

✓ Heat a small skillet over medium-low heat to toast the pecans. Cook the pecans until fragrant, about 3 minutes. Remove from the heat and set aside to cool.

✓ In a medium bowl, mix the chicken, onion, celery, pecans, and grapes.

✓ In a small bowl, whisk together the mayonnaise, yogurt, mustard, parsley, salt, and pepper. Spoon the sauce over the chicken mixture and stir until well combined.
Into each of 4 containers, place ¼ cup of lettuce and top with 1 cup of chicken salad. Store the pitas separately until ready to serve.

✓ When ready to eat, stuff the serving of salad and lettuce into 1 pita.

Nutrition: Calories: 418; Total Fat: 14g; Saturated Fat: 2g; Protein: 31g; Total Carbs: 43g; Fiber: 6g;

206) *Caprese Turkey Burgers*

Ingredients:

- 1/2 lb. 93% lean ground turkey
- 2 (1,5-oz) whole wheat hamburger buns (toasted)
- 1/4 cup shredded mozzarella cheese (part-skim)
- 1 egg

- *1 big tomato*
- *1 small clove garlic*
- *4 large basil leaves*
- *1/8 tsp. salt*
- *1/8 tsp. pepper*

Direction: •Preparation Time 10 Minutes Cooking Time: 10 Minutes Servings: 4

✓ *Combine turkey, white egg, Minced garlic, salt, and pepper (mix until combined);*

✓ *Shape into 2 cutlets. Put cutlets into a skillet; cook 5 to 7 minutes per side.*

✓ *Top cutlets properly with cheese and sliced tomato at the end of cooking.*
Put 1 cutlet on the bottom of each bun.

✓ *Top each patty with 2 basil leaves. Cover with bun tops.*

Nutrition: Calories 180 / Protein 7 g / Fat 4 g / Carbs 20 g

207) *Pasta Salad*

Ingredients:

- *8 oz. whole-wheat pasta*
- *2 tomatoes*
- *1 (5-oz) pkg spring mix*
- *9 slices bacon*
- *1/3 cup mayonnaise (reduced-fat)*
- *1 tbsp. Dijon mustard*
- *3 tbsp. apple cider vinegar*
- *1/4 tsp. salt*
- *1/2 tsp. pepper*

Direction: Preparation Time: 15 Minutes Cooking Time: 15 Minutes Servings: 4

✓ *Cook pasta.*

✓ *Chilled pasta, chopped tomatoes and spring mix in a bowl.*

✓ *Crumble-cooked bacon over pasta.*
Combine mayonnaise, mustard, vinegar, salt and pepper in a small bowl.

✓ *Pour dressing over pasta, stirring to coat.*

Nutrition: Calories 200 / Protein 15 g / Fat 3 g / Carbs 6 g

208) *Chicken, Strawberry, And Avocado Salad*

Ingredients:

- *1,5 cups chicken (skin removed)*
- *1/4 cup almonds*
- *2 (5-oz) pkg salad greens*
- *1 (16-oz) pkg strawberries*

- *1 avocado*
- *1/4 cup green onion*
- *1/4 cup lime juice*
- *3 tbsp. extra virgin olive oil*
- *2 tbsp. honey*
- *1/4 tsp. salt*
- *1/4 tsp. pepper*

Direction: Preparation Time: 10 Minutes

Cooking Time: 5 Minutes

✓ *Toast almonds until golden and fragrant.*

✓ *Mix lime juice, oil, honey, salt, and pepper. Mix greens, sliced strawberries, chicken, diced avocado, and sliced green onion and sliced almonds; drizzle with dressing. Toss to coat.*

Nutrition: Cals 150 / Protein 15 g /Fat 10 g /Carbs 5 g

209) *Lemon-Thyme Eggs*

Ingredients:

- *7 large eggs*
- *1/4 cup mayonnaise (reduced-fat)*
- *2 tsp. lemon juice*
- *1 tsp. Dijon mustard*
- *1 tsp. chopped fresh thyme*
- *1/8 tsp. cayenne pepper*

Direction: Preparation Time: 10 Minutes Cooking Time: 5 Minutes Servings: 4

✓ *Bring eggs to a boil.*

✓ *Peel and cut each egg in half lengthwise. Remove yolks to a bowl. Add mayonnaise, lemon juice, mustard, thyme, and cayenne to egg yolks; mash to blend. Fill egg white halves with yolk mixture.*

✓ *Chill until ready to serve.*

Nutrition: Calories 40 / Protein 10 g / Fat 6 g / Carbs 2 g

210) *Spinach Salad with Bacon*

Ingredients:

- *8 slices center-cut bacon*
- *3 tbsp. extra virgin olive oil*
- *1 (5-oz) pkg baby spinach*
- *1 tbsp. apple cider vinegar*
- *1 tsp. Dijon mustard*
- *1/2 tsp. honey*
- *1/4 tsp. salt*
- *1/2 tsp. pepper*

Direction: Preparation Time: 15 Minutes

Cooking Time: 0 Minutes Servings: 4

✓ *Mix vinegar, mustard, honey, salt and pepper in a bowl.*

✓ *Whisk in oil. Place spinach in a serving bowl; drizzle with dressing, and toss to coat. Sprinkle with cooked and crumbled bacon.*

Nutrition: Calories 110 / Protein 6 g / Fat 2 g / Carbs 1 g

211)   Pea and Collards Soup

Ingredients:

- *1/2 (16-oz) pkg black-eyed peas*
- *1 onion*
- *2 carrots*
- *1,5 cups ham (low-sodium)*
- *1 (1-lb) bunch collard greens (trimmed)*
- *1 tbsp. extra virgin olive oil*
- *2 cloves garlic*
- *1/2 tsp. black pepper*
- *Hot sauce*

Direction: Preparation Time: 10 Minutes Cooking Time: 50 Minutes Servings: 4

✓ *Cook chopped onion and carrots 10 Minutes.*

✓ *Add peas, diced ham, collards, and Minced garlic. Cook 5 Minutes.*

✓ *Add broth, 3 cups water, and pepper. Bring to a boil; simmer 35 Minutes, adding water if needed.*

Nutrition: Calories 86/Protein 15 g/Fat 2 g/Carbs 9 g

212)   Spanish Stew

Ingredients:

- *1.1/2 (12-oz) pkg smoked chicken sausage links*
- *1 (5-oz) pkg baby spinach*
- *1 (15-oz) can chickpeas*
- *1 (14.5-oz) can tomatoes with basil, garlic, and oregano*
- *1/2 tsp. smoked paprika*
- *1/2 tsp. cumin*
- *3/4 cup onions*
- *1 tbsp. extra virgin olive oil*

Direction: Preparation Time: 10 Minutes Cooking Time: 25 Minutes Servings: 4

✓ *Cook sliced the sausage in hot oil until browned. Remove from pot.*

✓ *Add chopped onions; cook until tender. Add sausage, drained and rinsed chickpeas, diced tomatoes, paprika, and ground cumin. Cook 15 Minutes.*

✓ *Add in spinach; cook for 1 to 2 Minutes.*

Nutrition: Calories 200 / Protein 10 g / Fat 20 g /

Carbs 1 g

213)   Creamy Taco Soup

Ingredients:

- *3/4 lb. ground sirloin*
- *1/2 (8-oz) cream cheese*
- *1/2 onion*
- *1 clove garlic*
- *1 (10-oz) can tomatoes and green chiles*
- *1 (14.5-oz) can beef broth*
- *1/4 cup heavy cream*
- *1,5 tsp. cumin*
- *1/2 tsp. chili powder*

Direction: Preparation Time: 10 Minutes Cooking Time: 20 Minutes Servings: 4

✓ *Cook beef, chopped onion, and Minced garlic until meat are browned and crumbly; drain and return to pot.*

✓ *Add ground cumin, chili powder, and cream cheese cut into small pieces and softened, stirring until cheese is melted.*
Add diced tomatoes, broth, and cream; bring to a boil, and simmer 10 Minutes—season with pepper and salt to taste.

Nutrition: Cal 60 / Protein 3 g / Fat 1 g /Carbs8 g

214)   Chicken with Caprese Salsa

Ingredients:

- *3/4 lb. boneless, skinless chicken breasts*
- *2 big tomatoes*
- *1/2 (8-oz) ball fresh mozzarella cheese*
- *1/4 cup red onion*
- *2 tbsp. fresh basil*
- *1 tbsp. balsamic vinegar*
- *2 tbsp. extra virgin olive oil (divided)*
- *1/2 tsp. salt (divided)*
- *1/4 tsp. pepper (divided)*

Direction: Preparation Time: 15 Minutes Cooking Time: 5 Minutes Servings: 4

✓ *Sprinkle cut in half lengthwise chicken with 1/4 tsp. salt and 1/8 tsp. pepper.*

✓ *Heat 1 tbsp. olive oil, cook chicken 5 Minutes. Meanwhile, mix chopped tomatoes, diced cheese, finely chopped onion, chopped basil, vinegar, 1 tbsp. oil, and 1/4 tsp. salt and 1/8 tsp. pepper.*

✓ *Spoon salsa over chicken.*

Nutrition: Calories 210 / Protein 28 g / Fat 17 g / Carbs 0, 1 g

215) *Balsamic-Roasted Broccoli*

Ingredients:

- 1 lb. broccoli
- 1 tbsp. extra virgin olive oil
- 1 tbsp. balsamic vinegar
- 1 clove garlic
- 1/8 tsp. salt
- Pepper to taste

Direction: Preparation Time: 10 Minutes

Cooking Time: 15 Minutes Servings: 4

✓ Preheat oven to 450F.
✓ Combine broccoli, olive oil, vinegar, Minced garlic, salt, and pepper; toss.
   Spread broccoli on a baking sheet.
✓ Bake 12 to 15 Minutes.

Nutrition: Calories 27 / Protein 3 g / Fat 0, 3 g / Carbs 4 g

216) *Hearty Beef and Vegetable Soup*

Ingredients:

- 1/2 lb. lean ground beef
- 2 cups beef broth
- 1,5 tbsp. vegetable oil (divided)
- 1 cup green bell pepper
- 1/2 cup red onion
- 1 cup green cabbage
- 1 cup frozen mixed vegetables
- 1/2 can tomatoes
- 1,5 tsp. Worcestershire sauce
- 1 small bay leaf
- 1,8 tsp. pepper
- 2 tbsp. ketchup

Direction: Preparation Time: 10 Minutes Cooking Time: 30 Minutes Servings: 4

✓ Cook beef in 1/2 tbsp. hot oil 2 Minutes.
✓ Stir in chopped bell pepper and chopped onion; cook 4 Minutes.
✓ Add chopped cabbage, mixed vegetables, stewed tomatoes, broth, Worcestershire sauce, bay leaf, and pepper; bring to a boil.
   Reduce heat to medium; cover, and cook 15 Minutes.
✓ Stir in ketchup and 1 tbsp. oil, and remove from heat. Let stand 10 Minutes.

Nutrition: Calories 170 / Protein 17 g / Fat 8 g / Carbs 3 g

217) *Cauliflower Muffin*

Ingredients:

- 2,5 cup cauliflower
- 2/3 cup ham
- 2,5 cups of cheese
- 2/3 cup champignon
- 1,5 tbsp. flaxseed
- 3 eggs
- 1/4 tsp. salt
- 1/8 tsp. pepper

Direction: Preparation Time: 15 Minutes Cooking Time: 30 Minutes Servings: 4

✓ Preheat oven to 375 F.
✓ Put muffin liners in a 12-muffin tin.
✓ Combine diced cauliflower, ground flaxseed, beaten eggs, cup diced ham, grated cheese, and diced mushrooms, salt, pepper.
   Divide mixture rightly between muffin liners.
✓ Bake 30 Minutes.

Nutrition: Cal 116 /Protein 10 g /Fat 7 g /Carbs 3 g

218) *Ham and Egg Cups*

Ingredients:

- 5 slices ham
- 4 tbsp. cheese
- 1,5 tbsp. cream
- 3 egg whites
- 1,5 tbsp. pepper (green)
- 1 tsp. salt
- pepper to taste

Direction: Preparation Time: 10 Minutes Cooking Time: 15 Minutes Servings: 4

✓ Preheat oven to 350 F.
✓ Arrange each slice of thinly sliced ham into 4 muffin tin.
✓ Put 1/4 of grated cheese into the ham cup.
   Mix eggs, cream, salt and pepper and divide it into 2 tins.
✓ Bake in oven 15 Minutes; after baking, sprinkle with green onions.

Nutrition: Calories 180 / Protein 13 g / Fat 13 g / Carbs 2 g

219) *Cauliflower Rice with Chicken*

Ingredients:

- 1/2 large cauliflower
- 3/4 cup cooked meat

- *1/2 bell pepper*
- *1 carrot*
- *2 ribs celery*
- *1 tbsp. stir fry sauce (low carb)*
- *1 tbsp. extra virgin olive oil*
- *Salt and pepper to taste*

Direction: Preparation Time: 15 Minutes Cooking Time: 15 Minutes Servings: 4

✓ *Chop cauliflower in a processor to "rice." Place in a bowl.*

✓ *Properly chop all vegetables in a food processor into thin slices.*
Chop cauliflower in a processor to "rice." Place in a bowl.

✓ *Properly chop all vegetables in a food processor into thin slices.*

✓ *Add cauliflower and other plants to WOK with heated oil. Fry until all veggies are tender.*

✓ *Add chopped meat and sauce to the wok and fry 10 Minutes and Serve. This dish is very mouth-watering!*

Nutrition: Calories 200 / Protein 10 g / Fat 12 g /Carbs 10 g

220) *Turkey with Fried Eggs*

Ingredients:

- *4 large potatoes*
- *1 cooked turkey thigh*
- *1 large onion (about 2 cups diced)*
- *butter*
- *Chile flakes*
- *4 eggs*
- *salt to taste*
- *pepper to taste*

Direction: Preparation Time: 10 Minutes Cooking Time: 20 Minutes Servings: 4

✓ *Rub the cold boiled potatoes on the coarsest holes of a box grater. Dice the turkey.*

✓ *Cook the onion in as much unsalted butter as you feel comfortable with until it's just fragrant and translucent.*
Add the rubbed potatoes and a cup of diced cooked turkey, salt and pepper to taste, and cook 20 Minutes.

Nutrition: Calories 170 / Protein 19 g / Fat 7 g /Carbs 6 g

DINNER

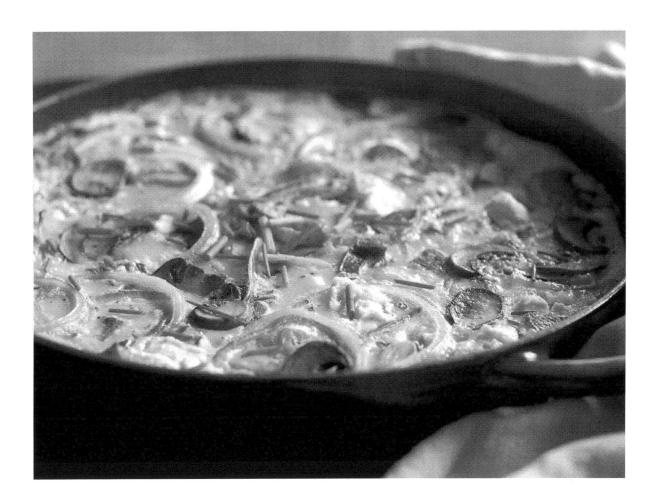

221) Pork Chop Diane

Ingredients:

- ¼ cup low-sodium chicken broth
- tbsp. freshly squeezed lemon juice
- 2 tsp. Worcestershire sauce
- tsp. Dijon mustard
- 4 (5 oz.) boneless pork top loin chops
- 1 tsp. extra-virgin olive oil
- 1 tsp. lemon zest
- 1 tsp. butter
- 2 tsp. chopped fresh chives

Direction: Preparation Time: 10 minutes Cooking Time: 20 minutes Servings: 4

- ✓ Blend together the chicken broth, lemon juice, Worcestershire sauce, and Dijon mustard and set it aside.
- ✓ Season the pork chops lightly.
- ✓ Situate large a skillet over medium-high heat and add the olive oil.
- ✓ Cook the pork chops, turning once, until they are no longer pink, about 8 minutes per side.
- ✓ Put aside the chops.
- ✓ Pour the broth mixture into the skillet and cook until warmed through and thickened, about 2 minutes.
- ✓ Blend lemon zest, butter, and chives.
- ✓ Garnish with a generous spoonful of sauce.

Nutrition: Calories: 200 Fat: 8g Carbohydrates: 1g

222) Autumn Pork Chops with Red Cabbage and Apples

Ingredients:

- ¼ cup apple cider vinegar
- 2 tbsp. granulated sweetener
- 4 (4 oz.) pork chops, about 1 inch thick
- 1 tbsp. extra-virgin olive oil
- ½ red cabbage, finely shredded
- 1 sweet onion, thinly sliced
- 1 apple, peeled, cored, and sliced
- 1 tsp. chopped fresh thyme

Direction: Preparation Time: 15 minutes Cooking Time: 30 minutes Servings: 4

- ✓ Scourge together the vinegar and sweetener. Set it aside.
- ✓ Season the pork with salt and pepper.
- ✓ Position a huge skillet over medium-high heat and add the olive oil.
- ✓ Cook the pork chops until no longer pink, turning once, about 8 minutes per side.
- ✓ Put chops aside.
- ✓ Add the cabbage and onion to the skillet and sauté until the vegetables have softened, about 5 minutes.
- ✓ Add the vinegar mixture and the apple slices to the skillet and bring the mixture to a boil.
- ✓ Adjust heat to low and simmer, covered, for 5 additional minutes.
- ✓ Return the pork chops to the skillet, along with any accumulated juices and thyme, cover, and cook for 5 more minutes.

Nutrition: Calories: 223 Carbohydrates: 12g Fiber: 3g

223) Chipotle Chili Pork Chops

Ingredients:

- Juice and zest 1 lime
- 1 tbsp. extra-virgin olive oil
- 1 tbsp. chipotle chili powder
- 2 tsp. minced garlic
- 1 tsp. ground cinnamon Pinch sea salt
- 4 (5 oz.) pork chops

Direction: Preparation Time: 4 hours Cooking Time: 20 minutes Servings: 4

- ✓ Combine the lime juice and zest, oil, chipotle chili powder, garlic, cinnamon, and salt in a resealable plastic bag. Add the pork chops. Remove as much air as possible and seal the bag.
- ✓ Marinate the chops in the refrigerator for at least 4 hours, and up to 24 hours, turning them several times.
- ✓ Ready the oven to 400°F and set a rack on a baking sheet. Let the chops rest at room temperature for 15 minutes, then arrange them on the rack and discard the remaining marinade.
- ✓ Roast the chops until cooked through, turning once, about 10 minutes per side.
- ✓ Serve with lime wedges.

Nutrition: Calories: 204 Carbohydrates: 1g Sugar: 1g

224) Orange-Marinated Pork Tenderloin

Ingredients:

- ¼ cup freshly squeezed orange juice
- 2 tsp. orange zest
- 2 tsp. minced garlic
- 1 tsp. low-sodium soy sauce
- 1 tsp. grated fresh ginger
- 1 tsp. honey
- 1½ pounds pork tenderloin roast
- 1 tbsp. extra-virgin olive oil

Direction: Preparation Time: 2 hours Cooking Time:

30 minutes Servings: 4

✓ *Blend together the orange juice, zest, garlic, soy sauce, ginger, and honey.*

✓ *Pour the marinade into a resealable plastic bag and add the pork tenderloin.*

✓ *Remove as much air as possible and seal the bag. Marinate the pork in the refrigerator, turning the bag a few times, for 2 hours.*

✓ *Preheat the oven to 400°F.*

✓ *Pull out tenderloin from the marinade and discard the marinade.*

✓ *Position big ovenproof skillet over medium-high heat and add the oil.*

✓ *Sear the pork tenderloin on all sides, about 5 minutes in total.*

✓ *Position skillet to the oven and roast for 25 minutes.*

✓ *Put aside for 10 minutes before serving*

Nutrition: Calories: 228 Carbs: 4g Sugar: 3g

225) *Homestyle Herb Meatballs*

Ingredients:

- *½ pound lean ground pork*
- *½ pound lean ground beef*
- *1 sweet onion, finely chopped*
- *¼ cup bread crumbs*
- *2 tbsp. chopped fresh basil*
- *2 tsp. minced garlic*
- *1egg*

Direction: Preparation Time: 10 minutes Cooking Time: 15 minutes Servings: 4

✓ *Preheat the oven to 350°F.*

✓ *Ready baking tray with parchment paper and set it aside.*

✓ *In a large bowl, mix together the pork, beef, onion, bread crumbs, basil, garlic, egg, salt, and pepper until very well mixed.*

✓ *Roll the meat mixture into 2-inch meatballs.*

✓ *Transfer the meatballs to the baking sheet and bake until they are browned and cooked through, about 15 minutes.*

✓ *Serve the meatballs with your favorite marinara sauce and some steamed green beans.*

Nutrition: Calories: 332 Carbs: 13g Sugar: 3g

226) *Lime-Parsley Lamb Cutlets*

Ingredients:

- *¼ cup extra-virgin olive oil*
- *¼ cup freshly squeezed lime juice*
- *2 tbsp. lime zest*

- *2 tbsp. chopped fresh parsley*
- *12 lamb cutlets (about 1½ pounds total)*

Direction: Preparation Time: 4 hours Cooking Time: 10 minutes Servings: 4

✓ *Scourge the oil, lime juice, zest, parsley, salt, and pepper.*

✓ *Pour marinade into a resealable plastic bag.*

✓ *Add the cutlets to the bag and remove as much air as possible before sealing.*

✓ *Marinate the lamb in the refrigerator for about 4 hours, turning the bag several times. Preheat the oven to broil.*

✓ *Remove the chops from the bag and arrange them on an aluminum foil-lined baking sheet. Discard the marinade.*

✓ *Broil the chops for 4 minutes per side for medium doneness.*

✓ *Let the chops rest for 5 minutes before serving.*

Nutrition: Calories: 413 Carbs: 1g Protein: 31g

227) *Mediterranean Steak Sandwiches*

Ingredients:

- *2 tbsp. extra-virgin olive oil*
- *2 tbsp. balsamic vinegar*
- *2 tsp. garlic*
- *2 tsp. lemon juice*
- *2 tsp. fresh oregano*
- *1 tsp. fresh parsley*
- *1 lb. flank steak*
- *4 whole-wheat pitas*
- *2 cups shredded lettuce*
- *1 red onion, thinly sliced*
- *1 tomato, chopped*
- *1-ounce low-sodium feta cheese*

Direction: Preparation Time: 1 hour Cooking Time: 10 minutes Servings: 4

✓ *Scourge olive oil, balsamic vinegar, garlic, lemon juice, oregano, and parsley.*

✓ *Add the steak to the bowl, turning to coat it completely.*

✓ *Marinate the steak for 1 hour in the refrigerator, turning it over several times.*

✓ *Preheat the broiler. Line a baking sheet with aluminum foil.*
Put steak out of the bowl and discard the marinade.

✓ *Situate steak on the baking sheet and broil for 5 minutes per side for medium.*

✓ *Set aside for 10 minutes before slicing.*

✓ *Stuff the pitas with the sliced steak, lettuce, onion, tomato, and feta.*

Nutrition: Calories: 344 Carbs: 22g Fiber: 3g

228) Roasted Beef with Peppercorn Sauce

Ingredients:

- ½ pounds top rump beef roast
- 3 tsp. extra-virgin olive oil
- 3 shallots, minced
- 2 tsp. minced garlic
- 1 tbsp. green peppercorns
- 2 tbsp. dry sherry
- tbsp. all-purpose flour
- cup sodium-free beef broth

Direction: Preparation Time: 10 minutes Cooking Time: 90 minutes Servings: 4

✓ Heat the oven to 300°F. Season the roast with salt and pepper.

✓ Position huge skillet over medium-high heat and add 2 tsp. of olive oil.

✓ Brown the beef on all sides, about 10 minutes in total, and transfer the roast to a baking dish.

✓ Roast until desired doneness, about 1½ hours for medium. When the roast has been in the oven for 1 hour, start the sauce.

✓ In a medium saucepan over medium-high heat, sauté the shallots in the remaining 1 tsp. of olive oil until translucent, about 4 minutes.
Stir in the garlic and peppercorns, and cook for another minute. Whisk in the sherry to deglaze the pan.

✓ Whisk in the flour to form a thick paste, cooking for 1 minute and stirring constantly.

✓ Fill in the beef broth and whisk for 4 minutes. Season the sauce.

✓ Serve the beef with a generous spoonful of sauce.

Nutrition: Calories: 330 Carbs: 4g Protein: 36g

229) Coffee-and-Herb-Marinated Steak

Ingredients:

- ¼ cup whole coffee beans
- 2 tsp. garlic
- 2 tsp. rosemary
- 2 tsp. thyme
- 1tsp. black pepper
- tbsp. apple cider vinegar
- 2 tbsp. extra-virgin olive oil
- 1 lb. flank steak, trimmed of visible fat

Direction: Preparation Time: 2 hours Cooking Time: 10 minutes Servings: 3

✓ Place the coffee beans, garlic, rosemary, thyme, and black pepper in a coffee grinder or food processor and pulse until coarsely ground.

✓ Transfer the coffee mixture to a resealable plastic bag and add the vinegar and oil. Shake to combine.

✓ Add the flank steak and squeeze the excess air out of the bag. Seal it. Marinate the steak in the refrigerator for at least 2 hours, occasionally turning the bag over.
Preheat the broiler. Line a baking sheet with aluminum foil.

✓ Pull the steak out and discard the marinade.

✓ Position steak on the baking sheet and broil until it is done to your liking.

✓ Put aside for 10 minutes before cutting it.

✓ Serve with your favorite side dish.

Nutrition: Calories: 313 Fat: 20g Protein: 31g

230) Traditional Beef Stroganoff

Ingredients:

- 1 tsp. extra-virgin olive oil
- 1 lb. top sirloin, cut into thin strips
- 1 cup sliced button mushrooms
- ½ sweet onion, finely chopped
- 1 tsp. minced garlic
- 1 tbsp. whole-wheat flour
- ½ cup low-sodium beef broth
- ¼ cup dry sherry
- ½ cup fat-free sour cream
- 1 tbsp. chopped fresh parsley

Direction: Preparation Time: 10 minutes Cooking Time: 30 minutes Servings: 4

✓ Position the skillet over medium-high heat and add the oil.

✓ Sauté the beef until browned, about 10 minutes, then remove the beef with a slotted spoon to a plate and set it aside.

✓ Add the mushrooms, onion, and garlic to the skillet and sauté until lightly browned about 5 minutes.

✓ Whisk in the flour and then whisk in the beef broth and sherry.

✓ Return the sirloin to the skillet and bring the mixture to a boil.

✓ Reduce the heat to low and simmer until the beef is tender, about 10 minutes.

✓ Stir in the sour cream and parsley. Season with salt and pepper

Nutrition: Calories: 257 Carbohydrates: 6g Fiber: 1g

231) Chicken and Roasted Vegetable Wraps

Ingredients:

- ½ small eggplant
- 1 red bell pepper
- 1 medium zucchini

- *½ small red onion, sliced*
- *tbsp. extra-virgin olive oil*
- *(8 oz.) cooked chicken breasts, sliced 4 whole-wheat tortilla wraps*

Direction: Preparation Time: 10 minutes Cooking Time: 20 minutes Servings: 4

✓ *Preheat the oven to 400°F.*
✓ *Wrap the baking sheet with foil and set it aside.*
✓ *In a large bowl, toss the eggplant, bell pepper, zucchini, and red onion with olive oil.*
✓ *Transfer the vegetables to the baking sheet and lightly season with salt and pepper.*
  Roast the vegetables until soft and slightly charred, about 20 minutes.
✓ *Divide the vegetables and chicken into 4 portions.*
✓ *Wrap 1 tortilla around each portion of chicken and grilled vegetables, and serve.*

Nutrition: Calories: 483 Carbohydrates: 45g Fiber: 3g

232)   *Spicy Chicken Cacciatore*

Ingredients:

- *(2 lb.) chicken*
- *¼ cup all-purpose flour*
- *2 tbsp. extra-virgin olive oil*
- *3 slices bacon*
- *1sweet onion*
- *2 tsp. minced garlic*
- *4 oz. button mushrooms halved*
- *1(28 oz.) can low-sodium stewed tomatoes*
- *½ cup red wine*
- *2 tsp. chopped fresh oregano*

Direction: Preparation Time: 20 minutes Cooking Time: 1 hour Servings: 6

✓ *Cut the chicken into pieces: 2 drumsticks, 2 thighs, 2 wings, and 4 breast pieces.*
✓ *Dredge the chicken pieces in the flour and season each piece with salt and pepper.*
✓ *Place a large skillet over medium-high heat and add the olive oil.*
✓ *Brown the chicken pieces on all sides, about 20 minutes in total.*
✓ *Transfer the chicken to a plate.*
✓ *Cook chopped bacon to the skillet for 5 minutes.*
✓ *With a slotted spoon, transfer the cooked bacon to the same plate as the chicken.*
  Pour off most of the oil from the skillet, leaving just a light coating.
✓ *Sauté the onion, garlic, and mushrooms in the skillet until tender, about 4 minutes.*
✓ *Stir in the tomatoes, wine, oregano, and red pepper flakes.*

✓ *Bring the sauce to a boil.*
✓ *Return the chicken and bacon, plus any accumulated juices from the plate, to the skillet.*
✓ *Reduce the heat to low and simmer until the chicken is tender,about 30 minutes.*
✓ *Serve!*

Nutrition: Calories: 230 Carbs: 14g Fiber: 2g

233)   *Ginger Citrus Chicken Thighs*

Ingredients:

- *4 chicken thighs, bone-in, skinless*
- *1 tbsp. grated fresh ginger*
- *1 tbsp. extra-virgin olive oil*
- *Juice and zest ½ lemon*
- *Juice and zest ½ orange*
- *2 tbsp. honey*
- *1 tbsp. reduced-sodium soy sauce*
- *1 tbsp. chopped fresh cilantro*

Direction: Preparation Time: 15 minutes Cooking Time: 30 minutes Servings: 4

✓ *Rub the chicken thighs with ginger and season lightly with salt.*
✓ *Place a large skillet over medium-high heat and add the oil.*
✓ *Brown the chicken thighs, turning once, for about 10 minutes.*
✓ *While the chicken is browning, stir together the lemon juice and zest, orange juice and zest, honey, soy sauce, and red pepper flakes in a small bowl.*
✓ *Add the citrus mixture to the skillet, cover, and reduce the heat to low.*
✓ *Braise chicken for 20 minutes, adding a couple of tbsp. water if the pan is too dry.*
✓ *Serve garnished with cilantro.*

Nutrition: Calories: 114 Carbs: 9g Protein: 9g

234)   *Chicken with Creamy Thyme Sauce*

Ingredients:

- *4 (4 oz.) chicken breasts*
- *1 tbsp. extra-virgin olive oil*
- *½ sweet onion, chopped*
- *1 cup low-sodium chicken broth*
- *2 tsp. chopped fresh thyme*
- *¼ cup heavy (whipping) cream*
- *1 tbsp. butter*
- *1 scallion*

Direction: Preparation Time: 15 minutes Cooking Time: 30 minutes Servings: 4

✓ *Preheat the oven to 375°F.*

✓ *Season the chicken breasts slightly.*

✓ *Position a large ovenproof skillet over medium-high heat and add the olive oil.*

✓ *Brown the chicken, turning once, about 10 minutes in total. Transfer the chicken to a plate.*

✓ *In the same skillet, sauté the onion until softened and translucent, about 3 minutes.*

✓ *Add the chicken broth and thyme, and simmer until the liquid has reduced by half, about 6 minutes.*

✓ *Stir in the cream and butter, and return the chicken and any accumulated juices from the plate to the skillet.*

✓ *Transfer the skillet to the oven. Bake until cooked through, about 10 minutes.*

✓ *Serve topped with the chopped scallion.*

Nutrition: Calories: 287 Carbohydrates: 4g Fiber: 1g

235) *One-Pot Roast Chicken Dinner*

Ingredients:

- *½ head cabbage*
- *1 sweet onion*
- *1 sweet potato*
- *4 garlic cloves*
- *2 tbsp. extra-virgin olive oil*
- *2 tsp. minced fresh thyme*
- *2½ pounds bone-in chicken thighs and drumsticks*

Direction: Preparation Time: 10 minutes Cooking Time: 40 minutes Servings: 6

✓ *Preheat the oven to 450°F.*

✓ *Lightly grease a large roasting pan and arrange the cabbage, onion, sweet potato, and garlic in the bottom. Drizzle with 1 tbsp. oil, sprinkle with the thyme, and season the vegetables lightly with salt and pepper.*

✓ *Season the chicken with salt and pepper. Place a large skillet over medium-high heat and brown the chicken on both sides in the remaining 1 tbsp. oil, about 10 minutes in total.*

✓ *Situate browned chicken on top of the vegetables in the roasting pan. Roast for 30 minutes.*

Nutrition: Calories: 540 Carbs: 14g Fiber: 4g

236) *Mushrooms with Bell Peppers*

Ingredients:

- *1 tbsp. grapeseed oil*
- *3 cups fresh button mushrooms, sliced*
- *¾ cups red bell peppers*
- *¾ cups green bell peppers strips*
- *1½ cup white onions strips*

- *2 tsp. fresh sweet basil*
- *2 tsp. fresh oregano*
- *½ tsp. cayenne powder Sea salt, as required*
- *2 tsp. onion powder*

Direction: Preparation Time: 15 minutes Cooking Time: 10 minutes Servings: 4

✓ *Cook the oil over medium-high heat and sauté the mushrooms, bell peppers, and onion for about 5-6 minutes.*

✓ *Add the herbs and spices and cook for about 2–3 minutes. Stir in the lime juice and serve hot.*

Nutrition: Calories: 80 Total Fat: 3.9g Protein: 2.8g

237) *Bell Peppers & Tomato Casserole*

Ingredients:

- *For Herb Sauce:*
- *4 garlic cloves, chopped*
- *½ cup fresh parsley, chopped*
- *½ cup fresh cilantro, chopped*
- *3 tbsp. avocado oil*
- *2 tbsp. fresh key lime juice*
- *½ tsp. ground cumin*
- *½ tsp. cayenne powder Sea salt, as required*

For Veggies:

- *1 large green bell pepper*
- *1 large yellow bell pepper*
- *1 large orange bell pepper*
- *1 large red bell pepper*
- *1 lb. plum tomatoes wedges*
- *2 tbsp. avocado oil*

Direction: Preparation Time: 15 minutes Cooking Time: 35 minutes Serves: 6

✓ *Lightly, grease the baking dish and preheat the oven to 350°F. For the sauce: transfer all ingredients in the food processor and pulse till smooth. In a large bowl, add the bell peppers and sauce and herb sauce and gently, toss to coat. Transfer the bell pepper mixture into the prepared baking dish. Drizzle with oil. Enclose the baking dish with foil and bake for about 35 minutes. Take off the cover of the baking dish and bake for another 20–30 minutes.*

✓ *Serve hot.*

Nutrition: Calories: 61 Total Fat: 2g Protein: 2g

238) *Veggies Casserole*

Ingredients:

- *3 plum tomatoes*

- *3 tbsp. spring water*
- *3 tbsp. avocado oil, divided*
- *½ onion, chopped*
- *3 tbsp. garlic, minced Sea salt, as required*
- *The cayenne powder as required*
- *1 zucchini*
- *1 yellow squash*
- *1 green bell pepper 1 red bell pepper*
- *1 yellow bell pepper*
- *1 tbsp. fresh thyme leaves*
- *1 tbsp. fresh key lime juice*

Direction: Preparation Time: 20 minutes Cooking Time: 45 minutes Servings: 5

✓ *Preheat oven to 375°F. Blend the tomatoes and water until pureed.*

✓ *In a bowl, add the tomato puree, 1 tbsp. oil, onion, garlic, salt, and black pepper and blend nicely. In the bottom of a 10x10-inch baking dish, spread the tomato paste mixture evenly.*
Arrange alternating vegetable slices, starting at the outer edge of the baking dish and working concentrically towards the center. Pour some remaining oil in the vegetables and sprinkle with salt and cayenne powder, followed by the thyme. Arrange a piece of parchment paper over the vegetables. Bake for about 45 minutes.

✓ *Serve hot.*

Nutrition: Calories: 77 Total Fat: 1.6g Protein: 3.2g

239) *Sweet & Spicy Chickpeas*

Ingredients:

- *6 plum tomatoes*
- *3 tbsp. agave nectar*
- *¼ cup date sugar*
- *tsp. onion powder*
- *½ tsp. ground ginger*
- *¼ tsp. cayenne powder*
- *Sea salt, as required*
- *cups cooked chickpeas*
- *¼ cup green bell peppers*
- *¼ cup white onions, chopped*

Direction: Preparation Time: 15 minutes Cooking Time: 1 hour 10 minutes Servings: 4

✓ *In a blender, add the tomatoes, agave, date sugar, and spices, and pulse until smooth. In a pan, add the tomato mixture, chickpeas, bell peppers, and onion over medium heat and bring to a boil.*

✓ *Cook for about 5 minutes. Reduce the heat to low and simmer for about 1 hour. Serve hot*

Nutrition: Calories: 327 Total Fat: 2g Protein: 13.3g

240) *Chickpeas & Veggie Stew*

Ingredients:

- *3 cups portabella mushrooms*
- *4 cups spring water*
- *1 cup cooked chickpeas*
- *1 cup fresh kale*
- *1 cup white onion*
- *½ cup red onion*
- *1 cup green bell peppers*
- *½ cup butternut squash*
- *2plum tomatoes, chopped*
- *2 tbsp. grapeseed oil*
- *1 tsp. dried oregano*
- *1 tsp. dried basil*
- *½ tsp. dried thyme*
- *2 tsp. onion powder*
- *1 tsp. cayenne powder*
- *½ tsp. ginger powder Sea salt, as required*

Direction: Preparation Time: 20 minutes Cooking Time: 1 hour 5 minutes Servings: 6

✓ *Transfer all the ingredients over high heat and bring to a boil.*

✓ *Reduce the heat to low and simmer, covered for about 1 hour, stirring occasionally.*

✓ *Serve hot.*

Nutrition: Calories: 138 Total Fat: 5.4g Protein: 5.1g

241) *Almond-Crusted Salmon*

Ingredients:

- *¼ cup almond meal*
- *¼ cup whole-wheat breadcrumbs*
- *¼ tsp. ground coriander*
- *⅛ tsp. ground cumin*
- *4 (6 oz.) boneless salmon fillets*
- *1 tbsp. fresh lemon juice*
- *Salt and pepper*

Direction: Preparation Time: 10 minutes Cooking Time: 15 minutes Servings: 4

✓ *Ready the oven at 500°F and line a small baking dish with foil.*

✓ *Combine the almond meal, breadcrumbs, coriander, and cumin in a small bowl.*

✓ *Rinse the fish in cool water then pat dry and brush with lemon juice.*
Season the fish with salt and pepper then dredge in the almond mixture on both sides.

✓ *Situate fish in the baking dish and bake for 15 minutes.*

Nutrition: Calories: 232 Carbs: 5.8g Sugar: 1.7g

242) Chicken & Veggie Bowl with Brown Rice

Ingredients:

- *1 cup instant brown rice*
- *¼ cup tahini*
- *¼ cup fresh lemon juice*
- *2 cloves minced garlic*
- *¼ tsp. ground cumin*
- *Pinch salt*
- *1 tbsp. olive oil*
- *4 (4 oz.) chicken breast halves*
- *½ medium yellow onion, sliced*
- *1 cup green beans, trimmed*
- *1 cup chopped broccoli*
- *4 cups chopped kale*

Direction: Preparation Time: 10 minutes Cooking Time: 20 minutes Servings: 4

- ✓ *Bring 1 cup of water to boil in a small saucepan.*
- ✓ *Stir in the brown rice and simmer for 5 minutes then cover and set aside.*
- ✓ *Meanwhile, whisk together the tahini with ¼-cup water in a small bowl.*
- ✓ *Stir in the lemon juice, garlic, and cumin with a pinch of salt and stir well.*
- ✓ *Heat up oil in a big cast-iron skillet over medium heat.*
- ✓ *Season the chicken with salt and pepper then add to the skillet.*
  Cook for 3 to 5 minutes on each side until cooked through then remove to a cutting board and cover loosely with foil.
- ✓ *Reheat the skillet and cook the onion for 2 minutes then stir in the broccoli and beans.*
- ✓ *Sauté for 2 minutes then stir in the kale and sauté 2 minutes more.*
- ✓ *Add 2 tbsp. Water then cover and steam for 2 minutes while you slice the chicken.*
- ✓ *Build the bowls with brown rice, sliced chicken, and sautéed veggies.*
- ✓ *Serve hot drizzled with the lemon tahini dressing.*

Nutrition: Calories: 435 Carbohydrates: 24g Fiber: 4.8g

243) Beef Steak Fajitas

Ingredients:

- *1 lb. lean beef sirloin, sliced thin*
- *1 tbsp. olive oil*
- *1 medium red onion, sliced*
- *1 red pepper, sliced thin*
- *1 green pepper, sliced thin*
- *½ tsp. ground cumin*
- *½ tsp. chili powder*
- *8 (6-inch) whole-wheat tortillas*
- *Fat-free sour cream*

Direction: Preparation Time: 10 minutes Cooking Time: 15 minutes Servings: 4

- ✓ *Preheat a huge cast-iron skillet over medium heat then add the oil.*
- ✓ *Add the sliced beef and cook in a single layer for 1 minute on each side.*
- ✓ *Remove the beef to a bowl and cover to keep warm.*
- ✓ *Reheat the skillet then add the onions and peppers—season with cumin and chili powder.*
- ✓ *Stir-fry the veggies to your liking then add to the bowl with the beef.*
- ✓ *Serve hot in small whole-wheat tortillas with sliced avocado and fat-free sour cream.*

Nutrition: Calories: 430 Carbohydrates: 30.5g Fiber: 17g

244) Italian Pork Chops

Ingredients:

- *4 pork chops, boneless*
- *3 garlic cloves, minced*
- *1 tsp. dried rosemary, crushed*
- *¼ tsp. pepper*
- *¼ tsp. sea salt*

Direction: Preparation Time: 5 minutes Cooking Time: 45 minutes Servings: 4

- ✓ *Prepare the oven to 425°F/218°C.*
- ✓ *Line baking tray with cooking spray and season pork chops with pepper and salt.*
- ✓ *Combine garlic and rosemary and rub all over pork chops.*
  Place pork chops in a prepared baking tray.
- ✓ *Roast pork chops in preheated oven for 10 minutes.*
- ✓ *Set temperature to 180ºC and roast for 25 minutes.*
- ✓ *Serve and enjoy*

Nutrition: Calories: 261 Carbs: 1g Protein: 18g

245) Chicken Mushroom Stroganoff

Ingredients:

- *1 cup fat-free sour cream.'*
- *2 tbsp. flour*
- *1 tbsp. Worcestershire sauce*
- *½ tsp. dried thyme*
- *1 chicken bouillon cube, crushed*
- *Salt and pepper*
- *½ cup water*

- *medium yellow onion*
- *8 oz. sliced mushrooms*
- *1 tbsp. olive oil*
- *2 cloves minced garlic*
- *12 oz. chicken breast*
- *6 oz. whole-wheat noodles, cooked*

Direction: Preparation Time: 5 minutes Cooking Time: 25 minutes Servings: 6

✓ *Whisk together 2/3 cup the sour cream with the flour, Worcestershire sauce, thyme, and crushed bouillon in a medium bowl.*

✓ *Season with salt and pepper then slowly stir in the water until well combined.*

✓ *Cook oil in a large skillet over medium-high heat.*

✓ *Sauté onions, mushrooms for 3 minutes. Cook garlic for 2 minutes more then add the chicken.*

✓ *Pour in the sour cream mixture and cook until thick and bubbling.*

✓ *Reduce heat and simmer for 2 minutes.*

✓ *Spoon the chicken and mushroom mixture over the cooked noodles and garnish with the remaining sour cream to serve.*

Nutrition: Calories: 295 Carbohydrates: 29.6g Fiber: 2.9g

246) Grilled Tuna Kebabs

Ingredients:

- *2 ½ tbsp. rice vinegar*
- *2 tbsp. freshly grated ginger*
- *2 tbsp. sesame oil*
- *2 tbsp. soy sauce*
- *2 tbsp. fresh chopped cilantro*
- *1 tbsp. minced green chili*
- *1 ½ pound fresh tuna*
- *1 large red pepper*
- *1 large red onion*

Direction: Preparation Time: 20 minutes Cooking Time: 10 minutes Servings: 4

✓ *Whisk together the rice vinegar, ginger, sesame oil, soy sauce, cilantro, and chili in a medium bowl—add a few drops of liquid stevia extract to sweeten.*

✓ *Toss in the tuna and chill for 20 minutes, covered. Meanwhile, grease a grill pan with cooking spray and soak wooden skewers in water.*

✓ *Slide the tuna cubes onto the skewers with red pepper and onion.*

✓ *Grill for 4 minutes per side and serve hot.*

Nutrition: Calories: 240 Carbohydrates: 8.5g Fiber: 1.7g

247) Cast-Iron Pork Loin

Ingredients:

- *(1 ½ pound) boneless pork loin*
- *Salt and pepper*
- *2 tbsp. olive oil*
- *2 tbsp. dried herb blend*

Direction: Preparation Time: 10 minutes Cooking Time: 20 minutes Servings: 6

✓ *Heat the oven to 425°F.*

✓ *Cut the excess fat from the pork and season.*

✓ *Heat the oil in a large cast-iron skillet over medium heat.*

✓ *Add the pork and cook for 2 minutes on each side. Sprinkle the herbs over the pork and transfer them to the oven.*

✓ *Roast for 10 to 15 minutes.*

✓ *Put aside for 10 minutes before cutting to serve.*

Nutrition: Calories: 205 Carbohydrates: 1g Protein: 29g

248) Crispy Baked Tofu

Ingredients:

- *1 (14 oz.) block extra-firm tofu*
- *1 tbsp. olive oil*
- *1 tbsp. cornstarch*
- *½ tsp. garlic powder*
- *Salt and pepper*

Direction: Preparation Time: 5 minutes Cooking Time: 25 minutes Servings: 4

✓ *Spread paper towels out on a flat surface.*

✓ *Cut the tofu into slices up to about ½-inch thick and lay them out.*

✓ *Cover the tofu with another paper towel and place a cutting board on top.*

✓ *Let the tofu drain for 10 to 15 minutes. Preheat the oven to 400°F and line a baking sheet with foil or parchment.*

✓ *Slice tofu into cubes and situate in a large bowl.*

✓ *Toss with olive oil, cornstarch, and garlic powder, salt, and pepper.*

✓ *Spread on the baking sheet and bake for 10 minutes.*

✓ *Flip the tofu and bake for another 10 to 15 minutes. Serve hot.*

Nutrition: Calories: 140 Carbs: 2.1g Fiber: 0.1g

249) Tilapia with Coconut Rice

Ingredients:

- *4 (6 oz.) boneless tilapia fillets*

- *1 tbsp. ground turmeric*
- *1tbsp. olive oil*
- *2 (8.8 oz.) packets precooked wholegrain rice*
- *1 cup light coconut milk*
- *½ cup fresh chopped cilantro*
- *1 ½ tbsp. fresh lime juice*

Direction: Preparation Time: 10 minutes Cooking Time: 15 minutes Servings: 4

✓ *Season the fish with turmeric, salt, and pepper.*

✓ *Cook oil in a large skillet at medium heat and add the fish.*

✓ *Cook for 2 to 3 minutes per side until golden brown.*

✓ *Remove the fish to a plate and cover to keep warm. Reheat the skillet and add the rice, coconut milk, and a pinch of salt.*

✓ *Simmer on high heat until thickened, about 3 to 4 minutes.*

✓ *Stir in the cilantro and lime juice.*

✓ *Spoon the rice onto plates and serve with the cooked fish.*

Nutrition: Calories: 460 Carbohydrates: 27.1g Fiber: 3.7g

250)   *Spicy Turkey Tacos*

Ingredients:

- *1 tbsp. olive oil*
- *1 medium yellow onion, diced*
- *2 cloves minced garlic*
- *1 pound 93% lean ground turkey*
- *1 cup tomato sauce, no sugar added*
- *1 jalapeno, seeded and minced*
- *8 low-carb multigrain tortillas*

Direction: Preparation Time: 5 minutes Cooking Time: 25 minutes Servings: 8

✓ *Heat up oil in a big skillet over medium heat.*

✓ *Add the onion and sauté for 4 minutes then stir in the garlic and cook 1 minute more.*

✓ *Stir in the ground turkey and cook for 5 minutes until browned, breaking it up with a wooden spoon.*

✓ *Sprinkle on the taco seasoning and cayenne then stir well.*

✓ *Cook for 30 seconds and mix in the tomato sauce and jalapeno.*

✓ *Simmer on low heat for 10 minutes while you warm the tortillas in the microwave.*

✓ *Serve the meat in the tortillas with your favorite taco toppings.*

Nutrition: Calories: 195 Carbohydrates: 15.4g Fiber: 8g

251)   *Quick and Easy Shrimp Stir-Fry*

Ingredients:

- *1 tbsp. olive oil*
- *1 lb. uncooked shrimp*
- *1 tbsp. sesame oil*
- *8 oz. snow peas*
- *4 oz. broccoli, chopped*
- *1 medium red pepper, sliced*
- *3 cloves minced garlic*
- *1 tbsp. fresh grated ginger*
- *½ cup soy sauce*
- *1 tbsp. Cornstarch*
- *tbsp. fresh lime juice*
- *¼ tsp. liquid stevia extract*

Direction: Preparation Time: 15 minutes Cooking Time: 15 minutes Servings: 5

✓ *Cook olive oil in a huge skillet over medium heat.*

✓ *Add the shrimp and season then sauté for 5 minutes.*

✓ *Remove the shrimp to a bowl and keep warm.*

✓ *Reheat the skillet with the sesame oil and add the veggies.*
Sauté until the veggies are tender, about 6 to 8 minutes.

✓ *Cook garlic and ginger for 1 minute more.*

✓ *Whisk together the remaining ingredients and pour them into the skillet.*

✓ *Toss to coat the veggies then add the shrimp and reheat. Serve hot.*

Nutrition: Calories: 220 Carbos: 12.7g Fiber: 2.6g

252)   *Chicken Burrito Bowl with Quinoa*

Ingredients:

- *1 tbsp. chipotle chills in adobo*
- *1 tbsp. olive oil*
- *½ tsp. garlic powder*
- *½ tsp. ground cumin*
- *1lb. boneless skinless chicken breast*
- *2 cups cooked quinoa*
- *2 cups shredded romaine lettuce*
- *1 cup black beans*
- *1 cup diced avocado*
- *3 tbsp. fat-free sour cream*

Direction: Preparation Time: 15 minutes Cooking Time: 10 minutes Servings: 6

✓ *Stir together the chipotle chills, olive oil, garlic powder, and cumin in a small bowl.*

✓ *Preheat a grill pan to medium-high and grease*

with cooking spray.
- ✓ Season the chicken with salt and pepper and add to the grill pan.
- ✓ Grill for 5 minutes then flip it and brush with the chipotle glaze.
  Cook for another 3 to 5 minutes until cooked through.
- ✓ Remove to a cutting board and chop the chicken.
- ✓ Assemble the bowls with 1/6 of the quinoa, chicken, lettuce, beans, and avocado.
- ✓ Top each with a half tbsp—fat-free sour cream to serve.

Nutrition: Calories: 410 Carbs: 37.4g Fiber: 8.5g

253) *Baked Salmon Cakes*

Ingredients:

- 15 oz. canned salmon, drained
- 1 large egg, whisked
- 2 tsp. Dijon mustard
- 1 small yellow onion, minced
- 1 ½ cups whole-wheat breadcrumbs
- ¼ cup low-fat mayonnaise
- ¼ cup nonfat Greek yogurt, plain
- 1 tbsp. fresh chopped parsley
- 1 tbsp. fresh lemon juice
- 2 green onions, sliced thin

Direction: Preparation Time: 10 minutes Cooking Time: 20 minutes Servings: 4

- ✓ Set the oven to 450°F and prep the baking sheet with parchment.
- ✓ Flake the salmon into a medium bowl then stir in the egg and mustard.
- ✓ Mix in the onions and breadcrumbs by hand, blending well, then shape into 8 patties.
- ✓ Grease a large skillet and heat it over medium heat. Fry patties for 2 minutes per side.
- ✓ Situate patties to the baking sheet and bake for 15 minutes.
- ✓ Meanwhile, whisk together the remaining ingredients.
- ✓ Serve the baked salmon cakes with creamy herb sauce.

Nutrition: Calories: 240 Carbs: 9.3g Fiber: 1.5g

254) *Rice and Meatball Stuffed Bell Peppers*

Ingredients:

- 4 bell peppers 1 tbsp. olive oil
- 1 small onion, chopped
- 2 garlic cloves, minced
- 1 cup frozen cooked rice, thawed
- 16 to 20 small frozen precooked meatballs
- ½ cup tomato sauce
- 2 tbsp. Dijon mustard

Direction: Preparation Time: 15 minutes Cooking Time: 20 minutes Serving: 4

- ✓ To prepare the peppers, cut off about ½ inch of the tops. Carefully take-out membranes and seeds from inside the peppers. Set aside.
- ✓ In a 6-by-6-by-2-inch pan, combine the olive oil, onion, and garlic—Bake in the air fryer for 2 to 4 minutes or until crisp and tender. Remove the vegetable mixture from the pan and set it aside in a medium bowl.
  Add the rice, meatballs, tomato sauce, and mustard to the vegetable mixture and stir to combine
- ✓ Stuff the peppers with the meat-vegetable mixture.
- ✓ Situate peppers in the air fryer basket and bake for 9 to 13 minutes or until the filling is hot and the peppers are tender.

Nutrition: Calories: 487 Carbs: 57g Fiber: 6g

255) *Stir-Fried Steak and Cabbage*

Ingredients:

- ½ lb. sirloin steak, cut into strips
- 2 tsp. cornstarch
- 1tbsp. peanut oil
- 2 cups chopped red or green cabbage
- 1 yellow bell pepper, chopped
- 2 green onions, chopped
- 2 garlic cloves, sliced
- ½-cup commercial stir-fry sauce

Direction: Preparation Time: 15 minutes Cooking Time: 10 minutes Servings: 4

- ✓ Toss the steak with the cornstarch and set aside
- ✓ In a 6-inch metal bowl, combine the peanut oil with the cabbage. Place in the basket and cook for 3 to 4 minutes.
- ✓ Remove the bowl from the basket and add the steak, pepper, onions, and garlic. Return to the air fryer and cook for 3 to 5 minutes.
- ✓ Add the stir-fry sauce and cook for 2 to 4 minutes. Serve over rice.

Nutrition: Calories: 180 Carbohydrates: 9g Fiber: 2g

256) *Nori-Burritos*

Ingredients:

- 1 avocado, ripe

- *450g cucumber (seeded)*
- *½ mango, ripe*
- *4 sheets nori seaweed*
- *1 zucchini, small*
- *Handful amaranth or dandelion greens*
- *Handful sprouted hemp seeds*
- *1 tsp. tahini*
- *Sesame seeds, to taste*

Direction: Preparation Time: 15 minutes Cooking Time: 20 minutes Servings: 2

✓ *Set the Nori sheet on a cutting board, the gleaming side facing down. Arrange all the ingredients on the nori sheet, leaving to the right 1-inch broad margin of exposed nori.*
Fold nori's sheet from the side nearest to you, roll it up and over the fillings, use both hands. Put some sesame seeds on top and slice them into thick pieces.

Nutrition: Calories: 201 Protein: 26g Fiber: 14g

257) *Grilled Zucchini Hummus Wrap*

Ingredients:

- *1 zucchini, ends removed and sliced*
- *1 plum tomato, sliced, or cherry tomatoes, halved*
- *¼ sliced red onion*
- *1 cup romaine lettuce or wild arugula*
- *4 tbsp. homemade hummus (mashed garbanzo beans)*
- *2 spelled flour tortillas*
- *tbsp. grapeseed oil*
- *Sea salt and cayenne pepper, to taste*

Direction: Preparation Time: 15 minutes Cooking Time: 25 minutes Servings: 4

✓ *Heat a skillet to medium heat or grill. In grapeseed oil, mix the sliced zucchini and sprinkle with sea salt and cayenne pepper. Place tossed, sliced zucchini directly on the grill and let cook for 3 minutes, flip over and cook for another 2 minutes. Set aside Zucchini.*

✓ *Place the tortillas on the grill for around a minute, or until the grill marks are noticeable and the tortillas are foldable. Remove tortillas from the grill and prepare wraps, 2 tbsp: hummus, slices of zucchini, ½ cup greens, slices of onion, and tomato. Wrap firmly, and instantly savor.*

Nutrition: Calories: 98 Protein: 20g Fiber: 12g

258) *Zucchini Bread Pancakes*

Ingredients:

- *cups spelled or Kamut flour*

- *2 tbsp. date sugar*
- *¼ cup mashed burro banana*
- *1 cup finely shredded zucchini*
- *2 cups homemade walnut milk*
- *½ cup chopped walnuts*
- *1 tbsp. grapeseed oil*

Direction: Preparation Time: 5 minutes Cooking Time: 20 minutes Servings: 5

✓ *Whisk flour in a large bowl with date sugar. Mix in walnut milk and mashed banana burro. Stir until just blended. Make sure the bowl's bottom is scraped so there are no dry mix pockets.*

✓ *Stir in shredded walnuts and Zucchini. Heat the grape seed oil over medium-high heat in a griddle or skillet.*

✓ *To make your pancakes, add batter onto the griddle. Cook on each side for 4-5 minutes. Serve with a syrup of agave and enjoy!*

Nutrition: Calories: 101 Protein: 27g Fiber: 14g

259) *Classic Homemade Hummus*

Ingredients:

- *cup cooked chickpeas*
- *¹/3 cup homemade tahini butter*
- *2 tbsp. olive oil*
- *tbsp. key lime juice*
- *A dash of onion powder*
- *Sea salt, to taste*

Direction: Preparation Time: 5 minutes Cooking Time: 10 minutes Servings: 3

✓ *Blend everything in a food processor or high powered blender and serve.*

Nutrition: Calories: 87 Protein: 16g Fiber: 8g

260) *Veggie Fajitas Tacos*

Ingredients:

- *1 onion*
- *Juice of ½ key lime*
- *2 bell peppers*
- *Your choice of approved seasonings (onion powder, cayenne pepper)*
- *6 corn-free tortillas*
- *1 tbsp. grapeseed oil*
- *Avocado*
- *2-3 large portobello mushrooms*

Direction: Preparation Time: 10 minutes Cooking Time: 15 minutes Servings: 3

✓ *Remove mushroom stems, spoon gills out if necessary, and clear tops clean. Slice into approximately ¹/₃ "thick slices. Slice the onion and bell peppers into thin slices.*

- ✓ *Pour 1 tbsp. Grapeseed oil into a big-size skillet on medium heat and onions and peppers. Cook for 2 minutes. Mix in seasonings and mushrooms. Stir frequently, and cook for another 7–8 minutes or until tender.*
  Heat the spoon and tortillas the fajita material into the middle of the tortilla. Serve with key lime juice and avocado.

Nutrition: Calories: 108 Protein: 20g Fiber: 14g

261) *Lemon Chicken with Peppers*

Ingredients:

- 1 tsp. cornstarch
- 1 tbsp. low sodium soy sauce
- 12 oz. chicken breast tenders, cut in thirds
- ¼ cup fresh lemon juice
- ¼ cup low sodium soy sauce
- ¼ cup fat-free chicken broth
- 1 tsp. fresh ginger, minced
- 2 garlic cloves, minced
- 1 tbsp. Splenda
- 1 tsp. cornstarch
- 1 tbsp. vegetable oil
- ¼ cup red bell pepper
- ¼ cup green bell pepper

Direction: Preparation Time: 5 minutes Cooking Time: 20 minutes Servings: 6

- ✓ *Scourge 1 tsp. cornstarch and 1 tbsp. soy sauce. Add sliced chicken tenders. Chill to marinate for 10 minutes.*
- ✓ *Stir the lemon juice, ¼ cup soy sauce, chicken broth, ginger, garlic, Splenda, and 1 tsp. Cornstarch together.*
  Warm up oil in a medium frying pan. Cook chicken over medium-high heat for 4 minutes.
- ✓ *Add sauce and sliced peppers. Cook 1 to 2 minutes more.*

Nutrition: Calories: 150 Fiber: 1g Carbohydrates: 6g

262) *Dijon Herb Chicken*

Ingredients:

- 4 skinless, boneless chicken breast halves
- 1 tbsp. butter
- 1tbsp. olive or vegetable oil
- 2 garlic cloves, finely minced
- ½ cup dry white wine
- ¼ cup water
- tbsp. Dijon-style mustard

- ½ tsp. dried dill weed
- ¼ tsp. coarsely ground pepper
- ¹/₃ cups chopped fresh parsley

Direction: Preparation Time: 7 minutes Cooking Time: 25 minutes Servings: 4

- ✓ *Situate chicken breasts between sheets of plastic wrap or waxed paper, and pound with a kitchen mallet until they are evenly about ¼-inch thick.*
- ✓ *Warm-up butter and oil over medium-high heat; cook chicken pieces for 3 minutes per side. Transfer chicken to a platter; keep warm and set aside. Sauté garlic for 15 seconds in skillet drippings; stir in wine, water, mustard, dill weed, salt, and pepper. Boil and reduce volume by ½, stirring up the browned bits at the bottom of the skillet.*
- ✓ *Drizzle sauce over chicken cutlets. Sprinkle with parsley and serve.*

Nutrition: Calories: 223 Fiber: 1g Carbohydrates: 6g

263) *Sesame Chicken Stir Fry*

Ingredients:

- 12 oz. skinless, boneless chicken breast
- 1 tbsp. vegetable oil
- 2 garlic cloves, finely minced
- 1 cup broccoli florets
- 1 cup cauliflowers
- ½ lb. fresh mushrooms, sliced
- 4 green onions, cut into 1-inch pieces
- 2 tbsp. low-sodium soy sauce
- 3 tbsp. dry sherry
- 1 tsp. finely minced fresh ginger
- 1 tsp. Cornstarch melted in 2 tbsp. water
- ¼ tsp. sesame oil
- ¼ cup dry-roasted peanuts

Direction: Preparation Time: 10 minutes Cooking Time: 30 minutes Servings: 6

- ✓ *Cut off fat from chicken and thinly slice diagonally into 1-inch strips.*
- ✓ *In a huge non-stick skillet, heat oil and stir-fry chicken for 4 minutes. Remove; put aside and keep warm.*
- ✓ *Stir-fry garlic for 15 seconds; then broccoli and cauliflower, stir-fry for 2 minutes. Then fry mushrooms, green onions, soy sauce, sherry, and ginger for 2 minutes.*
- ✓ *Pour dissolved arrowroot, sesame oil, peanuts, and the chicken. Cook until heated through and the sauce has thickened.*

Nutrition: Calories: 256 Carbos: 9g Protein: 30g

264) *Rosemary Chicken*

Ingredients:

- 1 (2 ½ to 3 lb.) broiler-fryer chicken
- Salt and ground black pepper to taste
- 4 garlic cloves, finely minced
- 1 tsp. dried rosemary
- ¼ cup dry white wine
- ¼ cup chicken broth

Direction: Preparation Time: 9 minutes Cooking Time: 30 minutes Servings: 4

✓ Preheat the broiler.

✓ Season chicken with salt and pepper. Place in the broiler pan. Broil 5 minutes per side.
Situate chicken, garlic, rosemary, wine, and broth in a Dutch oven. Cook, covered, at medium heat for about 30 minutes, turning once.

Nutrition: Calories: 176 Carbohydrates: 1g Fat: 1g

265) *Pepper Chicken Skillet*

Ingredients:

- 1 tbsp. vegetable oil
- 12 oz. skinless, boneless chicken breasts
- 2 garlic cloves, finely minced
- 3 bell peppers (red green and yellow)
- 2 medium onions, sliced
- 1 tsp. ground cumin
- 1 ½ tsp. dried oregano leaves
- tsp. chopped fresh jalapeño peppers
- 3 tbsp. fresh lemon juice
- 2 tbsp. chopped fresh parsley
- ¼ tsp. salt

Direction: Preparation Time: 10 minutes Cooking Time: 35 minutes Servings: 4

✓ In a big non-stick skillet, heat oil at medium-high heat; stir-fry chicken for 4 minutes.

✓ Cook garlic for 15 seconds, stirring constantly. Fry bell pepper strips, sliced onion, cumin, oregano, and chilies for 2 to 3 minutes.
Toss lemon juice, parsley, salt, and pepper and serve.

Nutrition: Calories: 174 Carbs: 6g Protein: 21g

266) *Dijon Salmon*

Ingredients:

- 1 tbsp. olive oil
- ½ pounds salmon fillets, cut into 6 pieces
- ¼ cup lemon juice
- tbsp. Equal (sugar substitute)
- 2 tbsp. Dijon mustard

- 1 tbsp. stick butter or margarine
- 1 tbsp. capers
- 1 garlic clove, minced
- 2 tbsp. chopped fresh dill

Direction: Preparation Time: 8 minutes Cooking Time: 26 minutes Servings: 3

✓ Heat up olive oil in a huge non-stick skillet over medium heat. Add salmon and cook for 5 minutes, turning once. Reduce heat to medium-low; cover. Cook 6 to 8 minutes or until salmon flakes easily with a fork.

✓ Remove salmon from skillet to serving plate; keep warm.
Add lemon juice, Equal, mustard, butter, capers, and garlic to skillet. Cook at medium heat for 3 minutes, stirring frequently.

✓ To serve, spoon sauce over salmon. Sprinkle with dill.

Nutrition: Calories: 252 Carbohydrates: 2g Protein: 23g

267) *Herb Lemon Salmon*

Ingredients:

- 2cups water 2/3 cup farro
- 1 medium eggplant 1
- red bell pepper
- 1 summer squash
- 1 small onion
- 1½ cups cherry tomatoes
- 3 tbsp. extra-virgin olive oil
- ¾ tsp. salt, divided
- ½ tsp. ground pepper
- 2 tbsp. capers
- tbsp. red-wine vinegar
- 2 tsp. honey
- 1¼ pounds salmon cut into 4 portions
- 1 tsp. lemon zest
- ½ tsp. Italian seasoning
- Lemon wedges for serving

Direction: Preparation Time: 10 minutes Cooking Time: 27 minutes Servings: 2

✓ Situate racks in the upper and lower thirds of the oven; set to 450°F. Prep 2 rimmed baking sheets with foil and coat with cooking spray.

✓ Boil water and farro. Adjust heat to low, cover, and simmer for 30 minutes. Drain if necessary.

✓ Mix eggplant, bell pepper, squash, onion, and tomatoes with oil, ½ tsp. salt and ¼ tsp. pepper. Portion between the baking sheets. Roast on the upper and lower racks, stir once halfway, for 25 minutes. Put them back to the bowl. Mix in capers, vinegar, and honey.

Rub salmon with lemon zest, Italian seasoning, and the remaining ¼ tsp. Each salt and pepper and situated on 1 of the baking sheets.

✓ *Roast on the lower rack for 12 minutes, depending on thickness. Serve with farro, vegetable caponata, and lemon wedges.*

Nutrition: Calories: 450 Fat: 17g Carbohydrates: 41g

268)   Ginger Chicken

Ingredients:

- *tbsp. vegetable oil - divided use*
- *1 lb. boneless, skinless chicken breasts*
- *1 cup red bell pepper strips*
- *1 cup sliced fresh mushrooms*
- *16 fresh pea pods, cut in half crosswise*
- *½ cup sliced water chestnuts*
- *¼ cup sliced green onions*
- *1 tbsp. grated fresh ginger root*
- *1 large garlic clove, crushed*
- *2/3 cup reduced-fat, reduced-sodium chicken broth*
- *2 tbsp. Equal (sugar substitute)*
- *2 tbsp. light soy sauce*
- *4 tsp. cornstarch*
- *2 tsp. dark sesame oil*

Direction: Preparation Time: 10 minutes Cooking Time: 25 minutes Servings: 5

✓ *Heat up 1 tbsp. vegetable oil in a huge skillet over medium-high heat. Stir fry chicken until no longer pink. Remove chicken from skillet.*

✓ *Heat remaining 1 tbsp. vegetable oil in the skillet. Add red peppers, mushrooms, pea pods, water chestnuts, green onion, ginger, and garlic. Sauté for 3–4 mins until vegetables are crisp-tender. Meanwhile, combine chicken broth, Equal, soy sauce, cornstarch, and sesame oil until smooth. Stir into skillet mixture. Cook at medium heat until thick and clear. Stir in chicken; heat through. Season with salt and pepper, if desired. Serve over hot cooked rice, if desired.*

Nutrition: Calories: 263 Fat: 11g Carbohydrates: 11g

269)   Salmon with Asparagus

Ingredients:

- *1 lb. Salmon, sliced into fillets*
- *1 tbsp. Olive Oil*
- *Salt & Pepper, as needed*
- *1 bunch of Asparagus, trimmed*
- *2 cloves of Garlic, minced*
- *Zest & Juice of 1/2 Lemon*

- *1 tbsp. Butter, salted*

Direction: Preparation Time: 5 Minutes Cooking Time: 10 Minutes Servings: 3

✓ *Spoon in the butter and olive oil into a large pan and heat it over medium-high heat.*

✓ *Once it becomes hot, place the salmon and season it with salt and pepper.*

✓ *Cook for 4 minutes per side and then cook the other side.*
Stir in the garlic and lemon zest to it.

✓ *Cook for further 2 minutes or until slightly browned.*

✓ *Off the heat and squeeze the lemon juice over it.*

✓ *Serve it hot.*

Nutrition: Calories: 409Kcal; Carbohydrates: 2.7g; Proteins: 32.8g; Fat: 28.8g; Sodium: 497mg

270)   Shrimp in Garlic Butter

Ingredients:

- *1 lb. Shrimp, peeled & deveined*
- *¼ tsp. Red Pepper Flakes*
- *6 tbsp. Butter, divided*
- *1/2 cup Chicken Stock*
- *Salt & Pepper, as needed*
- *2 tbsp. Parsley, minced*
- *5 cloves of Garlic, minced*
- *2 tbsp. Lemon Juice*

Direction: Preparation Time: 5 Minutes Cooking Time: 20 Minutes Servings: 4

✓ *Heat a large bottomed skillet over medium-high heat.*

✓ *Spoon in two tablespoons of the butter and melt it. Add the shrimp.*

✓ *Season it with salt and pepper. Sear for 4 minutes or until shrimp gets cooked.*

✓ *Transfer the shrimp to a plate and stir in the garlic.*

✓ *Sauté for 30 seconds or until aromatic.*
Pour the chicken stock and whisk it well. Allow it to simmer for 5 to 10 minutes or until it has reduced to half.

✓ *Spoon the remaining butter, red pepper, and lemon juice into the sauce. Mix.*

✓ *Continue cooking for another 2 minutes.*

✓ *Take off the pan from the heat and add the cooked shrimp to it.*

✓ *Garnish with parsley and transfer to the serving bowl.*

Nutrition: Calories: 307Kcal; Carbs: 3g; Proteins: 27g; Fat: 20g; Sodium: 522mg

271) *Cobb Salad*

Ingredients:

- 4 Cherry Tomatoes, chopped
- ¼ cup Bacon, cooked & crumbled
- 1/2 of 1 Avocado, chopped
- 2 oz. Chicken Breast, shredded
- 1 Egg, hardboiled
- 2 cups Mixed Green salad
- 1 oz. Feta Cheese, crumbled

Direction: Preparation Time: 5 Minutes Cooking Time: 5 Minutes Servings: 1

✓ Toss all the ingredients for the Cobb salad in a large mixing bowl and toss well.
   Serve and enjoy it.

Nutrition: Calories: 307Kcal; Carbs: 3g; Proteins: 27g; Fat: 20g; Sodium: 522mg

272) *Seared Tuna Steak*

Ingredients:

- 1 tsp. Sesame Seeds
- 1 tbsp. Sesame Oil
- 2 tbsp. Soya Sauce
- Salt & Pepper, to taste
- 2 × 6 oz. Ahi Tuna Steaks

Direction: Preparation Time: 10 Minutes Cooking Time: 10 Minutes Serving Size: 2

✓ Seasoning the tuna steaks with salt and pepper. Keep it aside on a shallow bowl.
✓ In another bowl, mix soya sauce and sesame oil.
✓ pour the sauce over the salmon and coat them generously with the sauce.
✓ Keep it aside for 10 to 15 minutes and then heat a large skillet over medium heat.
   Once hot, keep the tuna steaks and cook them for 3 minutes or until seared underneath.
✓ Flip the fillets and cook them for a further 3 minutes.
✓ Transfer the seared tuna steaks to the serving plate and slice them into 1/2 inch slices. Top with sesame seeds.

Nutrition: Calories: 255Kcal; Fat: 9g; Carbs: 1g; Proteins: 40.5g; Sodium: 293mg

273) *Beef Chili*

Ingredients:

- 1/2 tsp. Garlic Powder
- 1 tsp. Coriander, grounded
- 1 lb. Beef, grounded
- 1/2 tsp. Sea Salt
- 1/2 tsp. Cayenne Pepper
- 1 tsp. Cumin, grounded
- 1/2 tsp. Pepper, grounded
- 1/2 cup Salsa, low-carb & no-sugar

Direction: Preparation Time: 10 Minutes Cooking Time: 20 Minutes Serving Size: 4

✓ Heat a large-sized pan over medium-high heat and cook the beef in it until browned.
✓ Stir in all the spices and cook them for 7 minutes or until everything is combined.
   When the beef gets cooked, spoon in the salsa.
✓ Bring the mixture to a simmer and cook for another 8 minutes or until everything comes together.
✓ Take it from heat and transfer it to a serving bowl

Nutrition: Calories: 229 Carbs: 2g; Proteins: 33g;

274) *Greek Broccoli Salad*

Ingredients:

- 1 ¼ lb. Broccoli, sliced into small bites
- ¼ cup Almonds, sliced
- 1/3 cup Sun-dried Tomatoes
- ¼ cup Feta Cheese, crumbled
- ¼ cup Red Onion, sliced
- For the dressing:
- 1/4 cup Olive Oil
- Dash of Red Pepper Flakes
- 1 Garlic clove, minced
- ¼ tsp. Salt
- 2 tbsp. Lemon Juice
- 1/2 tsp. Dijon Mustard
- 1 tsp. Low Carb Sweetener Syrup
- 1/2 tsp. Oregano, dried

Direction: Preparation Time: 10 Minutes Cooking Time: 15 Minutes Servings: 4

✓ Mix broccoli, onion, almonds and sun-dried tomatoes in a large mixing bowl.
✓ In another small-sized bowl, combine all the dressing ingredients until emulsified.
   Spoon the dressing over the broccoli salad.
✓ Allow the salad to rest for half an hour before serving.

Nutrition: Calories: 272Kcal; Carbohydrates: 11.9g; Proteins: 8g; Fat: 21.6g; Sodium: 321mg

275) *Cheesy Cauliflower Gratin*

Ingredients:

- 6 deli slices Pepper Jack Cheese
- 4 cups Cauliflower florets

- *Salt and Pepper, as needed*
- *4 tbsp. Butter*
- *1/3 cup Heavy Whipping Cream*

Direction: Preparation Time: 5 Minutes Cooking Time: 25 Minutes Servings: 6

✓ *Mix the cauliflower, cream, butter, salt, and pepper in a safe microwave bowl and combine well.*

✓ *Microwave the cauliflower mixture for 25 minutes on high until it becomes soft and tender.*

✓ *Remove the ingredients from the bowl and mash with the help of a fork.*
Taste for seasonings and spoon in salt and pepper as required.

✓ *Arrange the slices of pepper jack cheese on top of the cauliflower mixture and microwave for 3 minutes until the cheese starts melting.*

✓ *Serve warm.*

Nutrition: Cal: 421; Carbs: 3g; Proteins: 19g;

276)   *Strawberry Spinach Salad*

Ingredients:

- *4 oz. Feta Cheese, crumbled*
- *8 Strawberries, sliced*
- *2 oz. Almonds*
- *6 Slices Bacon, thick-cut, crispy and crumbled*
- *10 oz. Spinach leaves, fresh*
- *2 Roma Tomatoes, diced*
- *2 oz. Red Onion, sliced thinly*

Direction: Preparation Time: 5 Minutes

Cooking Time: 10 Minutes Servings: 4

✓ *For making this healthy salad, mix all the ingredients needed to make the salad in a large-sized bowl and toss them well.*
Enjoy

Nutrition: Fat – 16g; Carbs – 8g; Proteins – 14g;

277)   *Cauliflower Mac & Cheese*

Ingredients:

- *1 Cauliflower Head, torn into florets*
- *Salt & Black Pepper, as needed*
- *¼ cup Almond Milk, unsweetened*
- *¼ cup Heavy Cream*
- *3 tbsp. Butter, preferably grass-fed*
- *1 cup Cheddar Cheese, shredded*

Direction: Preparation Time: 5 Minutes Cooking Time: 25 Minutes Serving Size: 4

✓ *Preheat the oven to 450 F.*

✓ *Melt the butter in a small microwave-safe bowl and heat it for 30 seconds.*

✓ *Pour the melted butter over the cauliflower florets along with salt and pepper. Toss them well.*

✓ *Place the cauliflower florets in a parchment paper-covered large baking sheet.*
Bake them for 15 minutes or until the cauliflower is crisp-tender.

✓ *Once baked, mix the heavy cream, cheddar cheese, almond milk, and the remaining butter in a large microwave-safe bowl and heat it on high heat*

✓ *for 2 minutes or until the cheese mixture is smooth. Repeat the procedure until the cheese has melted.*

✓ *Finally, stir in the cauliflower to the sauce mixture and coat well.*

Nutrition: Cal: 294; Fat: 23g; Carbs: 7g; Proteins: 11g

278)   *Easy Egg Salad*

Ingredients:

- *6 eggs, preferably free-range*
- *¼ tsp. Salt*
- *2 tbsp. Mayonnaise*
- *1 tsp. Lemon juice*
- *1 tsp. Dijon mustard*
- *Pepper, to taste*
- *Lettuce leaves, to serve*

Direction: Preparation Time: 5 Minutes

Cooking Time: 15 to 20 Minutes Servings: 4

✓ *Keep the eggs in a saucepan of water and pour cold water until it covers the egg by another 1 inch.*

✓ *Bring to a boil and then remove the eggs from heat.*

✓ *Peel the eggs under cold running water.*
Transfer the cooked eggs into a food processor and pulse them until chopped.

✓ *Stir in the mayonnaise, lemon juice, salt, Dijon mustard, and pepper and mix them well.*

✓ *Taste for seasoning and add more if required.*

✓ *Serve in the lettuce leaves.*

Nutrition: Calories – 166kcal; Fat – 14g; Carbs - 0.85g; Proteins – 10g; Sodium 132mg

279)   *Baked Chicken Legs*

Ingredients:

- *6 Chicken Legs*
- *¼ tsp. Black Pepper*
- *¼ cup Butter*
- *1/2 tsp. Sea Salt*
- *1/2 tsp. Smoked Paprika*
- *1/2 tsp. Garlic Powder*

Direction: Preparation Time: 10 Minutes Cooking Time: 40 Minutes Servings: 6

✓ Preheat the oven to 425 F.

✓ Pat the chicken legs with a paper towel to absorb any excess moisture.

✓ Marinate the chicken pieces by first applying the butter over them and then with the seasoning. Set it aside for a few minutes.
Bake them for 25 minutes. Turnover and bake for further 10 minutes or until the internal temperature reach 165 F.

✓ Serve them hot.

Nutrition: Calories – 236kL; Fat – 16g; Carbs – 0g; Protein – 22g; Sodium – 314mg

280)   Creamed Spinach

Ingredients:

- 3 tbsp. Butter
- ¼ tsp. Black Pepper
- 4 cloves of Garlic, minced
- ¼ tsp. Sea Salt
- 10 oz. Baby Spinach, chopped
- 1 tsp. Italian Seasoning
- 1/2 cup Heavy Cream
- 3 oz. Cream Cheese

Direction: Preparation Time: 5 Minutes Cooking Time: 10 Minutes Servings: 4

✓ Melt butter in a large sauté pan over medium heat.

✓ Once the butter has melted, spoon in the garlic and sauté for 30 seconds or until aromatic.
Spoon in the spinach and cook for 3 to 4 minutes or until wilted.

✓ Add all the remaining ingredients to it and continuously stir until the cream cheese melts and the mixture gets thickened.

✓ Serve hot

Nutrition: Calories – 274kL; Fat – 27g; Carbs – 4g; Protein – 4g; Sodium – 114mg

281)   Stuffed Mushrooms

Ingredients:

- 4 Portobello Mushrooms, large
- 1/2 cup Mozzarella Cheese, shredded
- 1/2 cup Marinara, low-sugar
- Olive Oil Spray

Direction: Preparation Time: 10 Minutes Cooking Time: 20 Minutes Servings: 4

✓ Preheat the oven to 375 F.

✓ Take out the dark gills from the mushrooms with the help of a spoon.
Keep the mushroom stem upside down and spoon it with two tablespoons of marinara sauce and mozzarella cheese.

✓ Bake for 18 minutes or until the cheese is bubbly.

Nutrition: Calories – 113kL; Fat – 6g; Carbs – 4g; Protein – 7g; Sodium – 14mg

282)   Cream Buns with Strawberries

Ingredients:

- 240g all-purpose flour
- 50g granulated sugar
- 8g baking powder
- 1g of salt
- 85g chopped cold butter
- 84g chopped fresh strawberries
- 120 ml whipping cream
- 2 large eggs
- 10 ml vanilla extract
- 5 ml of water

Direction: Preparation time: 10 minutes Cooking time: 12 minutes Servings: 6

✓ Sift flour, sugar, baking powder and salt in a large bowl. Put the butter with the flour with the use of a blender or your hands until the mixture resembles thick crumbs. Mix the strawberries in the flour mixture. Set aside for the mixture to stand. Beat the whipping cream, 1 egg and the vanilla extract in a separate bowl. Put the cream mixture in the flour mixture until they are homogeneous, and then spread the mixture to a thickness of 38 mm.
Use a round cookie cutter to cut the buns. Spread the buns with a combination of egg and water. Set aside

✓ Preheat the air fryer, set it to 180C. Place baking paper in the preheated inner basket. Place the buns on top of the baking paper and cook for 12 minutes at 180C, until golden brown.

Nutrition: Calories: 150Fat: 14g Carbs: 3g Protein: 11g Sugar: 8g Cholesterol: 0mg

283)   Blueberry Buns

Ingredients:

- 240g all-purpose flour
- 50g granulated sugar
- 8g baking powder
- 2g of salt
- 85g chopped cold butter
- 85g of fresh blueberries
- 3g grated fresh ginger
- 113 ml whipping cream
- 2 large eggs
- 4 ml vanilla extract
- 5 ml of water

Direction: Preparation time: 10 minutes Cooking

time: 12 minutes Servings: 6

✓ Put sugar, flour, baking powder and salt in a large bowl.
✓ Put the butter with the flour using a blender or your hands until the mixture resembles thick crumbs.
✓ Mix the blueberries and ginger in the flour mixture and set aside
✓ Mix the whipping cream, 1 egg and the vanilla extract in a different container.
Put the cream mixture with the flour mixture until combined.
✓ Shape the dough until it reaches a thickness of approximately 38 mm and cut it into eighths.
✓ Spread the buns with a combination of egg and water. Set aside. Preheat the air fryer set it to 180C.
✓ Place baking paper in the preheated inner basket and place the buns on top of the paper. Cook for 12 minutes at 180C, until golden brown

Nutrition: Calories: 105 Fat: 1.64g Carbs: 20.09g Protein: 2.43g Sugar: 2.1g Cholesterol: 0mg

284) *Vegetable Soup*

Ingredients:

* 8 cups Vegetable Broth
* 2 tbsp. Olive Oil
* 1 tbsp. Italian Seasoning
* 1 Onion, large & diced
* 2 Bay Leaves, dried
* 2 Bell Pepper, large & diced
* Sea Salt & Black Pepper, as needed
* 4 cloves of Garlic, minced
* 28 oz. Tomatoes, diced
* 1 Cauliflower head, medium & torn into florets
* 2 cups Green Beans, trimmed & chopped

Direction: Preparation Time: 10 Minutes

Cooking Time: 30 Minutes Servings: 5

✓ Heat oil in a Dutch oven over medium heat.
✓ Once the oil becomes hot, stir in the onions and pepper.
✓ Cook for 10 minutes or until the onion is softened and browned.
Spoon in the garlic and sauté for a minute or until fragrant.
✓ Add all the remaining ingredients to it. Mix until everything comes together.
✓ Bring the mixture to a boil. Lower the heat and cook for further 20 minutes or until the vegetables have softened.
✓ Serve hot.

Nutrition: Calories – 79kL; Fat – 2g; Carbs – 8g; Protein – 2g; Sodium – 187mg

285) *Misto Quente*

Ingredients:

* 4 slices of bread without shell
* 4 slices of turkey breast
* 4 slices of cheese
* 2 tbsp. cream cheese
* 2 spoons of butter

Direction: Preparation time: 5 minutes Cooking time: 10 minutes Servings: 4

✓ Preheat the air fryer. Set the timer of 5 minutes and the temperature to 200C.
✓ Pass the butter on one side of the slice of bread, and on the other side of the slice, the cream cheese. Mount the sandwiches are placing two slices of turkey breast and two slices of cheese between the bread, with the cream cheese inside and the side with butter.
✓ Place the sandwiches in the basket of the air fryer. Set the timer of the air fryer for 5 minutes and press the power button.

Nutrition: Calories: 340 Fat: 15g Carbs: 32g Protein: 15g Sugar: 0g Cholesterol: 0mg

286) *Garlic Bread*

Ingredients: Garlic Bread

* 2 stale French rolls
* 4 tbsp. crushed or crumpled garlic
* 1 cup of mayonnaise
* Powdered grated Parmesan
* 1 tbsp. olive oil

Direction: Preparation time: 10 minutes Cooking time: 15 minutes Servings: 4-5

✓ Preheat the air fryer. Set the time of 5 minutes and the temperature to 2000C.
✓ Mix mayonnaise with garlic and set aside.
✓ Cut the baguettes into slices, but without separating them completely.
Fill the cavities of equals. Brush with olive oil and sprinkle with grated cheese.
✓ Place in the basket of the air fryer. Set the timer to 10 minutes, adjust the temperature to 1800C and press the power button.

Nutrition: Calories: 340 Fat: 15g Carbs: 32g Protein: 15g Sugar: 0g Cholesterol: 0mg

287) *Bruschetta*

Ingredients:

* 4 slices of Italian bread
* 1 cup chopped tomato tea

- *1 cup grated mozzarella tea*
- *Olive oil*
- *Oregano, salt, and pepper*
- *4 fresh basil leaves*

**Direction: Preparation time: 5 minutes|
Cooking time: 10 minutes Servings: 2**

✓ *Preheat the air fryer. Set the timer of 5 minutes and the temperature to 2000C.*

✓ *Sprinkle the slices of Italian bread with olive oil. Divide the chopped tomatoes and mozzarella between the slices. Season with salt, pepper, and oregano.*

✓ *Put oil in the filling. Place a basil leaf on top of each slice.*
Put the bruschetta in the basket of the air fryer being careful not to spill the filling. Set the timer of 5 minutes, set the temperature to 180C, and press the power button.

✓ *Transfer the bruschetta to a plate and serve.*

Nutrition: Calories: 434 Fat: 14g Carbohydrates: 63g Protein: 11g Sugar: 8g Cholesterol: 0mg

288) *Cauliflower Potato Mash*

Ingredients:

- *2 cups potatoes, peeled and cubed*
- *2 tbsp. butter*
- *¼ cup milk*
- *10 oz. Cauliflower florets*
- *¾ tsp. salt*

Direction: Preparation Time: 30 minutes Servings: 4 Cooking Time: 5 minutes

✓ *Add water to the saucepan and bring to boil.*

✓ *Reduce heat and simmer for 10 minutes. Drain vegetables well. Transfer vegetables, butter, milk, and salt to a blender and blend until smooth.*

Nutrition: Calories 128 Fat 6.2 g, Sugar 3.3 g, Protein 3.2 g, Cholesterol 17 mg

289) *French toast in Sticks*

Ingredients:

- *4 slices of white bread, 38 mm thick, preferably hard*
- *2 eggs*
- *60 ml of milk*
- *15 ml maple sauce*
- *2 ml vanilla extract*
- *Nonstick Spray Oil*
- *38g of sugar*
- *3ground cinnamon*

- *Maple syrup, to serve*
- *Sugar to sprinkle*

**Direction: Preparation time: 5 minutes
Cooking time: 10 minutes Servings: 4**

✓ *Cut each slice of bread into thirds making 12 pieces. Place sideways*

✓ *Beat the eggs, milk, maple syrup and vanilla.*

✓ *Preheat the air fryer, set it to 175C.*

✓ *Dip the sliced bread in the egg mixture and place it in the preheated air fryer. Sprinkle French toast generously with oil spray.*
Cook French toast for 10 minutes at 175C. Turn the toast halfway through cooking.

✓ *Mix the sugar and cinnamon in a bowl.*

✓ *Cover the French toast with the sugar and cinnamon mixture when you have finished cooking.*

✓ *Serve with Maple syrup and sprinkle with powdered sugar*

Nutrition: Calories 128, Fat 6.2 g, Carbs 16.3 g, Sugar 3.3 g, Protein 3.2 g   Cholesterol 17 mg

290) *Muffins Sandwich*

Ingredients:

- *Nonstick Spray Oil*
- *1 slice of white cheddar cheese*
- *1 slice of Canadian bacon*
- *1 English muffin, divided*
- *15 ml hot water*
- *1 large egg*
- *Salt and pepper to taste*

Direction: Preparation time: 2 minutesCooking time: 10 minutes Servings: 1

✓ *Spray the inside of an 85g mold with oil spray and place it in the air fryer.*

✓ *Preheat the air fryer, set it to 160C.*

✓ *Add the Canadian cheese and bacon in the preheated air fryer.*

✓ *Pour the hot water and the egg into the hot pan and season with salt and pepper.*
Select Bread, set to 10 minutes.

✓ *Take out the English muffins after 7 minutes, leaving the egg for the full time.*

✓ *Build your sandwich by placing the cooked egg on top of the English muffins and serve*

Nutrition: Calories 400 Fat 26g, Carbs 26g, Sugar 15 g, Protein 3 g, Cholesterol 155 mg

291) *Bacon BBQ*

Ingredients:

- *13g dark brown sugar*

- *5g chili powder*
- *1g ground cumin*
- *1g cayenne pepper*
- *4 slices of bacon, cut in half*

Direction: Preparation time: 2 minutes

Cooking time: 8 minutes Servings: 2

✓ *Mix seasonings until well combined.*

✓ *Dip the bacon in the dressing until it is completely covered. Leave aside.*

✓ *Preheat the air fryer, set it to 160C. Place the bacon in the preheated air fryer*

✓ *Select Bacon and press Start/Pause.*

Nutrition: Calories: 1124 Fat: 72g Carbs: 59g Protein: 49g Sugar: 11g Cholesterol 77mg

292) *Stuffed French toast*

Ingredients:

- *1 slice of brioche bread,*
- *64 mm thick, preferably rancid*
- *113g cream cheese*
- *2 eggs*
- *15 ml of milk*
- *30 ml whipping cream*
- *38g of sugar*
- *3g cinnamon*
- *2 ml vanilla extract*
- *Nonstick Spray Oil*
- *Pistachios chopped to cover*
- *Maple syrup, to serve*

Direction: Preparation time: 4 minutes

Cooking time: 10 minutes Servings: 1

✓ *Preheat the air fryer, set it to 175C.*

✓ *Cut a slit in the middle of the muffin.*

✓ *Fill the inside of the slit with cream cheese. Leave aside.*

✓ *Mix the eggs, milk, whipping cream, sugar, cinnamon, and vanilla extract.*

✓ *Moisten the stuffed French toast in the egg mixture for 10 seconds on each side. Sprinkle each side of French toast with oil spray.*

✓ *Place the French toast in the preheated air fryer and cook for 10 minutes at 175C*

✓ *Stir the French toast carefully with a spatula when you finish cooking.*

✓ *Serve topped with chopped pistachios and acrid syrup.*

Nutrition: Calories: 159 Fat: 7.5g Carbs: 25.2g Protein: 14g Sugar: 0g Cholesterol 90mg

293) *Lean Lamb and Turkey Meatballs with Yogurt*

Ingredients:

- *1 egg white*
- *4 ounces ground lean turkey*
- *1 pound of lean ground lamb*
- *1 teaspoon each of cayenne pepper, ground coriander, red chili paste, salt, and ground cumin*
- *2 garlic cloves, minced*
- *1 1/2 tablespoons parsley, chopped*
- *1/4 cup of olive oil 1 tablespoon mint, chopped, For the yogurt*
- *2 tablespoons of buttermilk*
- *1 garlic clove, minced*
- *1/4 cup mint, chopped*
- *1/2 cup of Greek yogurt, non-fat*
- *Salt to taste*

Direction: Preparation Time: 10 minutes Servings: 4 Cooking Time: 8 minutes

✓ *Set the Air Fryer to 390 degrees.*

✓ *Mix all the ingredients for the meatballs in a bowl.*

✓ *Roll and mold them into golf-size round pieces.*

✓ *Arrange in the cooking basket—Cook for 8 minutes.*

✓ *While waiting, combine all the ingredients for the mint yogurt in a bowl. Mix well.*

✓ *Serve the meatballs with mint yogurt. Top with olives and fresh mint.*

Nutrition: Calorie: 154 Carbohydrate: 9g Fat: 2.5g Protein: 8.6g Fiber: 2.4g

294) *Scallion Sandwich*

Ingredients:

- *2 slices wheat bread*
- *2 teaspoons butter, low fat*
- *2 scallions, sliced thinly*
- *1 tablespoon of parmesan cheese, grated*
- *3/4 cup of cheddar cheese, reduced-fat, grated*

Direction: Preparation Time: 10 minutes Cooking Time: 10 minutes Servings: 1

✓ *Preheat the Air fryer to 356 degrees.*

✓ *Spread butter on a slice of bread. Place inside the cooking basket with the butter side facing down. Place cheese and scallions on top. Spread the rest of the butter on the other slice of bread Put it on top of the sandwich and sprinkle with parmesan cheese.*

✓ *Cook for 10 minutes.*

Nutrition: Calorie: 154 Carbohydrate: 9g Fat: 2.5g Protein: 8.6g Fiber: 2.4g

295) *Air Fried Section and Tomato*

Ingredients:

- *1 aubergine, sliced thickly into 4 disks*
- *1 tomato, sliced into 2 thick disks*
- *2 tsp. feta cheese, reduced fat*
- *2 fresh basil leaves, minced*
- *2 balls, small buffalo mozzarella, reduced-fat, roughly torn*
- *Pinch of salt*
- *Pinch of black pepper*

Direction: Preparation Time: 10 minutes Cooking Time: 5 minutes Servings: 2

✓ *Preheat Air Fryer to 330 degrees F.*

✓ *Spray small amount of oil into the air fryer basket. Fry aubergine slices for 5 minutes or until golden brown on both sides. Transfer to a plate.*

✓ *Fry tomato slices in batches for 5 minutes or until seared on both sides.*
To serve, stack salad starting with an aborigine base, buffalo mozzarella, basil leaves, tomato slice, and 1/2-teaspoon feta cheese.

✓ *Top of with another slice of aborigine and 1/2 tsp— feta cheese. Serve.*

Nutrition: Calorie: 140.3 Carbohydrate: 26.6 Fat: 3.4g Protein: 4.2g Fiber: 7.3g

296) *Cheesy Salmon Fillets*

Ingredients:

- *Ingredients: For the salmon fillets*
- *2 pieces, 4 oz. each salmon fillets, choose even cuts*
- *1/2 cup sour cream, reduced-fat*
- *¼ cup cottage cheese, reduced-fat*
- *¼ cup Parmigiano-Reggiano cheese, freshly grated*

Garnish:

- *Spanish paprika*
- *1/2 piece lemon, cut into wedges*

Direction: Preparation Time: 15 minutes Cooking Time: 20 minutes Servings: 2-3

✓ *Preheat Air Fryer to 330 degrees F.*

✓ *To make the salmon fillets, mix sour cream, cottage cheese, and Parmigiano-Reggiano cheese in a bowl. Layer salmon fillets in the Air fryer basket. Fry for 20 minutes or until cheese turns golden brown.*

✓ *To assemble, place a salmon fillet and sprinkle paprika. Garnish with lemon wedges and squeeze lemon juice on top. Serve.*

Nutrition: Calorie: 274 Carbohydrate: 1g Fat: 19g Protein: 24g Fiber: 0.5g

APPETIZERS AND SALADS

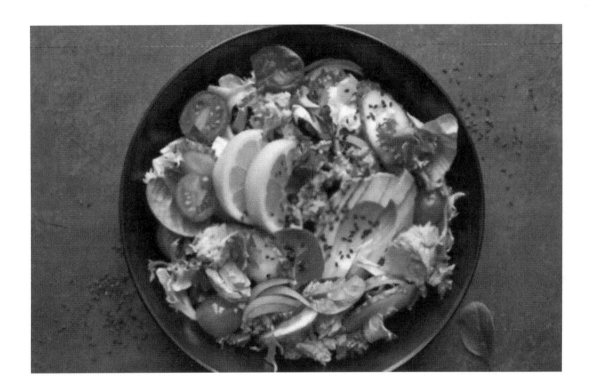

297) *Tuna Salad Recipe 1*

Ingredients:

- *1 can tuna (6 oz.)*
- *1/3 cup fresh cucumber, chopped*
- *1/3 cup fresh tomato, chopped*
- *1/3 cup avocado, chopped*
- *1/3 cup celery, chopped*
- *2 garlic cloves, minced*
- *4 tsp. olive oil*
- *2 tbsp. lime juice*
- *Pinch of black pepper*

Direction: Preparation Time: 10 minutes Cooking time: none Servings: 3

✓ *Prepare the dressing by combining olive oil, lime juice, minced garlic and black pepper.*
Mix the salad ingredients in a salad bowl and drizzle with the dressing.

Nutrition: Carbohydrates: 4.8 g Protein: 14.3 g Total sugars: 1.1 g Calories: 212 g

298) *Roasted Portobello Salad*

Ingredients:

- *11/2lb. Portobello mushrooms, stems trimmed*
- *3 heads Belgian endive, sliced*
- *1 small red onion, sliced*
- *4 oz. blue cheese*
- *8 oz. mixed salad greens*

Dressing:

- *3 tbsp. red wine vinegar*
- *1 tbsp. Dijon mustard*
- *2/3 cup olive oil*
- *Salt and pepper to taste*

Direction: Preparation Time: 10 minutes Cooking time: none Servings: 4

✓ *Preheat the oven to 450F.*

✓ *Prepare the dressing by whisking together vinegar, mustard, salt and pepper. Slowly add olive oil while whisking.*

✓ *Cut the mushrooms and arrange them on a baking sheet, stem-side up. Coat the mushrooms with some dressing and bake for 15 minutes.*
In a salad bowl toss the salad greens with onion, endive and cheese. Sprinkle with the dressing.

✓ *Add mushrooms to the salad bowl.*

Nutrition: Carbohydrates: 22.3 g Protein: 14.9 g Total sugars: 2.1 g Calories: 501

299) *Shredded Chicken Salad*

Ingredients:

- *2 chicken breasts, boneless, skinless*
- *1 head iceberg lettuce, cut into strips*
- *2 bell peppers, cut into strips*
- *1 fresh cucumber, quartered, sliced*
- *3 scallions, sliced*
- *2 tbsp. chopped peanuts*
- *1 tbsp. peanut vinaigrette*
- *Salt to taste*
- *1 cup water*

Direction: Preparation Time: 5 minutes Cooking time: 10 minutes Servings: 6

✓ *In a skillet simmer one cup of salted water.*

✓ *Add the chicken breasts, cover and cook on low for 5 minutes. Remove the cover. Then remove the chicken from the skillet and shred with a fork.*

✓ *In a salad bowl mix the vegetables with the cooled chicken, season with salt and sprinkle with peanut vinaigrette and chopped peanuts.*

Nutrition: Carbohydrates: 9 g Protein: 11.6 g Total sugars: 4.2 g Calories: 117

300) *Broccoli Salad*

Ingredients:

- *1 medium head broccoli, raw, florets only*
- *1/2 cup red onion, chopped*
- *12 oz. turkey bacon, chopped, fried until crisp*
- *1/2 cup cherry tomatoes, halved*
- *¼ cup sunflower kernels*
- *¾ cup raisins*
- *¾ cup mayonnaise*
- *2 tbsp. white vinegar*

Direction: Preparation Time: 10 minutes Cooking time: none Servings: 6

✓ *In a salad bowl combine the broccoli, tomatoes and onion.*

✓ *Mix mayo with vinegar and sprinkle over the broccoli.*

✓ *Add the sunflower kernels, raisins and bacon and toss well.*

Nutrition: Carbohydrates: 17.3 g Protein: 11 g Total sugars: 10 g Calories: 220

301) *Cherry Tomato Salad*

Ingredients:

- *40 cherry tomatoes, halved*
- *1 cup mozzarella balls, halved*

- *1 cup green olives, sliced*
- *1 can (6 oz.) black olives, sliced*
- *2 green onions, chopped*
- *3 oz. roasted pine nuts*

Dressing:

- *1/2 cup olive oil*
- *2 tbsp. red wine vinegar*
- *1 tsp. dried oregano*
- *Salt and pepper to taste*

Direction: Preparation Time: 10 minutes Cooking time: none Servings: 6

✓ *In a salad bowl, combine the tomatoes, olives and onions.*

✓ *Prepare the dressing by combining olive oil with red wine vinegar, dried oregano, salt and pepper. Sprinkle with the dressing and add the nuts.*

✓ *Let marinate in the fridge for 1 hour.*

Nutrition: Carbohydrates: 10.7 g Protein: 2.4 g Total sugars: 3.6 g

302) *Ground Turkey Salad*

Ingredients:

- *1 lb. lean ground turkey*
- *1/2 inch ginger, minced*
- *2 garlic cloves, minced*
- *1 onion, chopped*
- *1 tbsp. olive oil*
- *1 bag lettuce leaves (for serving)*
- *¼ cup fresh cilantro, chopped*
- *2 tsp. coriander powder*
- *1 tsp. red chili powder*
- *1 tsp. turmeric powder*
- *Salt to taste*
- *4 cups water*
- *Dressing:*
- *2 tbsp. fat free yogurt*
- *1 tbsp. sour cream, non-fat*
- *1 tbsp. low fat mayonnaise*
- *1 lemon, juiced*
- *1 tsp. red chili flakes*
- *Salt and pepper to taste*

Direction: Preparation Time: 10 minutes Cooking time: 35 minutes Servings: 6

✓ *In a skillet sauté the garlic and ginger in olive oil for 1 minute. Add onion and season with salt. Cook for 10 minutes over medium heat.*

✓ *Add the ground turkey and sauté for 3 more minutes. Add the spices (turmeric, red chili powder and coriander powder).*

✓ *Add 4 cups water and cook for 30 minutes, covered.*

Prepare the dressing by combining yogurt, sour cream, mayo, lemon juice, chili flakes, salt and pepper.

✓ *To serve arrange the salad leaves on serving plates and place the cooked ground turkey on them. Top with dressing.*

Nutrition: Carbohydrates: 9.1 g Protein: 17.8 g Total sugars: 2.5 g Calories: 176

303) *Asian Cucumber Salad*

Ingredients:

- *1 lb. cucumbers, sliced*
- *2 scallions, sliced*
- *2 tbsp. sliced pickled ginger, chopped*
- *¼ cup cilantro*
- *1/2 red jalapeño, chopped*
- *3 tbsp. rice wine vinegar*
- *1 tbsp. sesame oil*
- *1 tbsp. sesame seeds*

Direction: Preparation Time: 10 minutes

Cooking time: none Servings: 6

✓ *In a salad bowl combine all ingredients and toss together.*

✓ *Enjoy!*

Nutrition: Carbohydrates: 5.7 g Protein: 1 g Total sugars: 3.1 g Calories: 52

304) *Cauliflower Tofu Salad*

Ingredients:

- *2 cups cauliflower florets, blended*
- *1 fresh cucumber, diced*
- *1/2 cup green olives, diced*
- *1/3 cup red onion, diced*
- *2 tbsp. toasted pine nuts*
- *2 tbsp. raisins*
- *1/3 cup feta, crumbled*
- *1/2 cup pomegranate seeds*
- *2 lemons (juiced, zest grated)*
- *8 oz. tofu*
- *2 tsp. oregano*
- *2 garlic cloves, minced*
- *1/2 tsp. red chili flakes*
- *3 tbsp. olive oil*
- *Salt and pepper to taste*

Direction: Preparation time: 10 minutes Cooking time: 15 minutes Servings: 4

✓ *Season the processed cauliflower with salt and transfer it to a strainer to drain.*

✓ *Prepare the marinade for the tofu by combining 2 tbsp. lemon juice, 1.5 tbsp. olive oil, minced garlic, chili flakes, oregano, salt and pepper. Coat tofu in the marinade and set aside.*

✓ *Preheat the oven to 450F.*
Bake tofu on a baking sheet for 12 minutes.

✓ *In a salad bowl mix the remaining marinade with onions, cucumber, cauliflower, olives and raisins. Add in the remaining olive oil and grated lemon zest.*

✓ *Top with tofu, pine nuts, and feta and pomegranate seeds.*

Nutrition: Carbohydrates: 34.1 g Protein: 11.1 g Total sugars: 11.5 g Calories: 328

305)   Scallop Caesar Salad

Ingredients:

- 8 sea scallops
- 4 cups romaine lettuce
- 2 tsp. olive oil
- 3 tbsp. Caesar Salad Dressing
- 1 tsp. lemon juice
- Salt and pepper to taste

Direction: Preparation Time: 5 minutes

Cooking Time: 2 minutes Servings: 2

✓ *In a frying pan heat olive oil and cook the scallops in one layer no longer than 2 minutes per both sides—season with salt and pepper to taste. Arrange lettuce on plates and place scallops on top.*

✓ *Pour over the Caesar dressing and lemon juice.*

Nutrition: Carbohydrates: 14 g Protein: 30.7 g Total sugars: 2.2 g Calories: 340 g

306)   California Wraps

Ingredients:

- 4 slices turkey breast, cooked
- 4 slices ham, cooked
- 4 lettuce leaves
- 4 slices tomato
- 4 slices avocado
- 1 tsp. lime juice
- A handful watercress leaves
- 4 tbsp. Ranch dressing, sugar free

Direction: Preparation Time: 5 minutes Cooking Time: 15 minutes Servings: 4

✓ *Top a lettuce leaf with turkey slice, ham slice and tomato.*

✓ *In a bowl combine avocado and lime juice and place on top of tomatoes. Top with water cress and*

dressing.

✓ *Repeat with the remaining ingredients for 4. Topping each lettuce leaf with a turkey slice, ham slice, tomato and dressing.*

Nutrition: Carbohydrates: 4 g Protein: 9 g Total sugars: 0.5 g Calories: 140

307)   chicken Breast Salad

Ingredients:

- 1/2 chicken breast, skinless, boiled and shredded
- 2 long cucumbers, cut into 8 thick rounds each, scooped out (won't use in a).
- 1 tsp. ginger, minced
- 1 tsp. lime zest, grated
- 4 tsp. olive oil
- 1 tsp. sesame oil
- 1 tsp. lime juice
- Salt and pepper to taste

Direction: Preparation Time: 5 minutes Cooking Time: 15 minutes Servings: 4

✓ *In a bowl combine lime zest, juice, olive and sesame oils, ginger, and season with salt.*
Toss the chicken with the dressing and fill the cucumber cups with the salad.

Nutrition: Carbohydrates: 4 g Protein: 12 g Total sugars: 0.5 g Calories: 116 g

308)   Aromatic Toasted Pumpkin Seeds

Ingredients:

- cup pumpkin seeds
- 1 tsp. cinnamon
- packets stevia
- 1 tbsp. canola oil
- ¼ tsp. sea salt

Direction: Preparation Time: 5 minutes Cooking Time: 45 minutes Servings: 4

✓ *Prep the oven to 300°F (150°C).*

✓ *Combine the pumpkin seeds with cinnamon, stevia, canola oil, and salt in a bowl. Stir to mix well.*

✓ *Pour the seeds in a single layer on a baking sheet, then arrange the sheet in the preheated oven.*

✓ *Bake for 45 minutes or until well toasted and fragrant. Shake the sheet twice to bake the seeds evenly.*

✓ *Serve immediately.*

Nutrition: Calories: 202 Carbohydrates: 5.1g Fiber: 2.3g

309) *Easy Caprese Skewers*

Ingredients:

- *12 cherry tomatoes*
- *8 (1-inch) pieces Mozzarella cheese*
- *12 basil leaves*
- *¼ cup Italian Vinaigrette, for serving*

Direction: Preparation Time: 5 minutes Cooking Time: 0 minute Servings: 2

✓ *Thread the tomatoes, cheese, and basil leave alternatively through the skewers.*

✓ *Place the skewers on a huge plate and baste with the Italian Vinaigrette. Serve immediately.*

Nutrition: Calories: 230 Carbohydrates: 8.5g Fiber: 1.9g

310) *Sunflower Seeds and Arugula Garden Salad*

Ingredients:

- *¼ tsp. black pepper*
- *¼ tsp. salt*
- *1 tsp. fresh thyme, chopped*
- *2 tbsp. sunflower seeds, toasted*
- *2 cups red grapes, halved*
- *7 cups baby arugula, loosely packed*
- *1 tbsp. coconut oil*
- *2 tsp. honey*
- *3 tbsp. red wine vinegar*
- *1/2tsp. stone-ground mustard*

Direction: Preparation time: 5 minutes   Cooking time: 10 minutes Servings: 6

✓ *In a small bowl, whisk together mustard, honey and vinegar. Slowly pour oil as you whisk. In a large salad bowl, mix thyme, seeds, grapes and arugula.*

✓ *Drizzle with dressing and serve.*

Nutrition: Calories: 86.7g Protein: 1.6g Carbs: 13.1g Fat: 3.1g.

311) *Supreme Caesar Salad*

Ingredients:

- *¼ cup olive oil*
- *¾ cup mayonnaise*
- *1 head romaine lettuce, torn into bite-sized pieces*
- *1 tbsp. lemon juice*
- *1 tsp. Dijon mustard*
- *1 tsp. Worcestershire sauce*
- *3 cloves garlic, peeled and minced*
- *3 cloves garlic, peeled and quartered*

- *4 cups day-old bread, cubed*
- *5 anchovy filets, minced*
- *6 tbsp. grated parmesan cheese, divided*
- *Ground black pepper to taste*
- *Salt to taste*

Direction: Preparation time: 5 minutes Cooking time: 10 minutes Servings: 4

✓ *In a small bowl, whisk well lemon juice, mustard, Worcestershire sauce, 2 tbsp. parmesan cheese, anchovies, mayonnaise, and minced garlic. Season with pepper and salt to taste. Set aside in the ref.*

✓ *On medium fire, place a large nonstick saucepan and heat oil.*

✓ *Sauté quartered garlic until browned around a minute or two. Remove and discard. Add bread cubes in same pan, sauté until lightly browned. Season with pepper and salt. Transfer to a plate.*

✓ *In large bowl, place lettuce and pour in dressing. Toss well to coat. Top with remaining parmesan cheese.*

✓ *Garnish with bread cubes, serve, and enjoy.*

Nutrition: Calories: 443.3g Fat: 32.1g Protein: 11.6g Carbs: 27g

312) *Tabbouleh- Arabian Salad*

Ingredients:

- *¼ cup chopped fresh mint*
- *1 2/3 cups boiling water*
- *1 cucumber, peeled, seeded and chopped*
- *1 cup bulgur*
- *1 cup chopped fresh parsley*
- *1 cup chopped green onions*
- *1 tsp. salt*
- *1/3 cup lemon juice*
- *1/3 cup olive oil*
- *3 tomatoes, chopped*
- *Ground black pepper to taste*

Direction: Preparation time: 5 minutes

Cooking time: 10 minutes Servings: 6

✓ *In a large bowl, mix together boiling water and bulgur. Let soak and set aside for an hour while covered. After one hour, toss in cucumber, tomatoes, mint, parsley, onions, lemon juice and oil. Then season with black pepper and salt to taste. Toss well and refrigerate for another hour while covered before serving.*

Nutrition: Calories: 185.5g fat: 13.1g Protein: 4.1g Carbs: 12.8g

- *1 tbsp. gingerroot*

- 1 tbsp. no-sugar-added applesauce
- 2 tbsp. naturally brewed soy sauce
- ¼ tsp. dried red pepper flakes
- 2 tsp. sesame oil, toasted
- 1 (14 oz./397g) package extra-firm tofu
- 2 tbsp. fresh cilantro
- 1 tsp. sesame seeds

Direction: Preparation Time: 45 minutes Cooking Time: 20 minutes Servings: 6

✓ Combine the vinegar, scallion, ginger, applesauce, soy sauce, red pepper flakes, and sesame oil in a large bowl. Stir to mix well.

✓ Dunk the tofu pieces in the bowl, then refrigerate to marinate for 30 minutes.

✓ Preheat a grill pan over medium-high heat.

✓ Place the tofu on the grill pan with tongs, reserve the marinade, then grill for 8 minutes or until the tofu is golden brown and have deep grilled marks on both sides. Flip the tofu halfway through the cooking time. You may need to work in batches to avoid overcrowding.

✓ Transfer the tofu to a large plate and sprinkle with cilantro leaves and sesame seeds. Serve with the marinade alongside.

Nutrition: Calories: 90 Carbohydrates: 3g Fiber: 1g

313)   *Grilled Tofu with Sesame Seeds*

Ingredients:,

- 1½ tbsp. brown rice vinegar
- 1 scallion
- 1 tbsp. gingerroot
- 1 tbsp. no-sugar-added applesauce
- 2 tbsp. naturally brewed soy sauce,
- ¼ tsp. dried red pepper flakes
- 2 tsp. sesame oil, toasted
- 1 (14 oz./397g) package extra-firm tofu
- 2 tbsp. fresh cilantro
- 1 tsp. sesame seeds

Direction: Preparation Time: 45 minutes Cooking Time: 20 minutes Servings: 6

✓ Combine the vinegar, scallion, ginger, applesauce, soy sauce, red pepper flakes, and sesame oil in a large bowl. Stir to mix well.

✓ Dunk the tofu pieces in the bowl, then refrigerate to marinate for 30 minutes.

✓ Preheat a grill pan over medium-high heat., Place the tofu on the grill pan with tongs, reserve the marinade, then grill for 8 minutes or until the tofu is golden brown and have deep grilled marks on both sides.

✓ Flip the tofu halfway through the cooking time. You may need to work in batches to avoid overcrowding.

✓ Transfer the tofu to a large plate and sprinkle with cilantro leaves and sesame seeds.

✓ Serve with the marinade alongside.

Nutrition: Calories: 90 Carbohydrates: 3g Fiber: 1g

314)   *Kale Chips*

Ingredients:

- ¼ tsp. garlic powder
- Pinch cayenne to taste
- 1 tbsp. extra-virgin olive oil
- ½ tsp. sea salt, or to taste
- 1 (8 oz.) bunch kale

Direction: Preparation Time: 5 minutes Cooking Time: 15 minutes Servings: 1

✓ Prepare oven at 180ºC. Line 2 baking sheets with parchment paper.

✓ Toss the garlic powder, cayenne pepper, olive oil, and salt in a large bowl, then dunk the kale in the bowl.

✓ Situate kale in a single layer on 1 of the baking sheets.

✓ Arrange the sheet in the preheated oven and bake for 7 minutes. Remove the sheet from the oven and pour the kale into the single layer of the other baking sheet.

✓ Move the sheet of kale back to the oven and bake for another 7 minutes.

✓ Serve immediately.

Nutrition: Calories: 136 Carbohydrates: 3g Fiber: 1.1g

315)   *Simple Deviled Eggs*

Ingredients:

- 6 large eggs
- ⅛ tsp. mustard powder
- 2 tbsp. light mayonnaise

Direction: Preparation Time: 5 minutes Cooking Time: 8 minutes Servings: 12

✓ Sit the eggs in a saucepan, then pour in enough water to cover the egg. Bring to a boil, then boil the eggs for another 8 minutes. Turn off the heat and cover, then let sit for 15 minutes.

✓ Transfer the boiled eggs to a pot of cold water and peel them under the water.

✓ Transfer the eggs to a large plate, then cut in half. Remove the egg yolks and place them in a bowl, then mash with a fork.
Add the mustard powder, mayo, salt, and pepper to the bowl of yolks, then stir to mix well.

✓ Spoon the yolk mixture in the egg white on the plate. Serve immediately.

Nutrition: Calories: 45 Carbs: 1g Fiber: 0.9g

316) Sautéed Collard Greens and Cabbage

Ingredients:

- 2 tbsp. extra-virgin olive oil
- 1 collard greens bunch
- ½ small green cabbage
- 6 garlic cloves
- 1 tbsp. low-sodium soy sauce

Direction: Preparation Time: 10 minutes Cooking Time: 10 minutes Servings: 8

✓ Cook olive oil in a large skillet over medium-high heat.

✓ Sauté the collard greens in the oil for about 2 minutes, or until the greens start to wilt.

✓ Toss in the cabbage and mix well. Set to medium-low, cover, and cook for 5 to 7 minutes, stirring occasionally, or until the greens are softened. Fold in the garlic and soy sauce and stir to combine. Cook for about 30 seconds more until fragrant.

✓ Remove from the heat to a plate and serve.

Nutrition: Calories: 73 Carbs: 5.9g Fiber: 2.9g

317) Roasted Delicata Squash with Thyme

Ingredients:

- 1 (1½ lb.) Delicata squash
- 1 tbsp. extra-virgin olive oil
- ½ tsp. dried thyme
  ¼ tsp. salt
- ¼ tsp. freshly ground black pepper

Direction: Preparation Time: 10 minutes Cooking Time: 20 minutes Servings: 4

✓ Prep the oven to 400°F (205°C). Ready baking sheet with parchment paper and set aside.

✓ Add the squash strips, olive oil, thyme, salt, and pepper in a large bowl, and toss until the squash strips are fully coated.
Place the squash strips on the prepared baking sheet in a single layer. Roast for about 20 minutes, flipping the strips halfway through.

✓ Remove from the oven and serve on plates.

Nutrition: Calories: 78 Carbohydrates: 11.8g Fiber: 2.1g

318) Roasted Asparagus and Red Peppers

Ingredients:

- 1lb. (454g) asparagus
- 2 red bell peppers, seeded
- 1 small onion
- 2 tbsp. Italian dressing

Direction: Preparation Time: 5 minutes Cooking Time: 15 minutes Servings: 4

✓ Ready oven to (205°C). Wrap baking sheet with parchment paper and set aside.

✓ Combine the asparagus with the peppers, onion, dressing in a large bowl, and toss well.

✓ Arrange the vegetables on the baking sheet and roast for about 15 minutes. Flip the vegetables with a spatula once during cooking.

✓ Transfer to a large platter and serve.

Nutrition: Calories: 92 Carbs: 10.7g Fiber: 4g

319) Tarragon Spring Peas

Ingredients:

- 1 tbsp. unsalted butter
- ½ Vidalia onion
- 1 cup low-sodium vegetable broth
- 3 cups fresh shelled peas
- tbsp. minced fresh tarragon

Direction: Preparation Time: 10 minutes Cooking Time: 12 minutes Servings: 6

✓ Cook butter in a pan at medium heat.

✓ Sauté the onion in the melted butter for about 3 minutes, stirring occasionally.

✓ Pour in the vegetable broth and whisk well. Add the peas and tarragon to the skillet and stir to combine.

✓ Reduce the heat to low, cover, cook for about 8 minutes more, or until the peas are tender.

✓ Let the peas cool for 5 minutes and serve warm.

Nutrition: Calories: 82 Carbohydrates: 12g Fiber: 3.8g

320) Butter-Orange Yams

Ingredients:

- 2 medium jewel yams
- 2 tbsp. unsalted butter
- Juice of 1 large orange
- 1½ tsp. ground cinnamon
- ¼ tsp. ground ginger
- ¾ tsp. ground nutmeg
- ⅛ tsp. ground garlic cloves

Direction: Preparation Time: 7 minutes Cooking Time: 45 minutes Servings: 8

✓ Set oven at 180ºC.

✓ Arrange the yam dices on a rimmed baking sheet in a single layer. Set aside.

✓ Add the butter, orange juice, cinnamon, ginger, nutmeg, and garlic cloves to a medium saucepan over medium-low heat. Cook for 3 to 5 minutes, stirring continuously.

✓ Spoon the sauce over the yams and toss to coat well.

✓ Bake in the prepared oven for 40 minutes.

✓ Let the yams cool for 8 minutes on the baking sheet before removing and serving.

Nutrition: Calories: 129 Carbohydrates: 24.7g Fiber: 5g

321)   *Roasted Tomato Brussels Sprouts*

Ingredients:

- lb. (454 g) Brussels sprouts 1 tbsp. extra-virgin olive oil
- ½ cup sun-dried tomatoes
- 2 tbsp. lemon juice
- 1 tsp. lemon zest

Direction: Preparation Time: 15 minutes Cooking Time: 20 minutes Servings: 4

✓ Set oven 205ºC. Prep large baking sheet with aluminum foil.

✓ Toss the Brussels sprouts in the olive oil in a large bowl until well coated. Sprinkle with salt and pepper.

✓ Spread out the seasoned Brussels sprouts on the prepared baking sheet in a single layer. Roast for 20 minutes, shaking halfway through.

✓ Remove from the oven then situate in a bowl. Whisk tomatoes, lemon juice, and lemon zest, to incorporate. Serve immediately.

Nutrition: Calories: 111 Carbohydrates: 13.7g Fiber: 4.9g

322)   *Simple Sautéed Greens*

Ingredients:

- 2 tbsp. extra-virgin olive oil
- 1 pound (454 g) Swiss chard
- 1 lb. (454 g) kale
- ½ tsp. ground cardamom
- 1 tbsp. lemon juice

Direction: Preparation Time: 10 minutes Cooking Time: 10 minutes Servings: 4

✓ Heat up olive oil in a big skillet over medium-high

heat.

✓ Stir in Swiss chard, kale, cardamom, lemon juice to the skillet, and stir to combine. Cook for about 10 minutes, stirring continuously, or until the greens are wilted.

✓ Sprinkle with salt and pepper and stir well.

✓ Serve the greens on a plate while warm.

Nutrition: Calories: 139 Carbohydrates: 15.8g Fiber: 3.9g

323)   *Garlicky Mushrooms*

Ingredients:

- 1tbsp. butter
- 2tsp. extra-virgin olive oil
- 2 pounds' button mushrooms
- 2 tsp. minced fresh garlic
- 1 tsp. chopped fresh thyme

Direction: Preparation Time: 10 minutes Cooking Time: 12 minutes Servings: 4

✓ Warm up butter and olive oil in a huge skillet over medium-high heat.

✓ Add the mushrooms and sauté for 10 minutes,

✓ stirring occasionally.
  Stir in the garlic and thyme and cook for an additional 2 minutes.

✓ Season and serve on a plate.

Nutrition: Calories: 96 Carbs: 8.2g Fiber: 1.7g

324)   *Green Beans in Oven*

Ingredients:

- 12 oz. green bean pods
- 1 tbsp. olive oil
- ½ tsp. onion powder
- ⅛ tsp. Pepper
- ⅛ tsp. salt

Direction: Preparation Time: 5 minutes Cooking Time: 17 minutes Servings: 3

✓ Preheat oven to 350°F. Mix green beans with onion powder, pepper, and oil.

✓ Spread the seeds on the baking sheet.

✓ Bake for 17 minutes or until you have a delicious aroma in the kitchen.

Nutrition: Calories: 37 Protein: 1.4g Carbs: 5.5g

325)   *Parmesan Broiled Flounder*

Ingredients:

- 2 (4-oz) flounder
- ½ tbsp. Parmesan cheese

- *1 ½ tbsp. mayonnaise*
- *⅛ tsp. soy sauce*
- *¼ tsp. chili sauce*
- *⅛ tsp. salt-free lemon-pepper seasoning*

Direction: Preparation Time: 10 minutes Cooking Time: 7 minutes Servings: 2

✓ *Preheat flounder.*

✓ *Mix cheese, reduced-fat mayonnaise, soy sauce, chili sauce, seasoning.*

✓ *Put fish on a baking sheet coated with cooking spray, sprinkle with salt and pepper. Spread Parmesan mixture over flounder.*

✓ *Broil 6 to 8 minutes or until a crust appears on the fish.*

Nutrition: Calories: 200 Fat: 17g Carbohydrates: 7g

326) *Fish with Fresh Tomato - Basil Sauce*

Ingredients:

- *(4-oz) tilapia fillets*
- *1 tbsp. fresh basil, chopped*
- *⅛ tsp. salt*
- *1 pinch of crushed red pepper*
- *1 cup cherry tomatoes, chopped*
- *2 tsp. extra virgin olive oil*

Direction: Preparation Time: 10 minutes Cooking Time: 15 minutes Servings: 2

✓ *Preheat oven to 400°F.*

✓ *Arrange rinsed and patted dry fish fillets on foil (coat a foil baking sheet with cooking spray).*

✓ *Sprinkle tilapia fillets with salt and red pepper.*

✓ *Bake 12–15 minutes.*

✓ *Meanwhile, mix leftover ingredients in a saucepan.*

✓ *Cook over medium-high heat until tomatoes are tender.*

✓ *Top fish fillets properly with tomato mixture.*

Nutrition: Calories: 130 Protein: 30g Carbohydrates: 1g

327) *Seared Chicken with Roasted Vegetables*

Ingredients:

- *1 (8-oz) boneless, skinless chicken breasts*
- *¾ lb. small Brussels sprouts*
- *2 large carrots*
- *large red bell pepper*
- *1 small red onion*
- *2 garlic cloves halved*

- *2 tbsp. extra virgin olive oil*
- *½ tsp. dried dill*
- *¼ tsp. pepper*
- *¼ tsp. salt*

Direction: Preparation Time: 20 minutes Cooking Time: 30 minutes Servings: 1

✓ *Preheat oven to 425°F.*

✓ *Match Brussels sprouts cut in half, red onion cut into wedges, sliced carrots, bell pepper cut into pieces, and halved garlic on a baking sheet.*

✓ *Sprinkle with 1 tbsp. oil and with ⅛ tsp. salt and ⅛ tsp. pepper. Bake until well-roasted, cool slightly.*

✓ *In the Meantime, sprinkle chicken with dill, remaining ⅛ tsp. salt and*

✓ *⅛ tsp. pepper. Cook until the chicken is done. Put roasted vegetables with drippings over chicken.*

Nutrition: Calories: 170 Fat: 7g Protein: 12g

328) *Fish Simmered in Tomato-Pepper Sauce*

Ingredients:

- *2 (4-oz) cod fillets*
- *1 big tomato*
- *1/3 cup red peppers (roasted)*
- *3 tbsp. almonds*
- *2 garlic cloves*
- *2 tbsp. fresh basil leaves*
- *2 tbsp. extra virgin olive oil*
- *¼ tsp. salt*
- *⅛ tsp. pepper*

Direction: Preparation Time: 5 minutes Cooking Time: 10 minutes Servings: 2

✓ *Toast sliced almonds in a pan until fragrant.*

✓ *Grind almonds, basil, minced garlic, 1–2 tsp. oil in a food processor until finely ground.*

✓ *Add coarsely-chopped tomato and red peppers; grind until smooth. Season fish with salt and pepper.*

✓ *Cook in hot oil in a large pan over medium-high heat until fish is browned. Pour sauce around fish. Cook 6 minutes more.*

Nutrition: Calories: 90 Fat: 5g Carbohydrates: 7g

329) *Cheese Potato and Pea Casserole*

Ingredients:

- *1tbsp. olive oil*
- *¾ lb. red potatoes*
- *¾ cup green peas*
- *½ cup red onion*

- ¼ tsp. dried rosemary
- ¼ tsp. salt
- ⅛ tsp. pepper

Direction: Preparation Time: 10 minutes Cooking Time: 35 minutes Servings: 3

✓ Prepare oven to 350°F.

✓ Cook 1 tsp. oil in a skillet. Stir in thinly sliced onions and cook. Remove from pan.

✓ Situate half of the thinly sliced potatoes and onions in the bottom of the skillet; top with peas, crushed dried rosemary, and ⅛ tsp. Each salt and pepper. Place remaining potatoes and onions on top. Season with remaining ⅛ tsp. salt.

✓ Bake 35 minutes, pour the remaining 2 tsp. oil and sprinkle with cheese.

Nutrition: Calories: 80 Protein: 2g Carbs: 18g

330) Oven-Fried Tilapia

Ingredients:

- 2 (4-oz) tilapia fillets
- ¼ cup yellow cornmeal
- 2 tbsp. light ranch dressing
- 1 tbsp. canola oil
- 1 tsp. dill (dried)
- ⅛ tsp. salt

Direction: Preparation Time: 7 minutes Cooking Time: 15 minutes Servings: 2

✓ Preheat oven to 425°F. Brush both sides of rinsed and patted dry tilapia fish fillets with dressing.

✓ Combine cornmeal, oil, dill, and salt. Sprinkle fish fillets with cornmeal mixture.

✓ Put fish on a prepared baking sheet.

✓ Bake 15 minutes.

Nutrition: Calories: 96 Protein: 21g Fat: 2g

331) Chicken with Coconut Sauce

Ingredients:

- ½ lb. chicken breasts
- ⅓ cup red onion
- 1 tbsp. paprika (smoked)
- 2 tsp. cornstarch
- ½ cup light coconut milk
- 1 tsp. extra virgin olive oil
- l 2 tbsp. fresh cilantro
- 1(10-oz) can tomatoes and green chilis
- ¼ cup water

Direction: Preparation Time: 15 minutes Cooking Time: 20 minutes Servings: 2

✓ Cut chicken into little cubes; sprinkle with 1 ½ tsp. paprika.

✓ Heat oil, add chicken, and cook for 3 to 5 minutes.

✓ Remove from skillet, and fry the finely-chopped onion for 5 minutes.

✓ Return chicken to pan. Add tomatoes, 1 ½ tsp. paprika, and water. Bring to a boil, and then simmer for 4 minutes.

✓ Mix cornstarch and coconut milk; stir into the chicken mixture, and cook until it has done.

✓ Sprinkle with chopped cilantro.

Nutrition: Calories: 200 Protein: 10g Fat: 13g

332) Fish with Fresh Herb Sauce

Ingredients:

- 2 (4-oz) cod fillets
- ¹/3 cup fresh cilantro
- ¼ tsp. cumin
- 1tbsp. red onion
- tsp. extra virgin olive oil
- 1 tsp. red wine vinegar
- 1 small garlic clove
- ⅛ tsp. salt
- ⅛ black pepper

Direction: Preparation Time: 10 minutes Cooking Time: 10 minutes Servings: 2

✓ Combine chopped cilantro, finely chopped onion, oil, red wine vinegar, minced garlic, and salt.

✓ Sprinkle both sides of fish fillets with cumin and pepper.

✓ Cook fillets 4 minutes per side. Top each fillet with the cilantro mixture.

Nutrition: Calories: 90 Fat: 4g Carbohydrates: 2g

333) Skillet Turkey Patties

Ingredients:

- ½ lb. lean ground turkey
- ½ cup low-sodium chicken broth
- ¼ cup red onion
- ½ tsp. Worcestershire sauce
  1 tsp. extra virgin olive oil
- ¼ tsp. oregano (dried)
- ⅛ tsp. pepper

Direction: Preparation Time: 7 minutes Cooking Time: 8 minutes Servings: 2

✓ Combine turkey, chopped onion, Worcestershire sauce, dried oregano, and pepper; make 2 patties. Warm-up the oil and cook patties 4 minutes per side; set aside.

✓ *Add broth to skillet, bring to a boil. Boil 2 minutes, spoon sauce over patties.*

Nutrition: Calories: 180 Fat: 11g Carbohydrates: 9g

334) Turkey Loaf

Ingredients:

- *½ lb. 93% lean ground turkey*
- *1/3 cup panko breadcrumbs*
- *½ cup green onion*
- *1 egg*
- *½ cup green bell pepper*
- *1 tbsp. ketchup*
- *¼ cup sauce (spicy sauce)*
- *½ tsp. cumin, grounded*

Direction: Preparation Time: 10 minutes Cooking Time: 50 minutes Servings: 2

✓ *Preheat oven to 350°F. Mix lean ground turkey, 3 tbsp. Picante sauce, panko breadcrumbs, egg, chopped green onion, chopped green bell pepper, and cumin in a bowl (mix well);*

✓ *Put the mixture into a baking sheet; shape into an oval (about 1 ½ inches thick). Bake 45 minutes.*

✓ *Mix remaining Picante sauce and the ketchup; apply over the loaf. Bake 5 minutes longer. Let stand 5 minutes.*

Nutrition: Calories: 161 Protein: 20g Fat: 8g

335) Mushroom Pasta

Ingredients:

- *4 oz. wholegrain linguine*
- *1 tsp. extra virgin olive oil*
- *½ cup light sauce*
- *2 tbsp. green onion*
- *1 (8-oz) pkg mushrooms*
- *1 garlic clove*
- *⅛ tsp. salt*
- *⅛ tsp. pepper*

Direction: Preparation Time: 7 minutes Cooking Time: 10 minutes Servings: 4

✓ *Cook pasta according to package directions, drain.*

✓ *Fry sliced mushrooms for 4 minutes.*
Stir in fettuccine minced garlic, salt, and pepper. Cook 2 minutes.

✓ *Heat light sauce until heated; top pasta mixture properly with sauce and with finely-chopped green onion.*

Nutrition: Calories: 300 Fat: 1g Carbohydrates: 15g

336) Chicken Tikka Masala

Ingredients:

- *½ lb. chicken breasts*
- *¼ cup onion*
- *1 ½ tsp. extra virgin olive oil*
- *1 (14.5-oz) can tomatoes*
- *1 tsp. ginger*
- *1 tsp. fresh lemon juice*
- *1/3 cup plain Greek yogurt (fat-free)*
- *1 tbsp. garam masala*
- *¼ tsp. salt*
- *¼ tsp. pepper*

Direction: Preparation Time: 5 minutes Cooking Time: 15 minutes Servings: 2

✓ *Flavor chicken cut into 1-inch cubes with 1 ½ tsp. garam masala, ⅛ tsp. salt and pepper.*

✓ *Cook chicken and diced onion for 4 to 5 minutes. Add diced tomatoes, grated ginger, 1 ½ tsp. garam masala, ⅛ tsp. salt. Cook 8 to 10 minutes.*

✓ *Add lemon juice and yogurt until blended.*

Nutrition: Calories: 200 Protein: 26g Fat: 10g

337) Tomato and Roasted Cod

Ingredients:

- *2(4-oz) cod fillets*
- *cup cherry tomatoes*
- *2/3 cup onion*
- *tsp. orange rind*
- *1 tbsp. extra virgin olive oil*
- *1 tsp. thyme (dried)*
- *¼ tsp. salt, divided*
- *¼ tsp. pepper, divided*

Direction: Preparation Time: 10 minutes Cooking Time: 35 minutes Servings: 2

✓ *Preheat oven to 400°F. Mix in half tomatoes, sliced onion, grated orange rind, extra virgin olive oil, dried thyme, and ⅛ salt and pepper. Fry for 25 minutes. Remove from oven.*
Arrange fish on pan, and flavor with remaining ⅛ tsp. each salt and pepper. Put reserved tomato mixture over fish. Bake 10 minutes.

Nutrition: Calories: 120 Protein: 9g Fat: 2g

338) Ravioli

Ingredients:

- *8 oz. frozen vegan ravioli, thawed*
- *1 tsp. dried basil*

- 1 tsp. garlic powder
- ⅛ tsp. ground black pepper
- ¼ tsp. salt
- 1 tsp. dried oregano
- 2 tsp. nutritional yeast flakes
- ½ cup marinara sauce, unsweetened
- ½ cup panko bread crumbs
- ¼ cup liquid from chickpeas can

Direction: Preparation Time: 5 minutes Cooking Time: 16 minutes Servings: 4

✓ Place breadcrumbs in a bowl, sprinkle with salt, basil, oregano, and black pepper, add garlic powder and yeast and stir until mixed.

✓ Take a bowl and then pour in chickpeas liquid in it.

✓ Working on 1 ravioli at a time, first dip a ravioli in chickpeas liquid and then coat with breadcrumbs mixture.

✓ Prepare remaining ravioli in the same manner, then take a fryer basket, grease it well with oil, and place ravioli in it in a single layer.

✓ Switch on the air fryer, insert fryer basket, sprinkle oil on ravioli, shut with its lid, set the fryer at 390°F, then cook for 6 minutes, turn the ravioli and continue cooking 2 minutes until nicely golden and heated thoroughly.

✓ Cook the remaining ravioli in the same manner and serve with marinara sauce.

Nutrition: Calories: 150 Fat: 3g Protein: 5g

339) Onion Rings

Ingredients:

- 1 large white onion, peeled
- 2/3 cup pork rinds
- 3 tbsp. almond flour
- ½ tsp. garlic powder
- ½ tsp. paprika
- ¼ tsp. sea salt
- 3 tbsp. coconut flour
- 2 eggs, pastured

Direction: Preparation Time: 10 minutes Cooking Time: 32 minutes Servings: 4

✓ Switch on the air fryer, insert fryer basket, grease it with olive oil, then shut with its lid, set the fryer at 400°F, and preheat for 10 minutes.

✓ Meanwhile, slice the peeled onion into ½ inch thick rings.

✓ Take a shallow dish, add almond flour and stir in garlic powder, paprika, and pork rinds; take another shallow dish, add coconut flour and salt and stir until mixed.

✓ Crack eggs in a bowl and then whisk until combined.

Working on 1 onion ring at a time, first coat onion ring in coconut flour mixture, then it in egg, and coat with pork rind mixture by scooping over the onion until evenly coated.

✓ Open the fryer, place coated onion rings in it in a single layer, spray oil over onion rings, close with its lid, and cook for 16 minutes until nicely golden and thoroughly cooked, flipping the onion rings halfway through the frying.

✓ When the air fryer beeps, open its lid, transfer onion rings onto a serving plate and cook the remaining onion rings in the same manner. Serve straight away.

Nutrition: Calories: 135 Fat: 7g Protein: 8g

340) Cauliflower Fritters

Ingredients:

- 5 cups chopped cauliflower florets
- ½ cup almond flour
- ½ tsp. baking powder
- ½ tsp. ground black pepper
- ½ tsp. salt
- 2 eggs, pastured

Direction: Preparation Time: 10 minutes Cooking Time: 14 minutes Servings: 2

✓ Add chopped cauliflower in a blender or food processor, pulse until minced, and then tip the mixture in a bowl.

✓ Add remaining ingredients, stir well and then shape the mixture into ¹/₃-inch patties, an ice cream scoop of mixture per patty.

✓ Switch on the air fryer, insert fryer basket, grease it with olive oil, then shut with its lid, set the fryer at 390°F and preheat for 5 minutes.

✓ Then open the fryer, add cauliflower patties in it in a single layer, spray oil over patties, close with its lid and cook for 14 minutes at 375°F until nicely golden and cooked, flipping the patties halfway through the frying.

✓ Serve straight away with the dip.

Nutrition: Calories: 272 Fat: 0.3g Protein: 11g

341) Zucchini Fritters

Ingredients:

- 2 medium zucchinis, ends trimmed
- 3 tbsp. almond flour
- 1 tbsp. salt
- 1 tsp. garlic powder
- ¼ tsp. paprika
- ¼ tsp. ground black pepper
- ¼ tsp. onion powder 1 egg, pastured

Direction: Preparation Time: 20 minutes Cooking Time: 12 minutes Servings: 4

✓ *Wash and pat dry the zucchini, then cut its ends and grate the zucchini.*

✓ *Place grated zucchini in a colander, sprinkle with salt and let it rest for 10 minutes.*

✓ *Then wrap zucchini in a kitchen cloth and squeeze moisture from it as much as possible and place dried zucchini in another bowl.*

✓ *Add remaining ingredients into the zucchini and then stir until mixed.*

✓ *Take fryer basket, line it with parchment paper, grease it with oil, and drop zucchini mixture on it by a spoonful, about 1-inch apart and then spray well with oil.*

✓ *Switch on the air fryer, insert fryer basket, then shut with its lid, set the fryer at 360ºF, and cook the fritter for 12 minutes until nicely golden and cooked, flipping the fritters halfway through the frying.*

✓ *Serve straight away.*

Nutrition: Calories: 57 Protein: 1g Fat: 3g

342) *Air-Fried Kale Chips*

Ingredients:

- *1 large bunch of kale*
- *¾ tsp. red chili powder*
- *1 tsp. salt*
- *¾ tsp. ground black pepper*

Direction: Preparation Time: 5 minutes Cooking Time: 7 minutes Servings: 2

✓ *Remove the hard spines from the kale leaves, then cut kale into small pieces and place them in a fryer basket.*

✓ *Spray oil over kale, then sprinkle with salt, chili powder, and black pepper and toss until well mixed.*

✓ *Switch on the air fryer, insert fryer basket, then shut with its lid, set the fryer at 375ºF, and cook for 7 minutes until kale is crispy, shaking halfway through the frying.*

✓ *When the air fryer beeps, open its lid, transfer kale chips onto a serving plate and serve.*

Nutrition: Calories: 66.2 Fat: 4g Protein: 2.5g

343) *Radish Chips*

Ingredients:

- *8 oz. radish slices*
- *½ tsp. garlic powder*
- *1 tsp. salt*
- *½ tsp. onion powder*

- *½ tsp. ground black pepper*

Direction: Preparation Time: 5 minutes Cooking Time: 20 minutes Servings: 2

✓ *Wash the radish slices, pat them dry, place them in a fryer basket, and then spray oil on them until well coated.*

✓ *Sprinkle salt, garlic powder, onion powder, and black pepper over radish slices and then toss until well coated.*

✓ *Switch on the air fryer, insert fryer basket, then shut with its lid, set the fryer at 370ºF, and cook for 10 minutes, stirring the slices halfway through.*

✓ *Then spray oil on radish slices, shake the basket and continue frying for 10 minutes, stirring the chips halfway through.*

✓ *Serve straight away.*

Nutrition: Calories: 21 Protein: 0.2g Fat: 1.8g

344) *Avocado Fries*

Ingredients:

- *1 medium avocado, pitted*
- *1 egg*
- *½ cup almond flour*
- *¼ tsp. salt*
- *¼ tsp. ground black pepper*
- *½ tsp. salt*

Direction: Preparation Time: 10 minutes Cooking Time: 20 minutes Servings: 2

✓ *Switch on the air fryer, insert fryer basket, grease it with olive oil, then shut with its lid, set the fryer at 400ºF and preheat for 10 minutes.*

✓ *Meanwhile, cut the avocado in half and then cut each half into wedges, each about ½-inch thick.*

✓ *Place flour in a shallow dish, add salt and black pepper, and stir until mixed.*

✓ *Crack the egg in a bowl and then whisk until blended.*
  Working on 1 avocado piece at a time, first dip it in the egg, then coat it in the almond flour mixture and place it on a wire rack.

✓ *Open the fryer, add avocado pieces to it in a single layer, spray oil over avocado, close with its lid and cook for 10 minutes until nicely golden and crispy, shaking halfway through the frying.*

✓ *When the air fryer beeps, open its lid, transfer avocado fries onto a serving plate and serve.*

Nutrition: Calories: 251 Fat: 17g Protein: 6g

345) *Roasted Peanut Butter Squash*

Ingredients:

- *1 butternut squash, peeled*

- 1 tsp. cinnamon
- 1 tbsp. olive oil

Direction: Preparation Time: 5 minutes Cooking Time: 22 minutes Servings: 4

✓ Switch on the air fryer, insert fryer basket, grease it with olive oil, then shut with its lid, set the fryer at 220°F, and preheat for 5 minutes.

✓ Meanwhile, peel the squash cut it into 1-inch pieces, and then place them in a bowl.

✓ Drizzle oil over squash pieces, sprinkle with cinnamon, and then toss until well coated.

✓ Open the fryer, add squash pieces in it, close with its lid and cook for 17 minutes until nicely golden and crispy, shaking every 5 minutes.

✓ When the air fryer beeps, open its lid, transfer squash onto a serving plate and serve.

Nutrition: Calories: 116 Fat: 3g Protein: 1g

346)   *Cabbage Wedges*

Ingredients:

- 1 small head of green cabbage
- 6 bacon strips, thick-cut, pastured
- 1 tsp. onion powder
- ½ tsp. ground black pepper
- 1 tsp. garlic powder
- ¾ tsp. salt
- ¼ tsp. red chili flakes
- ½ tsp. fennel seeds
- 3 tbsp. olive oil

Direction: Preparation Time: 10 minutes Cooking Time: 29 minutes Servings: 6

✓ Switch on the air fryer, insert the fryer basket, grease it with olive oil, then shut with its lid, set the fryer at 350°F and preheat for 5 minutes.

✓ Open the fryer, add bacon strips in it, close with its lid and cook for 10 minutes until nicely golden and crispy, turning the bacon halfway through the frying.

✓ Meanwhile, prepare the cabbage and for this, remove the outer leaves of the cabbage and then cut it into eight wedges, keeping the core intact.

✓ Prepare the spice mix and for this, place onion powder in a bowl, add black pepper, garlic powder, salt, red chili, and fennel and stir until mixed.

✓ Drizzle cabbage wedges with oil and then sprinkle with spice mix until well coated.
When the air fryer beeps, open its lid, transfer bacon strips to a cutting board and let it rest.

✓ Add seasoned cabbage wedges into the fryer basket, close with its lid, then cook for 8 minutes at 400°F, flip the cabbage, spray with oil and continue air frying for 6 minutes until nicely golden

and cooked.

✓ When done, transfer cabbage wedges to a plate.

✓ Chop the bacon, sprinkle it over cabbage and serve.

Nutrition: Calories: 123 Fat: 11g Protein: 4g

347)   *Buffalo Cauliflower Wings*

Ingredients:

- 1 tbsp. almond flour
- 1 medium head of cauliflower
- 1 ½ tsp. salt
- 4 tbsp. hot sauce
- 1 tbsp. olive oil

Direction: Preparation Time: 5 minutes Cooking Time: 30 minutes Servings: 6

✓ Switch on the air fryer, insert fryer basket, grease it with olive oil, then shut with its lid, set the fryer at 400°F, and preheat for 5 minutes.

✓ Meanwhile, cut cauliflower into bite-size florets and set aside.

✓ Place flour in a large bowl, whisk in salt, oil, and hot sauce until combined, add cauliflower florets and toss until combined.

✓ Open the fryer, add cauliflower florets in it in a single layer, close with its lid and cook for 15 minutes until nicely golden and crispy, shaking halfway through the frying.

✓ When the air fryer beeps, open its lid, transfer cauliflower florets onto a serving plate and keep warm.

✓ Cook the remaining cauliflower florets in the same manner and serve.

Nutrition: Calories: 48 Fat: 4g Protein: 1g

348)   *Sweet Potato Cauliflower Patties*

Ingredients:

- 1 green onion, chopped
- 1 large sweet potato, peeled
- 1 tsp. minced garlic
- 1 cup cilantro leaves
- 2 cup cauliflower florets
- ¼ tsp. ground black pepper
- ¼ tsp. salt
- ¼ cup sunflower seeds
- ¼ tsp. cumin
- ¼ cup ground flaxseed
- ½ tsp. red chili powder
- 2 tbsp. ranch seasoning mix
- 2 tbsp. arrowroot starch

Direction: Preparation Time: 20 minutes Cooking

Time: 40 minutes Servings: 7

✓ *Cut peeled sweet potato into small pieces, then place them in a food processor and pulse until pieces are broken up.*

✓ *Then add onion, cauliflower florets, and garlic, pulse until combined, add remaining ingredients and pulse more until incorporated.*

✓ *Tip the mixture in a bowl, shape the mixture into seven 1 ½ inch thick patties, each about ¼ cup, then place them on a baking sheet and freeze for 10 minutes.*

✓ *Switch on the air fryer, insert fryer basket, grease it with olive oil, then shut with its lid.*
Set the fryer at 400°F and preheat for 10 minutes.

✓ *Open the fryer, add patties to it in a single layer, close with its lid and cook for 20 minutes until nicely golden and cooked, flipping the patties halfway through the frying.*

✓ *When the air fryer beeps, open its lid, transfer patties onto a serving plate, and keep them warm.*

✓ *Cook the remaining patties in the same manner and serve.*

Nutrition: Calories: 88 Fat: 4.4g Protein: 3.9g

349) *Okra*

Ingredients:

- *1 cup almond flour*
- *8 oz. fresh okra*
- *½ tsp. sea salt*
- *1 cup milk, reduced-fat*
- *1 egg, pastured*

Direction: Preparation Time: 10 minutes Cooking Time: 10 minutes Servings: 4

✓ *Crack the egg in a bowl, pour in the milk, and whisk until blended.*

✓ *Cut the stem from each okra, then cut it into ½-inch pieces, add them into the egg mixture and stir until well coated.*

✓ *Mix flour and salt and add it into a large plastic bag.*

✓ *Working on 1 okra piece at a time, drain the okra well by letting excess egg drip off, add it to the flour mixture, then seal the bag and shake well until okra is well coated.*
Place the coated okra on a grease air fryer basket, coat the remaining okra pieces in the same manner, and place them into the basket.

✓ *Switch on the air fryer, insert fryer basket, spray okra with oil, then shut with its lid, set the fryer at 390°F, and cook for 10 minutes until nicely golden and cooked, stirring okra halfway through the frying.*

✓ *Serve straight away.*

Nutrition: Calories: 250 Fat: 9g Protein: 3g

350) *Air-Fried Brussels Sprouts*

Ingredients:

- *2 cups Brussels sprouts*
- *¼ tsp. sea salt*
- *1 tbsp. olive oil*
- *1 tbsp. apple cider vinegar*

Direction: Preparation Time: 5 minutes Cooking Time: 10 minutes Servings: 2

✓ *Switch on the air fryer, insert the fryer basket, grease it with olive oil, then shut with its lid, set the fryer at 400°F, and preheat for 5 minutes.*

✓ *Meanwhile, cut the sprouts lengthwise into ¼-inch thick pieces, add them to a bowl, add remaining ingredients and toss until well coated.*
Open the fryer, add sprouts to it, close with its lid and cook for 10 minutes until crispy and cooked, shaking halfway through the frying.

✓ *When the air fryer beeps, open its lid, transfer sprouts onto a serving plate, and serve.*

Nutrition: Calories: 88 Fat: 4.4g Protein: 3.9g

351) *Asparagus Avocado Soup*

Ingredients:

- *1 avocado, peeled, pitted, cubed*
- *12 oz. Asparagus*
- *½ tsp. ground black pepper*
- *1 tsp. garlic powder*
- *tsp. sea salt*
- *tbsp. olive oil, divided*
- *½ lemon juice*
- *2 cups vegetable stock*

Direction: Preparation Time: 10 minutes Cooking Time: 20 minutes Servings: 4

✓ *Switch on the air fryer, insert fryer basket, grease it with olive oil, then shut with its lid, set the fryer at 425°F and preheat for 5 minutes.*

✓ *Meanwhile, place asparagus in a shallow dish, drizzle with 1 tbsp. oil, sprinkle with garlic powder, salt, and black pepper, and toss until well mixed.*

✓ *Open the fryer, add asparagus to it, close with its lid and cook for 10 minutes until nicely golden and roasted, shaking halfway through the frying.*
When the air fryer beeps, open its lid and transfer asparagus to a food processor.

✓ *Add remaining ingredients into a food processor and pulse until well combined and smooth.*

✓ *Tip the soup in a saucepan, pour in water if the soup is too thick, and heat it over medium-low heat for 5 minutes until thoroughly heated.*

✓ *Ladle soup into bowls and serve.*

Nutrition: Calories: 208 Fat: 16g Protein: 6g

352) *Broccoli Salad*

Ingredients:

- *8 cups broccoli florets*
- *3 strips of bacon, cooked and crumbled*
- *¼ cup sunflower kernels*
- *1 bunch of green onion, sliced*

What you will need from the store cupboard:

- *3 tablespoons seasoned rice vinegar*
- *3 tablespoons canola oil*
- *1/2 cup dried cranberries*

Direction: Preparation Time: 10 minutes, Cooking Time: 10 minutes; Servings: 10

- ✓ *Combine the green onion, cranberries, and broccoli in a bowl.*
- ✓ *Whisk the vinegar, and oil in another bowl. Blend well.*
- ✓ *Now drizzle over the broccoli mix. Coat well by tossing.*
- ✓ *Sprinkle bacon and sunflower kernels before serving.*

Nutrition: Calories 121, Carbs 14g, Cholesterol 2mg, Fiber 3g, Sugar 1g, Fat 7g, Protein 3g, Sodium 233mg

353) *Tenderloin Grilled Salad*

Ingredients:

- *1 lb. pork tenderloin*
- *10 cups mixed salad greens*
- *2 oranges, seedless, cut into bite-sized pieces*
- *1 tablespoon orange zest, grated*

What you will need from the store cupboard:

- *2 tablespoons of cider vinegar*
- *2 tablespoons olive oil*
- *2 teaspoons Dijon mustard*
- *1/2 cup juice of an orange*
- *2 teaspoons honey*
- *1/2 teaspoon ground pepper*

Direction: Preparation Time: 25-30 minutes, minutes; Servings: 2-4

- ✓ *Bring together all the dressing ingredients in a bowl.*
- ✓ *Grill each side of the pork covered over medium heat for 9 minutes.*
- ✓ *Slice after 5 minutes.*
- ✓ *Slice the tenderloin thinly.*
- ✓ *Keep the greens on your serving plate.*
- ✓ *Top with the pork and oranges.*
- ✓ *Sprinkle nuts (optional).*

Nutrition: Calories 211, Carbs 13g, Cholesterol 51mg,

Fiber 3g, Sugar 0.8g, Fat 9g, Protein 20g, Sodium 113mg

354) *Barley Veggie Salad*

Ingredients:

- *1 tomato, seeded and chopped*
- *2 tablespoons parsley, minced*
- *1 yellow pepper, chopped*
- *1 tablespoon basil, minced*
- *¼ cup almonds, toasted*

What you will need from the store cupboard:

- *1-1/4 cups vegetable broth*
- *1 cup barley*
- *1 tablespoon lemon juice*
- *2 tablespoons of white wine vinegar*
- *3 tablespoons olive oil*
- *¼ teaspoon pepper*
- *1/2 teaspoon salt*
- *1 cup of water*

Direction: Preparation Time: 10 minutes, minutes; Servings: 6

- ✓ *Boil the broth, barley, and water in a saucepan.*
- ✓ *Reduce heat. Cover and let it simmer for 10 minutes.*
- ✓ *Take out from the heat.*
- ✓ *In the meantime, bring together the parsley, yellow pepper, and tomato in a bowl. Stir the barley in.*
- ✓ *Whisk the vinegar, oil, basil, lemon juice, water, pepper and salt in a bowl.*
- ✓ *Pour this over your barley mix. Toss to coat well.*
- ✓ *Stir the almonds in before serving.*

Nutrition: Calories 211, Carbs 27g, Cholesterol 0mg, Fiber 7g, Sugar 0g, Fat 10g, Protein 6g, Sodium 334mg

355) *Spinach Shrimp Salad*

Ingredients:

- *1 lb. uncooked shrimp, peeled and deveined*
- *2 tablespoons parsley, minced*
- *¾ cup halved cherry tomatoes*
- *1 medium lemon*
- *4 cups baby spinach*

What you will need from the store cupboard:

- *2 tablespoons butter*
- *3 minced garlic cloves*
- *¼ teaspoon pepper*
- *¼ teaspoon salt*

Direction: Preparation Time: 15-20 minutes;

Servings: 2-3

✓ Melt the butter over the medium temperature in a nonstick skillet.

✓ Add the shrimp.

✓ Now cook the shrimp for 3 minutes until your shrimp becomes pink.

✓ Add the parsley and garlic.

✓ Cook for another minute. Take out from the heat. Keep the spinach in your salad bowl.

✓ Top with the shrimp mix and tomatoes.

✓ Drizzle lemon juice on the salad.

✓ Sprinkle pepper and salt.

Nutrition: Calories 201, Carbs 6g, Cholesterol 153mg, Fiber 2g, Sugar 0g, Fat 10g, Protein 21g, Sodium 350mg

356) *Sweet Potato and Roasted Beet Salad*

Ingredients:

- 2 beets
- 1 sweet potato, peeled and cubed
- 1 garlic clove, minced
- 2 tablespoons walnuts, chopped and toasted
- 1 cup fennel bulb, sliced

What you will need from the store cupboard:

- 3 tablespoons balsamic vinegar
- 1 teaspoon Dijon mustard
- 1 tablespoon honey
- 3 tablespoons olive oil
- ¼ teaspoon pepper
- ¼ teaspoon salt
- 3 tablespoons water

Direction: Preparation Time: 15 minutes, Servings: 2-3

✓ Scrub the beets. Trim the tops to 1 inch.

✓ Wrap in foil and keep on a baking sheet.

✓ Bake until tender. Take off the foil.

✓ Combine water and sweet potato in a bowl.

✓ Cover. Microwave for 5 minutes. Drain off.

✓ Now peel the beets. Cut into small wedges. Arrange the fennel, sweet potato and beets on 4 salad plates.

✓ Sprinkle nuts.

✓ Whisk the honey, mustard, vinegar, water, garlic, pepper and salt.

✓ Whisk in oil gradually.

✓ Drizzle over the salad.

Nutrition: Calories 270, Carbs 37g, Cholesterol 0mg, Fiber 6g, Sugar 0.3g, Fat 13g, Protein 5g, Sodium 309mg

357) *Potato Calico Salad*

Ingredients:

- 4 red potatoes, peeled and cooked
- 1-1/2 cups kernel corn, cooked
- 1/2 cup green pepper, diced
- 1/2 cup red onion, chopped
- 1 cup carrot, shredded

What you will need from the store cupboard:

- 1/2 cup olive oil
- ¼ cup vinegar
- 1-1/2 teaspoons chili powder
- 1 teaspoon salt
- Dash of hot pepper sauce

Direction: Preparation Time: 15 minutes, Cooking Time: 5 minutes; Servings: 14

✓ Keep all the ingredients together in a jar.

✓ Close it and shake well.

✓ Cube the potatoes. Combine with the carrot, onion, and corn in your salad bowl.
Pour the dressing over.

✓ Now toss lightly.

Nutrition: Calories 146, Carbs 17g, Cholesterol 0mg, Fiber 0g, Sugar 0g, Fat 9g, Protein 2g, Sodium 212mg

358) *Mango and Jicama Salad*

Ingredients:

- 1 jicama, peeled
- 1 mango, peeled
- 1 teaspoon ginger root, minced
- 1/3 cup chives, minced
- 1/2 cup cilantro, chopped

What you will need from the store cupboard:

- ¼ cup canola oil
- 1/2 cup white wine vinegar
- 2 tablespoons of lime juice
- ¼ cup honey
- 1/8 teaspoon pepper
- ¼ teaspoon salt

Direction: Preparation Time: 15 minutes, Cooking Time: 5 minutes; Servings: 8

✓ Whisk together the vinegar, honey, canola oil, gingerroot, paper, and salt.

✓ Cut the mango and jicama into matchsticks.

✓ Keep in a bowl.
Now toss with the lime juice.

✓ Add the dressing and herbs. Combine well by

tossing.

Nutrition: Calories 143, Carbs 20g, Cholesterol 0mg, Fiber 3g, Sugar 1.6g, Fat 7g, Protein 1g, Sodium 78mg

359)   Asian Crispy Chicken Salad

Ingredients:

- *2 chicken breast halved, skinless*
- *1/2 cup panko bread crumbs*
- *4 cups spring mix salad greens*
- *4 teaspoons of sesame seeds*
- *1/2 cup mushrooms, sliced*

What you will need from the store cupboard:

- *1 teaspoon sesame oil*
- *2 teaspoons of canola oil*
- *2 teaspoons hoisin sauce*
- *¼ cup sesame ginger salad dressing*

Direction: Preparation Time: 12 minutes, Cooking Time: 10 minutes; Servings: 2

- ✓ *Flatten the chicken breasts to half-inch thickness.*
- ✓ *Mix the sesame oil and hoisin sauce. Brush over the chicken.*
- ✓ *Combine the sesame seeds and panko in a bowl.*
- ✓ *Now dip the chicken mix in it.*
  Cook each side of the chicken for 5 minutes.
- ✓ *In the meantime, divide the salad greens between two plates.*
- ✓ *Top with mushroom.*
- ✓ *Slice the chicken and keep on top. Drizzle the dressing.*

Nutrition: Calories 386, Carbs 29g, Cholesterol 63mg, Fiber 6g, Sugar 1g, Fat 17g, Protein 30g, Sodium 620mg

360)   Kale, Grape and Bulgur Salad

Ingredients:

- *1 cup bulgur*
- *1 cup pecan, toasted and chopped*
- *¼ cup scallions, sliced*
- *1/2 cup parsley, chopped*
- *2 cups California grapes, seedless and halved*

What you will need from the store cupboard:

- *2 tablespoons of extra virgin olive oil*
- *¼ cup of juice from a lemon*
- *Pinch of kosher salt*
- *Pinch of black pepper*
- *2 cups of water*

Direction: Preparation Time: 12 minutes, Cooking Time: 14 minutes; Servings: 2

- ✓ *Boil 2 cups of water in a saucepan*
- ✓ *Stir the bulgur in and 1/2 teaspoon of salt.*
- ✓ *Take out from the heat.*
- ✓ *Keep covered. Drain.*
  Stir in the other ingredients.
- ✓ *Season with pepper and salt.*

Nutrition: Calories 289, Carbs 33g, Fat 17g, Protein 6g,

361)   Strawberry Salsa

Ingredients:

- *4 tomatoes, seeded and chopped*
- *1-pint strawberry, chopped*
- *1 red onion, chopped*
- *2 tablespoons of juice from a lime*

What you will need from the store cupboard:

- *1 tablespoon olive oil*
- *2 garlic cloves, minced*
- *1 jalapeno pepper, minced*

Direction: Preparation Time: 15 minutes, Cooking Time: 14 minutes; Servings: 2

- ✓ *Bring together the strawberries, tomatoes, jalapeno, and onion in the bowl.*
- ✓ *Stir in the garlic, oil, and lime juice. Refrigerate. Serve with separately cooked pork or poultry.*

Nutrition: Calories 19, Carbs 3g, Fiber 1g, Sugar 0.2g, Cholesterol 0mg, Total Fat 1g

362)   Garden Wraps

Ingredients:

- *1 cucumber, chopped*
- *1 sweet corn*
- *1 cabbage, shredded*
- *1 tablespoon lettuce, minced*
- *1 tomato, chopped*
- *2 teaspoons of low-sodium soy sauce*

What you will need from the store cupboard:

- *3 tablespoons of rice vinegar*
- *2 teaspoons peanut butter*
- *1/3 cup onion paste*
- *1/3 cup chili sauce*

Direction: Preparation Time: 20 minutes, Cooking Time: 10 minutes; Servings: 8

- ✓ *Cut corn from the cob. Keep in a bowl.*
- ✓ *Add the tomato, cabbage, cucumber, and onion paste.*
- ✓ *Now whisk the vinegar, peanut butter, and chili*

sauce together.
- ✓ Pour this over the vegetable mix. Toss for coating. Let this stand for 10 minutes.
- ✓ Take your slotted spoon and place 1/2 cup salad in every lettuce leaf.
- ✓ Fold the lettuce over your filling.

Nutrition: Calories 64, Carbs 13g, Fiber 2g, Sugar 1g, Cholesterol 0mg, Total Fat 1g, Protein 2g

363) *Party Shrimp*

Ingredients:

- 16 oz. uncooked shrimp, peeled and deveined
- 1-1/2 teaspoons of juice from a lemon
- 1/2 teaspoon basil, chopped
- 1 teaspoon coriander, chopped
- 1/2 cup tomato

What you will need from the store cupboard:
- 1 tablespoon of olive oil
- 1/2 teaspoon Italian seasoning
- 1/2 teaspoon paprika
- 1 sliced garlic clove
- ¼ teaspoon pepper

Direction: Preparation Time: 15 minutes, Cooking Time: 10 minutes; Servings: 30

- ✓ Bring together everything except the shrimp in a dish or bowl.
- ✓ Add the shrimp. Coat well by tossing. Set aside.
- ✓ Drain the shrimp. Discard the marinade. Keep them on a baking sheet. It should not be greased.
- ✓ Broil each side for 4 minutes. The shrimp should become pink.

Nutrition: Calories 14, Carbs 0g, Fiber 0g, Sugar 0g, Cholesterol 18mg, Total Fat 0g, Protein 2g

364) *Zucchini Mini Pizzas*

Ingredients:

- 1 zucchini, cut into ¼ inch slices diagonally
- 1/2 cup pepperoni, small slices
- 1 teaspoon basil, minced
- 1/2 cup onion, chopped
- 1 cup tomatoes

What you will need from the store cupboard:
- 1/8 teaspoon pepper
- 1/8 teaspoon salt
- 3/4 cup mozzarella cheese, shredded
- 1/3 cup pizza sauce

Direction: Preparation Time: 24 mins Servings: 2

- ✓ Preheat your broiler. Keep the zucchini in 1 layer on your greased baking sheet.
- ✓ Add the onion and tomatoes. Broil each side for 1 to 2 minutes till they become tender and crisp.
- ✓ Now sprinkle pepper and salt. Top with cheese, pepperoni, and sauce.
- ✓ Broil for a minute. The cheese should melt.
- ✓ Sprinkle basil on top.

Nutrition: Calories 29, Carbs 1g, Fiber 0g, Sugar 1g, Cholesterol 5mg, Total Fat 2g, Protein 2g

365) *Garlic-Sesame Pumpkin Seeds*

Ingredients:

- 1 egg white
- 1 teaspoon onion, minced
- 1/2 teaspoon caraway seeds
- 2 cups pumpkin seeds
- 1 teaspoon sesame seeds

What you will need from the store cupboard:
- 1 garlic clove, minced
- 1 tablespoon of canola oil
- ¾ teaspoon of kosher salt

Direction: Preparation Time: 10 minutesCooking Time: 20 minutes Servings: 2

- ✓ Preheat your oven to 350 °F .
- ✓ Whisk together the oil and egg white in a bowl.
- ✓ Include pumpkin seeds. Coat well by tossing.
- ✓ Now stir in the onion, garlic, sesame seeds, caraway seeds, and salt
Spread in 1 layer in your parchment-lined baking pan.
- ✓ Bake for 15 minutes until it turns golden brown.

Nutrition: Calories 95, Carbs 9g, Fiber 3g, Sugar 0g, Cholesterol 0mg, Total Fat 5g, Protein 4g

366) *Tuna Salad Recipe 2*

Ingredients:

- 2 (5-ounce) cans water-packed tuna, drained
- 2 tablespoons fat-free plain Greek yogurt
- Salt and ground black pepper, as required
- 2 medium carrots, peeled and shredded
- 2 apples, cored and chopped
- 2 cups fresh spinach, torn

Direction: Preparation Time: 15 minutes Servings: 2

- ✓ In a large bowl, add the tuna, yogurt, salt and black pepper and gently, stir to combine.
Add the carrots and apples and stir to combine.

✓ *Serve immediately.*

Nutrition: Calories 306; Total Fat 1.8g ; Saturated Fat 0 g ; Cholesterol 63 mg ; Total Carbs 38 g Sugar 26 g ; Fiber 7.6 g ; Sodium 324 mg ; Potassium 602 mg ; Protein 35.8 g

POULTRY

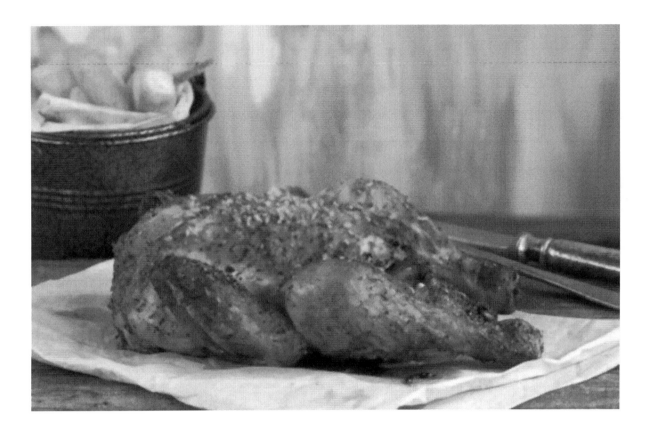

367)   *Chicken & Broccoli Bake*

Ingredients:

- 6 (6-ounce) boneless, skinless chicken breasts
- 3 broccoli heads, cut into florets
- 4 garlic cloves, minced
- ¼ cup olive oil
- 1 teaspoon dried oregano, crushed
- 1 teaspoon dried rosemary, crushed
- Sea Salt and ground black pepper, as required

Direction: Preparation Time: 15 minutes Cooking Time: 45 minutes Servings: 6

✓ Preheat the oven to 375 degrees F. Grease a large baking dish. In a large bowl, add all the ingredients and toss to coat well.

✓ In the bottom of the prepared baking dish, arrange the broccoli florets and top with chicken breasts in a single layer.

✓ Bake for about 45 minutes
Remove from the oven and set aside for about 5 minutes before serving.

✓ **Meal Prep Tip:**

✓ Remove the baking dish from the oven and set it aside to cool completely. In 6 containers, divide the chicken breasts and broccoli evenly and refrigerate for about 2 days.

✓ Reheat in microwave before serving.

Nutrition: Calories 443 Total Fat 21.5 g Saturated Fat 4.7 g Cholesterol 151 mg Total Carbs 9.4 g Sugar 2.2g Fiber 3.6 g Sodium 189 mg Potassium 831 mg Protein 53 g

368)   *Chicken Chili*

Ingredients:

- 4 cups low-sodium chicken broth, divided
- 3 cups boiled black beans, divided 1 tablespoon extra-virgin olive oil
- 1 large onion, chopped 1 jalapeño pepper, seeded and chopped
- 4 garlic cloves, minced 1 teaspoon dried thyme, crushed
- 1½ tablespoons ground coriander
- 1 tablespoon ground cumin
- ½ tablespoon red chili powder
- 4 cups cooked chicken, shredded
- 1 tablespoon fresh lime juice
- ¼ cup fresh cilantro, chopped

Direction: Preparation Time: 15 minutes Cooking Time: 40 minutes Servings: 6

✓ In a food processor, add 1 cup of broth and 1 can of black beans and pulse until smooth. Transfer the beans puree into a bowl and set aside.

✓ In a large pan, heat the oil over medium heat and sauté the onion and jalapeño for about 4-5 minutes.

✓ Add the garlic, spices and sea salt and sauté for about 1 minute.

✓ Add the beans puree and remaining broth and bring to a boil. Now, reduce the heat to low and simmer for about 20 minutes.
Stir in the remaining can of beans, chicken and lime juice and bring to a boil.

✓ Now, reduce the heat to low and simmer for about 5-10 minutes.

✓ Serve hot with the garnishing of cilantro.

✓ **Meal Prep Tip:** Transfer the chili into a large bowl and set aside to cool.

✓ Divide the chili into 6 containers evenly. Cover the containers and refrigerate for 1-2 days.

✓ Reheat in the microwave before serving.

Nutrition: Calories 356 Total Fat 7.1 g Saturated Fat 1.2 g Cholesterol 72 mg Total Carbs 33 g Sugar 2.7 g Fiber 11.6 g Protein 39.6 g

369)   *Chicken with Chickpeas*

Ingredients:

- 2 tablespoons olive oil
- 1 pound skinless, boneless chicken breast, cubed
- 2 carrots, peeled and sliced 1 onion, chopped
- 2 celery stalks, chopped 2 garlic cloves, chopped
- 1 tablespoon fresh ginger root, minced
- ½ teaspoon dried oregano, crushed
- ¾ teaspoon ground cumin
- ¼-13 teaspoon cayenne pepper
- ¼ teaspoon ground turmeric
- 1 cup tomatoes, crushed
- 1½ cups low-sodium chicken broth
- 1 zucchini, sliced
- 1 cup boiled chickpeas, drained
- 1 tablespoon fresh lemon juice
- ½ teaspoon paprika

Direction: Preparation Time: 15 minutes Cooking Time: 36 minutes Servings: 4

✓ In a large nonstick pan, heat the oil over medium heat and cook the chicken cubes for about 4-5 minutes.

✓ With a slotted spoon, transfer the chicken cubes onto a plate.

✓ In the same pan, add the carrot, onion, celery and garlic and sauté for about 4-5 minutes.

✓ Add the ginger, oregano and spices and sauté for

about 1 minute.
Add the chicken, tomato and broth and bring to a boil. Now, reduce the heat to low and simmer for about 10 minutes.

✓ Add the zucchini and chickpeas and simmer, covered for about 15 minutes. Stir in the lemon juice and serve hot.

✓ **Meal Prep Tip:**

✓ Transfer the chicken mixture into a large bowl and set it aside to cool. Divide the mixture into 4 containers evenly. Cover the containers and refrigerate for 1-2 days. Reheat in the microwave before serving.

Nutrition: Calories 308 Total Fat 12.3 g Saturated Fat 2.7 g Cholesterol 66 mg Total Carbs 19 g Sugar 5.3g Fiber 4.7 g Sodium 202 mg Potassium 331 mg Protein 30.7 g

370) *Chicken Soup*

Ingredients:

* 1 tablespoon olive oil
* 1 small carrot, peeled and chopped
* ½ cup onion, chopped
* 1 celery stalk, chopped 2 garlic cloves, minced
* 1 tablespoon fresh thyme, chopped
* 1 tablespoon fresh rosemary, chopped
* ½ teaspoon ground cumin
* ¼ teaspoon red pepper flakes, crushed lime zest, grated finely
* 5 cups low-sodium chicken broth
* 1¼ cups cooked chicken, chopped
* 2 cups fresh spinach, torn
* 1¼ cups zucchini, chopped
* Ground black pepper, as required
* 2 tablespoons fresh lime juice
* 1 teaspoon fresh

Direction: Preparation Time: 15 minutes Cooking Time: 23 minutes Servings: 4

✓ In a large soup pan, heat the oil over medium heat and sauté the carrot, onion and celery for about 8-9 minutes.

✓ Add the garlic, rosemary and spices and sauté for about 1 minute.

✓ Add the broth and bring to a boil over high heat.

✓ Now, reduce the heat to medium-low and simmer for about 5 minutes.
Add the cooked chicken, spinach and zucchini and simmer for about 6-8 minutes.

✓ Stir in the black pepper and lime juice and remove from heat.

✓ Serve hot with the garnishing of lime zest. **Meal Prep Tip:** Transfer the soup into a large bowl and set it aside to cool.

✓ Divide the soup into 4 containers evenly. Cover the containers and refrigerate for 1-2 days. Reheat in the microwave before serving.

Nutrition: Calories 224 Total Fat 6.8g Saturated Fat 1.4 g Cholesterol 74 mg Total Carbs 7.5 g Sugar 2 g Protein 31.8 g

371) *Chicken & Peanut Stir-Fry*

Ingredients:

Nutrition: Calories 224 Total Fat 6.8g Saturated Fat 1.4 g Cholesterol 74 mg Total Carbs 7.5 g Sugar 2 g Protein 31.8 g

* 3 tablespoons lime juice
* ½ teaspoon lime zest
* 4 cloves garlic, minced
* 2 teaspoons chili bean sauce
* 1 tablespoon fish sauce
* 1 tablespoon water
* 2 tablespoons peanut butter
  3 teaspoons oil, divided
* 1 lb. chicken breast, sliced into strips
* 1 red sweet pepper, sliced into strips
* 3 green onions, sliced thinly
* 2 cups broccoli, shredded
* 2 tablespoons peanuts, chopped

Direction: Preparation Time: 15 minutes Cooking Time: 15 minutes Servings: 4

✓ In a bowl, mix the lime juice, lime zest, garlic, chili bean sauce, fish sauce, water and peanut butter.

✓ Mix well. In a pan over medium high heat, add 2 teaspoons of oil.
Cook the chicken until golden on both sides.

✓ Pour in the remaining oil. Add the pepper and green onions.

✓ Add the chicken, broccoli and sauce. Cook for 2 minutes. Top with peanuts before serving.

Nutrition: Calories 368 Total Fat 11 g Saturated Fat 2 g Cholesterol 66 mg Sodium 556 mg Total Carbohydrate 34 g Dietary Fiber 3 g Total Sugars 4 g Protein 32 g Potassium 482 mg

372) *Chicken, Oats & Chickpeas Meatloaf*

Ingredients:

* ½ cup cooked chickpeas
* 2 egg whites
* 2½ teaspoons poultry seasoning
* Ground black pepper, as required
* 10 ounce lean ground chicken
* 1 cup red bell pepper, seeded and minced
* 1 cup celery stalk, minced

- *1/3 cup steel-cut oats 1 cup tomato puree, divided*
- *2 tablespoons dried onion flakes, crushed*
- *1 tablespoon prepared mustard*

Direction: Preparation Time: 20 minutes Cooking Time: 1¼ hours Servings: 4

✓ *Preheat the oven to 350 degrees F. Grease a 9x5-inch loaf pan. In a food processor, add chickpeas, egg whites, poultry seasoning and black pepper and pulse until smooth.*

✓ *Transfer the mixture into a large bowl. Add the chicken, veggies oats, ½ cup of tomato puree and onion flakes and mix until well combined.*

✓ *Transfer the mixture into prepared loaf pan evenly.*

✓ *With your hands, press, down the mixture slightly. In another bowl mix together mustard and remaining tomato puree. Place the mustard mixture over loaf pan evenly.*
Bake for about 1-1¼ hours or until desired doneness. Remove from the oven and set aside for about 5 minutes before slicing..

✓ *Cut into desired sized slices and serve.*

Meal Prep Tip:

✓ *In a resealable plastic bag, place the cooled meatloaf slices and seal the bag. Refrigerate for about 2-4 days. Reheat in the microwave on High for about 1 minute before serving.*

Nutrition: Calories 229 Total Fat 5.6 g Saturated Fat 1.4 g Cholesterol 50 mg Total Carbs 23.7 g Sugar 5.2 g Fiber 4.7 g Sodium 227 mg Potassium 509 mg Protein 21.4 g

373) *Meatballs Curry*

Ingredients:

- *For Meatballs:*
- *1 pound lean ground chicken*
- *1 tablespoon onion paste*
- *1 teaspoon fresh ginger paste*
- *1 teaspoon garlic paste*
- *1 green chili, chopped finely*
- *1 tablespoon fresh cilantro leaves, chopped*
- *1 teaspoon ground coriander*
- *½ teaspoon cumin seeds*
- *½ teaspoon red chili powder*
- *½ teaspoon ground turmeric*
- *1/8 teaspoon salt*

For Curry:
- *3 tablespoons olive oil*
- *½ teaspoon cumin seeds*
- *1 (1-inch) cinnamon stick*
- *2 onions, chopped 1 teaspoon fresh ginger, minced*
- *1 teaspoons garlic, minced*

- *4 tomatoes, chopped finely*
- *2 teaspoons ground coriander*
- *1 teaspoon garam masala powder*
- *½ teaspoon ground nutmeg*
- *½ teaspoon red chili powder*
- *½ teaspoon ground turmeric*
- *Salt, as required 1 cup filtered water*
- *3 tablespoons fresh cilantro, chopped*

Direction: Preparation Time: 20 minutes Cooking Time: 25 minutes Servings: 6

For meatballs:

✓ *In a large bowl, add all ingredients and mix until well combined.*

✓ *Make small equal-sized meatballs from mixture. In a large deep skillet, heat the oil over medium heat and cook the meatballs for about 3-5 minutes or until browned from all sides.*

✓ *Transfer the meatballs into a bowl. In the same skillet, add the cumin seeds and cinnamon stick and sauté for about 1 minute.*

✓ *Add the onions and sauté for about 4-5 minutes.*

✓ *Add the ginger and garlic paste and sauté for about 1 minute.*
Add the tomato and spices and cook, crushing with the back of spoon for about 2-3 minutes.

✓ *Add the water and meatballs and bring to a boil.*

✓ *Now, reduce the heat to low and simmer for about 10 minutes.*

✓ *Serve hot with the garnishing of cilantro.*

Meal Prep Tip:

✓ *Transfer the curry into a large bowl and set it aside to cool. Divide the curry into 5 containers evenly.*

✓ *Cover the containers and refrigerate for 1-2 days. Reheat in the microwave before serving.*

Nutrition: Calories 196 Total Fat 11.4 g Saturated Fat 2.4 g Cholesterol 53 mg Total Carbs 7.9 g Sugar 3.9 g Fiber 2.1 g Sodium 143 mg Potassium 279 mg Protein 16.7 g

374) *Herbed Turkey Breast*

Ingredients:

- *½ cup olive oil*
- *2 tablespoons fresh lemon juice*
- *1 tablespoon scallion, chopped*
- *½ teaspoon dried marjoram, crushed*
- *½ teaspoon dried sage, crushed*
- *½ teaspoon dried thyme, crushed*
- *Salt and ground black pepper, as required*
- *1 (2-pound) boneless, skinless turkey breast half*

Direction: Preparation Time: 15 minutes Cooking Time: 1 hour 50 minutes Servings: 6

✓ *Preheat the oven to 325 degrees F. Arrange a rack*

into a greased shallow roasting pan. In a small pan, all the ingredients except turkey breast over medium heat and bring to a boil, stirring frequently.

✓ Remove from the heat and set aside to cool. Place turkey breast into the prepared roasting pan. Place some of the herb mixtures over the top of the turkey breast.

✓ Cover the roasting pan and bake for about 1¼-1¾ hours, basting with the remaining herb mixture occasionally.
Remove from the oven and set aside for about 10-15 minutes before slicing.

✓ With a sharp knife, cut into desired slices and serve.

✓ **Meal Prep Tip:**

✓ Transfer the turkey breast slices onto a wire rack to cool completely.

✓ With foil pieces, wrap the turkey breast slices and refrigerate for about 1-2 days. Reheat in the microwave before serving.

Nutrition: Calories 319 Total Fat 17.5 g Saturated Fat 2.4 g Cholesterol 93 mg Total Carbs 0.3 g Protein 27.4 g

375) <u>Turkey with Lentils</u>

Ingredients:

- 3 tablespoons olive oil, divided 1 onion, chopped
- 1 tablespoon fresh ginger, minced
- 4 garlic cloves, minced
- 3 plum tomatoes, chopped finely
- 2 cups dried red lentils, soaked for 30 minutes and drained
- 2 teaspoons cumin seeds
- ½ teaspoon cayenne pepper
- 1 pound lean ground turkey
- 1 jalapeño pepper, seeded and chopped
- 2 scallions, chopped
- ¼ cup fresh cilantro, chopped
- 2 cups filtered water

Direction: Preparation Time: 15 minutes Cooking Time: 51 minutes Servings: 7

✓ In a Dutch oven, heat 1 tablespoon of oil over medium heat and sauté the onion, ginger and garlic for about 5 minutes.

✓ Stir in tomatoes, lentils and water and bring to a boil. Now, reduce the heat to medium-low and simmer, covered for about 30 minutes.

✓ Meanwhile, in a skillet, heat the remaining oil over medium heat and sauté the cumin seeds and cayenne pepper for about 1 minute.

✓ Transfer the mixture into a small bowl and set aside. In the same skillet, add turkey and cook for about 4-5 minutes

Add the jalapeño and scallion and cook for about 4-5 minutes. Add the spiced oil mixture and stir to combine well.

✓ Transfer the turkey mixture to simmering lentils and simmer for about 10-15 minutes or until desired doneness.

✓ Serve hot. **Meal Prep Tip:** Transfer the turkey mixture into a large bowl and set aside to cool. Divide the mixture into 4 containers evenly. Cover the containers and refrigerate for 1-2 days. Reheat in the microwave before serving.

Nutrition: Calories 361 Total Fat 11.5.4 g Saturated Fat 2.4 g

376) <u>Stuffed Chicken Breasts Greek-style</u>

Ingredients:

- 4 oz. chicken breasts, skinless and boneless
- ¼ cup onion, minced
- 4 artichoke hearts, minced
- 1 teaspoon oregano, crushed
- 4 lemon slices

What you will need from the store cupboard:

- 1 cup canned chicken broth, fat-free
- 1-1/2 lemon juice
- 1 tablespoon olive oil
- 2 teaspoons of cornstarch
- Ground pepper Salt, optional

Direction: Servings: 4 Cooking Time: 20 Minutes

✓ Take out all the fat from the chicken. Wash and pat dry. Season your chicken with pepper and salt.

✓ Pound the chicken to make it flat and thin. Bring together the oregano, onion, and artichoke hearts.

✓ Now spoon equal amounts of the mix at the center of your chicken.

✓ Roll up the log and secure it using a skewer or toothpick—heat oil in your skillet over medium temperature.
Add the chicken. Brown all sides evenly.

✓ Pour the lemon juice and broth.

✓ Add lemon slices on top of the chicken.

✓ Simmer covered for 10 minutes. Transfer to a platter.

✓ Remove the skewers or toothpick.

✓ Mix cornstarch with a fork. Transfer to skillet and stir over high temperature. Put lemon sauce on the chicken.

Nutrition: Calories 224, Carbohydrates 8g, Fiber 1g, Cholesterol 82mg, Total Fat 5g, Protein 21g, Sodium 339mg

377) Chicken & Tofu

Ingredients:

- 2 tablespoons olive oil, divided 2 tablespoons orange juice
- 1 tablespoon Worcestershire sauce 1 tablespoon low-sodium soy sauce
- 1 teaspoon ground turmeric 1 teaspoon dry mustard
- 8 oz. chicken breast, cooked and sliced into cubes
- 8 oz. extra-firm tofu, drained and sliced into cubed
- 2 carrots, sliced into thin strips 1 cup mushroom, sliced
- 2 cups fresh bean sprouts
- 3 green onions, sliced
- 1 red sweet pepper, sliced into strips

Direction: Preparation Time: 1 hour and 15 minutes Cooking Time: 25 minutes Servings: 6

- ✓ In a bowl, mix half of the oil with the orange juice, Worcestershire sauce, soy sauce, turmeric and mustard.
- ✓ Coat all sides of chicken and tofu with the sauce.
- ✓ Marinate for 1 hour. In a pan over medium heat, add 1 tablespoon oil.
Add carrot and cook for 2 minutes.
- ✓ Add mushroom and cook for another 2 minutes.
- ✓ Add bean sprouts, green onion and sweet pepper.
- ✓ Cook for two to three minutes. Stir in the chicken and heat through.

Nutrition: Calories 285 Fat 9 g Carbs 30 g Protein 20 g

378) Honey Mustard Chicken

Ingredients:

- 2 tablespoons honey mustard
- 2 teaspoons olive oil
- Salt to taste
- 1 lb. chicken tenders
- 1 lb. baby carrots, steamed
- Chopped parsley

Direction: Preparation Time: 15 minutes Cooking Time: 12 minutes Servings: 4

- ✓ Preheat your oven to 450 degrees F.
- ✓ Mix honey mustard, olive oil and salt.
- ✓ Coat the chicken tenders with the mixture. Place the chicken on a single layer on the baking pan.
Bake for 10 to 12 minutes. Serve with steamed carrots and garnish with parsley.

Nutrition: Calories 366 Total Fat 8 g Saturated Fat 2 g Total Carbs 46 g Total Sugars 13 g Protein 33 g

379) Lemon Garlic Turkey

Ingredients:

- 4 turkey breasts fillet
- 2 cloves garlic, minced
- 1 tablespoon olive oil
- 3 tablespoons lemon juice
- 1 oz. Parmesan cheese, shredded Pepper to taste
- 1 tablespoon fresh sage, snipped 1 teaspoon lemon zest

Direction: Preparation Time: 1 hour and 10 minutes Cooking Time: 5 minutes Servings: 4

- ✓ Pound the turkey breast until flat. In a bowl, mix the olive oil, garlic and lemon juice.
- ✓ Add the turkey to the bowl. Marinate for 1 hour.
- ✓ Broil for 5 minutes until the turkey is fully cooked. Sprinkle cheese on top on the last minute of cooking. In a bowl, mix the pepper, sage and lemon zest.
- ✓ Sprinkle this mixture on top of the turkey before serving.

Nutrition: Calories 188 Total Fat 7 g Saturated Fat 2 g Cholesterol 71 mg Sodium 173 mg Total Carbohydrate 2 g Dietary Fiber 0 g Total Sugars 0 g Protein 29 g Potassium 264 mg

380) Chicken & Spinach

Ingredients:

- 2 tablespoons olive oil
- 1 lb. chicken breast fillet, sliced into small pieces
- Salt and pepper to taste
- 4 cloves garlic, minced
- 1 tablespoon lemon juice
- ½ cup dry white wine
- 1 teaspoon lemon zest
- 10 cups fresh spinach, chopped
- 4 tablespoons Parmesan cheese, grated

Direction: Preparation Time: 15 minutes Cooking Time: 13 minutes Servings: 4

- ✓ Pour oil in a pan over medium heat. Season chicken with salt and pepper.
- ✓ Cook in the pan for 7 minutes until golden on both sides.
Add the garlic and cook for 1 minute. Stir in the lemon juice and wine.
- ✓ Sprinkle lemon zest on top. Simmer for 5 minutes.
- ✓ Add the spinach and cook until wilted.
- ✓ Serve with Parmesan cheese.

Nutrition: Calories 334 Total Fat 12 g Saturated Fat 3 g Cholesterol 67 mg Sodium 499 mg Total Carbohydrate 25 g Dietary Fiber 2 g Total Sugars 1 g Protein 29 g

381) Balsamic Chicken

Ingredients:

- 6 chicken breast halves, skin removed
- 1 onion, sliced into wedges 1 tablespoon tapioca (quick-cooking), crushed
- Salt and pepper to taste
- 1 teaspoon dried thyme, crushed
- 1 teaspoon dried rosemary, crushed
- ¼ cup balsamic vinegar
- 2 tablespoons chicken broth
- 9 oz. frozen Italian green beans
- 1 red sweet pepper, sliced into strips

Direction: Preparation Time: 15 minutes Cooking Time: 5 hours Servings: 6

✓ Put the chicken, onion and tapioca inside a slow cooker. Season with the salt, pepper, thyme and rosemary.

✓ Seal the pot and cook on low setting for 4 hours and 30 minutes.
  Add the sweet pepper and green beans.

✓ Cook for 30 more minutes.

✓ Pour sauce over the chicken and vegetables before serving.

Nutrition: Calories 234 Total Fat 2 g Saturated Fat 1 g Cholesterol 100 mg Sodium 308 mg Total Carbohydrate 10 g Dietary Fiber 2 g Total Sugars 5 g Protein 41 g Potassium 501 mg

382) Greek Chicken Lettuce Wraps

Ingredients:

- 2 tablespoons freshly squeezed lemon juice
- 1 teaspoon lemon zest
- 5 teaspoons olive oil, divided
- 3 teaspoons garlic, minced and divided
- 1 teaspoon dried oregano
- ¼ teaspoon red pepper, crushed
- 1 lb. chicken tenders
- 1 cucumber, sliced in half and grated
- Salt and pepper to taste
- ¾ cup non-fat Greek yogurt
- 2 teaspoons fresh mint, chopped
- 2 teaspoons fresh dill, chopped
- 4 lettuce leaves
- ½ cup red onion, sliced 1 cup tomatoes, chopped

Direction: Preparation Time: 1 hour and 15 minutes Cooking Time: 8 minutes Servings: 4

✓ In a bowl, mix the lemon juice, lemon zest, half of oil, half of garlic, and red pepper. Coat the chicken with the marinade.

✓ Marinate it for 1 hour. Toss grated cucumber in salt. Squeeze to release liquid.

✓ Add the yogurt, dill, salt, pepper, remaining garlic and remaining oil.

✓ Grill the chicken for 4 minutes per side. Shred the chicken and put on top of the lettuce leaves.

✓ Top with the yogurt mixture, onion and tomatoes.

✓ Wrap the lettuce leaves and secure with a toothpick.

Nutrition: Calories 353 Total Fat 9 g Saturated Fat 1 g Cholesterol 58 mg Sodium 559 mg Total Carbohydrate 33 g Dietary Fiber 6 g Total Sugars 6 g Protein 37 g Potassium 459 mg

383) Lemon Chicken with Kale

Ingredients:

- 1 tablespoon olive oil
- 1 lb. chicken thighs, trimmed
- Salt and pepper to taste
- ½ cup low-sodium chicken stock
- 1 lemon, sliced
- 1 tablespoon fresh tarragon, chopped
- 4 cloves garlic, minced
- 6 cups baby kale

Direction: Preparation Time: 10 minutes Cooking Time: 19 minutes Servings: 4

✓ Pour olive oil in a pan over medium heat. Season chicken with salt and pepper.

✓ Cook until golden brown on both sides. Pour in the stock. Add the lemon, tarragon and garlic. Simmer for 15 minutes.

✓ Add the kale and cook for 4 minutes.

Nutrition: Calories 374 Total Fat 19 g Saturated Fat 4 g Cholesterol 76 mg Sodium 378 mg Total Carbohydrate 26 g Dietary Fiber 3 g Total Sugars 2 g Protein 25 g Potassium 677 mg

MEAT

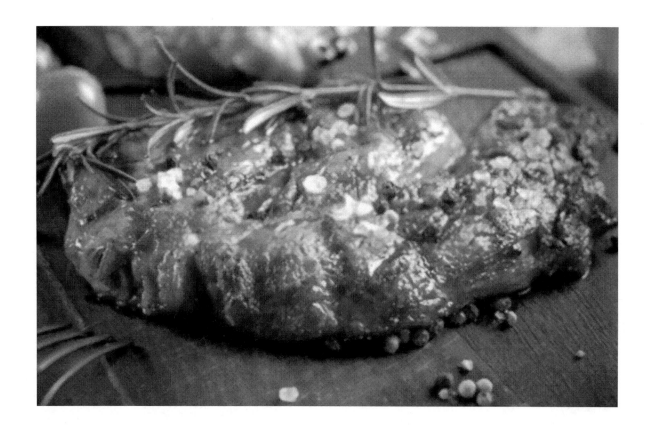

384)   *Pork Chops with Grape Sauce*

Ingredients:,

- Cooking spray
- 4 pork chops
- ¼ cup onion, sliced
- 1 clove garlic, minced
- 1/2 cup low-sodium chicken broth,
- ¾ cup apple juice
- 1 tablespoon cornstarch
- 1 tablespoon balsamic vinegar
- 1 teaspoon honey
- 1 cup seedless red grapes, sliced in half

Direction: Preparation Time: 15 minutesCooking Time: 25 minutes Servings: 4

- ✓ Spray oil on your pan.
- ✓ Put it over medium heat.
- ✓ Add the pork chops to the pan.
- ✓ Cook for 5 minutes per side.
- ✓ Remove and set aside.
- ✓ Add onion and garlic.
- ✓ Cook for 2 minutes.
- ✓ Pour in the broth and applejuice.
- ✓ Bring to a boil.,Reduce heat to simmer.
- ✓ Put the pork chops back to theskillet.
- ✓ Simmer for 4 minutes.
- ✓ In a bowl, mix the cornstarch,vinegar and honey.
- ✓ Add to the pan.
- ✓ Cook until the sauce hasthickened.
- ✓ Add the grapes.
- ✓ Pour sauce over the porkchops before serving.

Nutrition: Calories 188; Total Fat 4 g; Saturated Fat 1 g; Cholesterol 47 mg; Sodium 117 mg; Total Carbohydrate 18 g;Dietary Fiber 1 g; Total Sugars 13 g; Protein 19 g; Potassium 759 mg

385)   *Pork with Cranberry Relish,*

Ingredients:,,

- 12 oz. pork tenderloin, fat trimmed and sliced crosswise
- Salt and pepper to taste
- ¼ cup all-purpose flour
- 2 tablespoons olive oil,1 onion, sliced thinly
- ¼ cup dried cranberries
- ¼ cup low-sodium chickenbroth
- 1 tablespoon balsamic vinegar,

Direction: Preparation Time: 30 minutesCooking Time: 30 minutes Servings: 4,

- ✓ Flatten each slice of porkusing a mallet.

- ✓ In a dish, mix the salt, pepperand flour.
- ✓ Dip each pork slice into theflour mixture.
- ✓ Add oil to a pan over mediumhigh heat.
- ✓ Cook pork for 3 minutes perside or until golden crispy.,Transfer to a serving plate andcover with foil.
- ✓ Cook the onion in the pan for4 minutes.
- ✓ Stir in the rest of theingredients.
- ✓ Simmer until the sauce hasthickened.,

Nutrition: Calories 211; Total Fat 9 g; Saturated Fat 2 g; Cholesterol 53 mg; Sodium 116 mg; Total Carbohydrate 15 g;Dietary Fiber 1 g; Total Sugars 6 g; Protein 18 g; Potassium 378 mg,

386)   *Roasted Pork & Apples*

Ingredients:,

- Salt and pepper to taste
- 1/2 teaspoon dried, crushed
- 1 lb. pork tenderloin
- 1 tablespoon canola oil,1 onion, sliced into wedges
- 3 cooking apples, sliced intowedges
- 2/3 cup apple cider
- Sprigs fresh sage

Direction: Preparation Time: 15 minutesCooking Time: 30 minutes Servings: 4

- ✓ In a bowl, mix salt, pepper andsage.
- ✓ Season both sides of pork withthis mixture.
- ✓ Place a pan over medium heat.
- ✓ Brown both sides.
- ✓ Transfer to a roasting pan.
- ✓ Add the onion on top andaround the pork.,Drizzle oil on top of the porkand apples.
- ✓ Roast in the oven at 425 degrees F for 10 minutes.
- ✓ Add the apples, roast foranother 15 minutes.
- ✓ In a pan, boil the apple ciderand then simmer for 10 minutes.
- ✓ Pour the apple cider sauce over the pork before serving.

Nutrition: Calories 239; Total Fat 6 g; Saturated Fat 1 g; Cholesterol 74 mg; Sodium 209 mg; Total Carbohydrate 22g; Dietary Fiber 3 g; Total Sugars 16 g; Protein 24 g; Potassium 655 mg

387)   *Sesame Pork with Mustard Sauce*

Ingredients:,

- 2 tablespoons low-sodiumteriyaki sauce
- ¼ cup chili sauce
- 2 cloves garlic, minced
- 2 teaspoons ginger, grated

- *2 pork tenderloins,2 teaspoons sesame seeds*
- *¼ cup low fat sour cream*
- *1 teaspoon Dijon mustard*
- *Salt to taste*
- *1 scallion, chopped*

Direction: Preparation Time: 25 minutesCooking Time: 25 minutes Servings: 4

✓ *Preheat your oven to 425degrees F.*

✓ *Mix the teriyaki sauce, chilisauce, garlic and ginger.*

✓ *Put the pork on a roasting pan.*

✓ *Brush the sauce on both sidesof the pork.*

✓ *Bake in the oven for 15minutes.,Brush with more sauce.*

✓ *Top with sesame seeds.*

✓ *Roast for 10 more minutes.*

✓ *Mix the rest of the ingredients.*

✓ *Serve the pork with mustardsauce.*

Nutrition: Calories 135 ; Total Fat 3 g; Saturated Fat 1 g; Cholesterol 56X mg; Sodium 302 mg; Total Carbohydrate 7g; Dietary Fiber 1 g; Total Sugars 15 g; Protein 20 g;Potassium 755 mg

388) *Steakwith Mushroom Sauce*

Ingredients:,

- *12 oz. sirloin steak, sliced andtrimmed*
- *2 teaspoons grilling seasoning*
- *2 teaspoons oil*
- *6 oz. broccoli, trimmed*
- *2 cups frozen peas,3 cups fresh mushrooms, sliced*
- *1 cup beef broth (unsalted)*
- *1 tablespoon mustard*
- *2 teaspoons cornstarch*
- *Salt to taste*

Direction: Preparation Time: 20 minutesCooking Time: 5 minutes Servings: 4

✓ *Preheat your oven to 350degrees F.*

✓ *Season meat with grillingseasoning.*

✓ *In a pan over medium highheat, cook the meat and broccoli for 4 minutes.*

✓ *Sprinkle the peas around thesteak.*

✓ *Put the pan inside the ovenand bake for 8 minutes.*

✓ *Remove both meat and vegetables from the pan.,Add the mushrooms to thepan.*

✓ *Cook for 3 minutes.*

✓ *Mix the broth, mustard, saltand cornstarch.*

✓ *Add to the mushrooms.*

✓ *Cook for 1 minute.*

✓ *Pour sauce over meat andvegetables before*

serving.

Nutrition: Calories 226; Total Fat 6 ; Saturated Fat 2 g; Cholesterol 51 mg ; Sodium 356 mg; Total Carbohydrate 16g; Dietary Fiber 5 g; Total Sugars 6 g; Protein 26 g;

389) *Steakwith Tomato& Herbs*

Ingredients:,

- *8 oz. beef loin steak, sliced inhalf*
- *Salt and pepper to taste*
- *Cooking spray,1 teaspoon fresh basil, snipped*
- *¼ cup green onion, sliced*
- *1/2 cup tomato, chopped*

Direction: Preparation Time: 30 minutesCooking Time: 30 minutes Servings: 2

✓ *Season the steak with salt andpepper.*

✓ *Spray oil on your pan.*

✓ *Put the pan over medium highheat.*

✓ *Once hot, add the steaks.*

✓ *Reduce heat to medium.*

✓ *Cook for 10 to 13 minutes formedium, turning once.,Add the basil and green onion.*

✓ *Cook for 2 minutes.*

✓ *Add the tomato.*

✓ *Cook for 1 minute.*

✓ *Let cool a little before slicing.*

Nutrition: Calories 170; Total Fat 6 g; Saturated Fat 2 g; Cholesterol 66 mg; Sodium 207 mg; Total Carbohydrate 3 g;Dietary Fiber 1 g; Total Sugars 5 g; Protein 25 g; Potassium 477 mg

390) *Barbecue Beef Brisket*

Ingredients:,

- *4 lb. beef brisket (boneless),trimmed and sliced*
- *1 bay leaf*
- *2 onions, sliced into rings*
- *1/2 teaspoon dried thyme,crushed*
- *¼ cup chili sauce,1 clove garlic, minced*
- *Salt and pepper to taste*
- *2 tablespoons light brownsugar*
- *2 tablespoons cornstarch*
- *2 tablespoons cold water*

Direction: Preparation Time: 25 minutesCooking Time: 10 hours Servings: 10

✓ *Put the meat in a slow cooker.*

✓ *Add the bay leaf and onion.*

✓ *In a bowl, mix the thyme, chilisauce, salt, pepper and sugar.*

✓ *Pour the sauce over the meat.*

✓ Mix well.

✓ Seal the pot and cook on low heat for 10 hours.,Discard the bay leaf.

✓ Pour cooking liquid in a pan.

✓ Add the mixed water and cornstarch.

✓ Simmer until the sauce has thickened.

✓ Pour the sauce over the meat.

Nutrition: Calories 182; Total Fat 6 g; Saturated Fat 2 g; Cholesterol 57 mg; Sodium 217 mg; Total Sugars 4 g; Protein 20 g; Potassium 383 mg

391) *Steak with Tomato & Herbs*

Ingredients:,

- 8 oz. beef loin steak, sliced in half
- Salt and pepper to taste
- Cooking spray,1 teaspoon fresh basil, snipped
- ¼ cup green onion, sliced
- 1/2 cup tomato, chopped

Direction: Preparation Time: 30 minutesCooking Time: 30 minutes Servings: 2

✓ Season the steak with salt and pepper.

✓ Spray oil on your pan.

✓ Put the pan over medium high heat.

✓ Once hot, add the steaks.

✓ Reduce heat to medium.

✓ Cook for 10 to 13 minutes for medium, turning once.,Add the basil and green onion.

✓ Cook for 2 minutes.

✓ Add the tomato.

✓ Cook for 1 minute.

✓ Let cool a little before slicing.

Nutrition: Calories 170; Total Fat 6 g; Saturated Fat 2 g; Cholesterol 66 mg; Sodium 207 mg; Total Carbohydrate 3 g;Dietary Fiber 1 g; Total Sugars 5 g; Protein 25 g; Potassium 477 mg

391) *Beef & Asparagus*

Ingredients:,

- 2 teaspoons olive oil
- 1 lb. lean beef sirloin, trimmed and sliced
- 1 carrot, shredded
- Salt and pepper to taste,
- 12 oz. asparagus, trimmed and sliced
- 1 teaspoon dried herbs de Provence, crushed
- 1/2 cup Marsala
- ¼ teaspoon lemon zest

Direction: Preparation Time: 15 minutesCooking Time: 10 minutes Servings: 4

✓ Pour oil in a pan over medium heat.

✓ Add the beef and carrot.

✓ Season with salt and pepper.

✓ Cook for 3 minutes.,Add the asparagus and herbs.

✓ Cook for 2 minutes.

✓ Add the Marsala and lemon zest.

✓ Cook for 5 minutes, stirring frequently.

Nutrition: Calories 327; Total Fat 7 g; Saturated Fat 2 g; Cholesterol 69 mg ; Sodium 209 mg; Total Carbohydrate 29g; Dietary Fiber 2 g; Total Sugars 3 g; Protein 28 g;Potassium 576 mg

392) *Italian Beef,*

Ingredients:,

- Cooking spray
- 1 lb. beef round steak,trimmed and sliced
- 1 cup onion, chopped
- 2 cloves garlic, minced
- 1 cup green bell pepper,chopped
- 1/2 cup celery, chopped,2 cups mushrooms, sliced
- 14 1/2 oz. canned diced tomatoes
- 1/2 teaspoon dried basil
- ¼ teaspoon dried oregano
- 1/8 teaspoon crushed red pepper
- 2 tablespoons Parmesan cheese, grated

Direction: Preparation Time: 20 minutesCooking Time: 1 hour and 20 minutes Servings: 4

✓ Spray oil on the pan over medium heat.

✓ Cook the meat until brown on both sides.

✓ Transfer meat to a plate.

✓ Add the onion, garlic, bell pepper, celery and mushroom to the pan.

✓ Cook until tender.,Add the tomatoes, herbs, and pepper.

✓ Put the meat back to the pan.

✓ Simmer while covered for 1hour and 15 minutes.

✓ Stir occasionally.

✓ Sprinkle Parmesan cheese on top of the dish before serving.

Nutrition: Calories 212; Total Fat 4 g; Saturated Fat 1 g;Cholesterol 51 mg; Sodium 296 mg; Total Sugars 6 g; Protein 30 g; Potassium 876 mg

393) *Lamb with Broccoli & Carrots*

Ingredients:,

- 2 cloves garlic, minced
- 1 tablespoon fresh ginger,grated
- ¼ teaspoon red pepper,crushed

- 2 tablespoons low-sodium soysauce
- 1 tablespoon white vinegar
- 1 tablespoon cornstarch,
- 12 oz. lamb meat, trimmedand sliced
- 2 teaspoons cooking oil
- 1 lb. broccoli, sliced intoflorets
- 2 carrots, sliced into strips
- ¾ cup low-sodium beef broth
- 4 green onions, chopped
- 2 cups cooked spaghettisquash pasta

Direction: Preparation Time: 20 minutes Cooking Time: 10 minutes Servings: 4

✓ Combine the garlic, ginger, redpepper, soy sauce, vinegar andcornstarch in a bowl.
✓ Add lamb to the marinade.
✓ Marinate for 10 minutes.
✓ Discard marinade.
✓ In a pan over medium heat,add the oil.
✓ Add the lamb and cook for 3minutes.,Transfer lamb to a plate.
✓ Add the broccoli and carrots.
✓ Cook for 1 minute.
✓ Pour in the beef broth.
✓ Cook for 5 minutes.
✓ Put the meat back to the pan.
✓ Sprinkle with green onion andserve on top of spaghetti squash.

Nutrition: Cal 205; Total Fat 6 g; Saturated Fat 1 g; Cholesterol 40 mg; Sodium 659 mg; Total Carb. 17 g

394) *Rosemary Lamb,*

Ingredients:

- Salt and pepper to taste
- 2 teaspoons fresh rosemary,snipped,
- 5 lb. whole leg of lamb, trimmed and cut with slits onall sides
- 3 cloves garlic, slivered
- 1 cup water

Direction: Preparation Time: 15 minutesCooking Time: 2 hours Servings: 14

✓ Preheat your oven to 375degrees F.
✓ Mix salt, pepper and rosemaryin a bowl.
✓ Sprinkle mixture all over thelamb.
✓ Insert slivers of garlic into theslits.
✓ ✓☞Put the lamb on a roastingpan.
✓ Add water to the pan.
✓ Roast for 2 hours.

Nutrition: Calories 136; Total Fat 4 g; Saturated Fat 1g cholesterol 71 mg; Sodium 218 mg; Protein 23 g;

395) *Mediterranean Lamb Meatballs*

Ingredients:,

- 12 oz. roasted red peppers
- 1 1/2 cups whole wheatbreadcrumbs
- 2 eggs, beaten
- 1/3 cup tomato sauce,1/2 cup fresh basil
- ¼ cup parsley, snipped
- Salt and pepper to taste
- 2 lb. lean ground lamb

Direction: Preparation Time: 10 minutesCooking Time: 20 minutes Servings: 8

✓ Preheat your oven to 350degrees F.
✓ In a bowl, mix all the ingredients and then form intomeatballs.,Put the meatballs on a bakingpan.
✓ Bake in the oven for 20minutes.

Nutrition: Calories 94; Total Fat 3 g; Saturated Fat 1 g; Cholesterol 35 mg Sodium 170 mg; Total Carbohydrate 2 g; Dietary Fiber 1 g; Total Sugars 0 g

396) *Shredded Beef,*

Ingredients:,

- 1.5lb lean steak
- 1 cup lowsodium gravy,
- 2tbsp mixed spices

Direction: Servings: 2 Cooking Time: 35 Minutes

✓ Mix all the ingredients in yourInstant Pot. Cook on Stew for 35 minutes.,
✓ Release the pressure naturally.Shred the beef.

Nutrition: Calories: 200 Carbs: 2 Sugar: 0 Fat: 5 Protein: 48 GL: 1

397) *Classic Mini Meatloaf*

Ingredients:,

- 1 pound 80/20 ground beef
- ¼ medium yellow onion,peeled and diced
- ½ medium green bell pepper,seeded and diced
- 1 large egg
- 3 tablespoons blanched finelyground almond flour,1 tablespoon
- Worcestershire sauce
- ½ teaspoon garlic powder
- 1 teaspoon dried parsley
- 2 tablespoons tomato paste
- ¼ cup water
- 1 tablespoon powderederythritol

Direction: Servings: 6 Cooking Time: 25 Minutes

✓ In a large bowl, combine ground beef, onion,

pepper, egg, and almond flour. Pour inthe

✓ Worcestershire sauce and addthe garlic powder and parsleyto the bowl.

✓ Mix until fully combined. Divide the mixture into two and place it into two (4") loafbaking pans.,In a small bowl, mix the tomato paste, water, and erythritol. Spoon half themixture over each loaf.

✓ Working in batches if necessary, place loaf pans intothe air fryer basket.

✓ Adjust the temperature to 350°F and set the timer for 25minutes or until the internal

✓ temperature is 180°F. Servewarm.

Nutrition: Calories: 170 Protein: 14.9 G Fiber: 0.9 G NetCarbohydrates: 2.6 G Sugar Alcohol: 1.5 G Fat: 9.4 G Sodium: 85 Mg Carbohydrates: 5.0 G Sugar: 1.5 G

398) *Skirt Steak With Asian Peanut Sauce*

Ingredients:,

- ⅓ cup light coconut milk
- 1 teaspoon curry powder
- 1 teaspoon coriander powder
- 1 teaspoon reduced-sodiumsoy sauce,
- 1¼ pound skirt steak Cooking spray
- ½ cup Asian Peanut Sauce

Direction: Servings: 4 Cooking Time: 15 Minutes

✓ In a large bowl, whisk together the coconut milk, curry powder, coriander powder, and soy sauce.

✓ Add the steak and turn tocoat.

✓ Cover the bowl and refrigerate for at least 30 minutes and no longer than24 hours.

✓ Preheat the barbecue or coat agrill pan with cooking spray and place the steak over medium-high heat.,Grill the meat until it reachesan internal temperature of 145°F, about 3 minutes per side.

✓ Remove the steak from the grilland let it rest for 5 minutes. Slice the steak into 5-ounce pieces and serve each with 2 tablespoons of the Asian Peanut Sauce.

✓ REFRIGERATE: Store the cooled steak in a reseal ablecontainer for up to 1 week. Reheat each piece in the

✓ microwave for 1 minute.

Nutrition: Calories: 361 Fat: 22g Saturated Fat: 7g Protein:36g Total Carbs: 8g Fiber: 2g Sodium: 349mg

399) *Roasted Pork Loin With Grainy Mustard Sauce*

Ingredients:,

- (2-pound) boneless pork loinroast Sea salt

- Freshly ground black pepper
- 3 tablespoons olive oil,
- 1½ cups heavy (whipping)cream
- 3 tablespoons grainy mustard,such as Pommery

Direction: Servings: 8 Cooking Time: 70 Minutes

✓ Preheat the oven to 375°F. Season the pork roast all overwith sea salt and pepper.

✓ Place a large skillet over medium-high heat and addthe olive oil.

✓ Brown the roast on all sides inthe skillet, about 6 minutes intotal, and place the roast in a baking dish.

✓ Roast until a meat thermometer inserted in the thickest part of the roast reads155°F, about 1 hour.,When there is approximately 15 minutes of roasting time left, place a small saucepan over medium heat and add theheavy cream and mustard. Stirthe sauce until it simmers, then reduce the heat to low.

✓ Simmer the sauce until it isvery rich and thick, about 5minutes.

✓ Remove the pan from the heatand set it aside. Let the pork rest for 10 minutes before slicing and serve with thesauce.

Nutrition: Calories 368 Fat: 29g Protein: 25g Carbs: 2gFiber: 0g Net Carbs: 2g Fat 70%/Protein 25%/Carbs 5%

400) *Meatballs In Tomato Gravy*

Ingredients:,

For Meatballs:

- 1 pound lean ground lamb
- 1 tablespoon homemadetomato paste
- ¼ cup fresh cilantro leaves,chopped
- 1 small onion, chopped finely
- 2 garlic cloves, minced
- ½ teaspoon ground cumin
- 1/8 teaspoon salt Groundblack pepper, as required
- 1½ cups warm low-sodiumchicken broth,

For Tomato Gravy:

- 3 tablespoons olive oil, divided 2 medium onions, chopped finely
- 2 garlic cloves, minced
- ½ tablespoon fresh ginger,minced
- 1 teaspoon dried thyme,crushed
- 1 teaspoon dried oregano,crushed
- 3 large tomatoes, chopped
- finely Ground black pepper, asrequired

Direction: Servings: 6 Cooking Time: 30 Minutes

✓ For meatballs: in a large bowl,add all the ingredients and mix until well combined. Make small equal-sized balls from the mixture and set themaside.

✓ For the gravy: in a large pan,heat 1 tablespoon of oil over medium heat.

✓ Add the meatballs and cook for about 4-5 minutes or until lightly browned from all sides.With a slotted spoon, transfer the meatballs onto a plate.

✓ In the same pan, heat the remaining oil over medium heat and sauté the onion forabout 8-10 minutes. Add thegarlic, ginger and herbs and sauté for about 1 minute.,. Add the tomatoes and cookfor about 3-4 minutes, crushing with the back of spoon. Add the warm broth and bring to a boil.

✓ Carefully, place the meatballsand cook for 5 minutes, without stirring.

✓ Now, reduce the heat to low and cook partially covered forabout 15-20 minutes, stirringgently 2-3 times. Serve hot.

✓ Meal Prep Tip:

✓ Transfer the meatballs mixture into a large bowl andset aside to cool. Divide the mixture into 6 containers evenly. Cover the containers and refrigerate for 1-2 days.

✓ Reheat in the microwavebefore serving.

Nutrition: Calories 248 Total Fat 12.9 g Saturated Fat 3 g Cholesterol 68 mg Total Carbs 10 g Sugar 4.8 g Fiber 2.5 g Sodium 138 mg Potassium 591 mg Protein 23.4 g

401) Garlic-braisedShortRib

Ingredients:,

• 4 (4-ounce) beef short ribs
• Sea salt
• Freshly ground black pepper
• 1 tablespoon olive oil,2 teaspoons minced garlic
• ½ cup dry red wine
• 3 cups Rich Beef Stock (here)

Direction: Servings: 4 Cooking Time: 2 Hours, 20 Minutes

✓ Preheat the oven to 325°F.Season the beef ribs on all sides with salt and pepper.

✓ Place a deep ovenproof skilletover medium-high heat and add the olive oil.

✓ Sear the ribs on all sides untilbrowned, about 6 minutes in total.

✓ Transfer the ribs to a plate.Add the garlic to the skillet and sauté until translucent,about 3 minutes.

✓ Whisk in the red wine todeglaze the pan.,Be sure to scrape all the browned bits from the meatfrom the bottom of the pan.

✓ Simmer the wine until it isslightly reduced, about 2 minutes.

✓ Add the beef stock, ribs, and any accumulated juices on theplate back to the skillet and bring the

liquid to a boil.

✓ Cover the skillet and place it inthe oven to braise the ribs until the meat is fall-off-the- bone tender, about 2 hours.

✓ Serve the ribs with a spoonfulof the cooking liquid drizzledover each serving.

Nutrition: Calories: 481 Fat: 38g Protein: 29g Carbs: 5gFiber: 3g Net Carbs: 2g Fat 70%/Protein 25%/Carbs 5%

402) Pulled Pork,

Ingredients:,

• 2 tablespoons chili powder
• 1 teaspoon garlic powder
• ½ teaspoon onion powder,½ teaspoon ground black pepper
• ½ teaspoon cumin

Direction: Servings: 8 Cooking Time: 2½ Hours

✓ (4-pound) pork shoulder In a small bowl, mix chili powder, garlic powder, onion powder, pepper, and cumin.

✓ Rub the spice mixture over the pork shoulder, patting it into the skin.

✓ Place the pork shoulder into the air fryer basket.

✓ Adjust the temperature to 350°F and set the timer for 150 minutes.,Pork skin will be crispy and meat easily shredded with two forks when done.

✓ The internal temperature should be at least 145°F.

Nutrition: Calories: 537 Protein: 42.6 G Fiber: 0.8 G Net Carbohydrates: 0.7 G Fat: 35.5 G Sodium: 180 MgCarbohydrates: 1.5 G Sugar: 0.2 G

403) Rosemary-garlic Lamb Racks

Ingredients:,

• 4 tablespoons extra-virgin olive oil
• 2 tablespoons finely chopped fresh rosemary,
• 2 teaspoons minced garlic Pinch sea salt
• 2 (1-pound) racks
• French-cut lamb chops (8 bones each)

Direction: Servings: 4 Cooking Time: 25 Minutes

✓ In a small bowl, whisk together the olive oil, rosemary, garlic, and salt. Place the racks in a sealable freezer bag and pour the olive oil mixture into the bag.

✓ Massage the meat through the bag so it is coated with the marinade. Press the air out of the bag and seal it.

✓ Marinate the lamb racks in the refrigerator for 1 to 2 hours— Preheat the oven to 450°F. Place a large ovenproof skillet over medium-high heat.,Take the lamb racks out of the bag and sear them in the skillet on all sides, about 5 minutes in total.

✓ Arrange the racks upright in the skillet, with the bones interlaced, and roast them in the oven until they reach your desired doneness, about 20 minutes for medium-rare or until the internal temperature reaches 125°F.

✓ Let the lamb rest for 10 minutes and then cut the racks into chops. Serve 4 chops per person.

Nutrition: Calories: 354 Fat: 30g Protein: 21g Carbs: 0g Fiber: 0g Net Carbs: 0g Fat 70%/Protein 30%/Carbs 0%

404) *Irish Pork Roast,*

Ingredients:,

- 1 ½ lb. parsnips, peeled and sliced into small pieces
- 1 ½ lb. carrots, sliced into small pieces
- 3 tablespoons olive oil,,divided 2 teaspoons fresh thyme leaves, divided
- Salt and pepper to taste
- 2 lb. pork loin roast
- 1 teaspoon honey
- 1 cup dry hard cider Applesauce

Direction: Preparation Time: 40 minutes Cooking Time: 1 hour Servings: 8

✓ Preheat your oven to 400 degrees F.

✓ Drizzle half of the oil over the parsnips and carrots. Season with half of the thyme, salt and pepper.

✓ Arrange on a roasting pan. Rub the pork with the remaining oil.

✓ Season with the remaining thyme.

✓ Season with salt and pepper.

✓ Put it on the roasting pan on top of the vegetables.,Roast for 65 minutes.

✓ Let cool before slicing.

✓ Transfer the carrots and parsnips in a bowl and mix with honey.

✓ Add the cider. Place in a pan and simmer over low heat until the sauce has thickened.

✓ Serve the pork with vegetables and applesauce.

Nutrition: Calories 272 Total Fat 8 g Saturated Fat 2 g Cholesterol 61 mg Sodium 327 mg Total Carbohydrate 23 g Dietary Fiber 6 g Total Sugars 10 g Protein 24 g

405) *Barbecue Beef Brisket*

Ingredients:,

- 4 lb. beef brisket (boneless),trimmed and sliced
- 1 bay leaf
- 2 onions, sliced into rings

- ½ teaspoon dried thyme,crushed
- ¼ cup chili sauce,1 clove garlic, minced Salt andpepper to taste
- 2 tablespoons light brownsugar
- 2 tablespoons cornstarch
- 2 tablespoons cold water

Direction: Preparation Time: 25 minutes Cooking Time: 10hours Servings: 10

✓ Put the meat in a slow cooker.Add the bay leaf and onion. Ina bowl, mix the thyme, chili sauce, salt, pepper and sugar.

✓ Pour the sauce over the meat.Mix well. Seal the pot and cook on low heat for 10 hours.

✓ Discard the bay leaf. Pourcooking liquid in a pan.,Add the mixed water andcornstarch.

✓ Simmer until the sauce hasthickened.

✓ Pour the sauce over the meat.

Nutrition: Calories 182 Total Fat 6 g Saturated Fat 2 g Cholesterol 57 mg Sodium 217 mg Total Carbohydrate 9 gDietary Fiber 1 g Total Sugars 4 g Protein 20 g

406) *Lamb&Chickpeas*

Ingredients:,

- 1 lb. lamb leg (boneless), trimmed and sliced into smallpieces
- 2 tablespoons olive oil
- 1 teaspoon ground coriander
- Salt and pepper to taste
- ½ teaspoon ground cumin
- ¼ teaspoon red pepper,crushed
- ¼ cup fresh mint, chopped
- 2 teaspoons lemon zest,2 cloves garlic, minced
- 30 oz. unsalted chickpeas,rinsed and drained
- 1 cup tomatoes, chopped
- 1 cup English cucumber,chopped
- ¼ cup fresh parsley, snipped 1tablespoon red wine vinegar

Direction: Preparation Time: 30 minutes Cooking Time: 30minutes Servings: 4

✓ Preheat your oven to 375degrees F.

✓ Place the lamb on a bakingdish.

✓ Toss in half of the following:oil, cumin and coriander.

✓ Season with red pepper, saltand pepper.,Mix well— roast for 20 minutes. In a bowl, combine the rest of the ingredients withthe remaining seasonings.

✓ Add salt and pepper. Serve lamb with chickpea mixture.

Nutrition: Calories 366 Total Fat 15 g Saturated Fat 3 g Cholesterol 74 mg Sodium 369 mg Total Carbohydrate 27 gDietary Fiber 7 g Protein 32 g

407)   *Braised Lamb with Vegetables*

Ingredients:,

- Salt and pepper to taste
- 2 ½ lb. boneless lamb leg, trimmed and sliced into cubes
- 1 tablespoon olive oil
- 1 onion, chopped
- 1 carrot, chopped
- 14 oz. canned diced tomatoes 1 cup low-sodium beef broth
- 1 tablespoon fresh rosemary, chopped 4 cloves garlic, minced
- 1 cup pearl onions
- 1 cup baby turnips, peeled and sliced into wedges
- 1 ½ cups baby carrots
- 1 ½ cups peas
- 2 tablespoons fresh parsley, chopped

Direction: Preparation Time: 30 minutes Cooking Time: 2 hours and 15 minutes Servings: 6

- ✓ Sprinkle salt and pepper on both sides of the lamb. Pour oil into a deep skillet.
- ✓ Cook the lamb for 6 minutes. Transfer lamb to a plate.
- ✓ Add onion and carrot—Cook for 3 minutes. Stir in the tomatoes, broth, rosemary and garlic. Simmer for 5 minutes., Add the lamb back to the skillet.
- ✓ Reduce heat to low. Simmer for 1 hour and 15 minutes. Add the pearl onion, baby carrot and baby turnips.
- ✓ Simmer for 30 minutes. Add the peas.
- ✓ Cook for 1 minute. Garnish with parsley before serving.

Nutrition: Calories 420 Total Fat 14 g Saturated Fat 4 g holesterol 126 mg Sodium 529 mg Total Carbohydrate 16 g Dietary Fiber 4 g Total Sugars 7 g Protein 43 g Potassium 988 mg

408)   *Beef Salad,*

Ingredients:,

- For Steak:
- 1½ pounds skirt steak, trimmed and cut into 4 pieces
- Salt and ground black pepper, as required

For Salad:

- 2 medium green bell pepper, seeded and sliced thinly
- 2 large tomatoes, sliced
- 1 cup onion, sliced thinly, 8 cups mixed fresh baby greens

For Dressing:

- 2 teaspoons Dijon mustard
- 4 tablespoons balsamic vinegar
- ½ cup olive oil
- Salt and ground black pepper, as required

Direction: Preparation Time: 20 minutes Cooking Time: 8 minutes Servings: 6

- ✓ Preheat the grill to medium- high heat. Grease the grill grate. Sprinkle the beef steak with a little salt and black pepper. Place the steak onto the grill and cook, covered for about 3-4 minutes per side. Transfer the steak onto a cutting board for about 10 minutes before slicing. With a sharp knife, cut the beef steaks into thin slices.
- ✓ Meanwhile, in a large bowl, mix together all salad ingredients. For the dressing: in another bowl, add all the ingredients and beat until well
- ✓ combined., Pour the dressing over the salad and gently toss to coat well. Divide the salad onto serving plates evenly. Top each plate with the steak slices and serve.
- ✓ Meanwhile, in a large bowl, mix together all salad ingredients. For the dressing: in another bowl, add all the ingredients and beat until well combined. Pour the dressing over salad and gently toss to coat well. Divide the salad onto serving plates evenly. Top each plate with the steak slices and serve.

Nutrition: Calories 313 Total Fat 21.4 g Saturated Fat 5.1 g Cholesterol 50 mg Total Carbs 6.4 g Sugar 3.4 g Protein 24 g

409)   *Beef Curry,*

Ingredients:,

- 1 cup fat-free plain Greek yogurt
- ½ teaspoon garlic paste
- ½ teaspoon ginger paste
- ½ teaspoon ground cloves
- ½ teaspoon ground cumin
- 2 teaspoons red pepper flakes, crushed,
- ¼ teaspoon ground turmeric
- Salt, as required
- 2 pounds round steak, cut into pieces
- ¼ cup olive oil
- 1 medium yellow onion, thinly sliced
- 1½ tablespoons fresh lemon juice
- ¼ cup fresh cilantro, chopped

Direction: Preparation Time: 20 minutes Cooking Time: 40 minutes Servings: 6

- ✓ In a large bowl, add the yogurt, garlic paste, ginger paste and spices and mix well.
- ✓ Add the steak pieces and generously coat with the yogurt mixture. Set aside for at least 15 minutes.
- ✓ In a large skillet, heat the oil over medium-high heat and sauté the onion for about 4-5 minutes.

✓ Add the steak pieces with marinade and stir to combine.Immediately, adjust the heat to low and simmer, covered,Stir in the lemon juice andsimmer for about 10 moreminutes.

✓ Garnish with fresh cilantroand serve hot.

✓ Meal Prep Tip:

✓ Transfer the curry into a largebowl and set it aside to cool.

✓ Divide the curry into 6containers evenly.

✓ Cover the containers andrefrigerate for 1-2 days.

✓ Reheat in the microwavebefore serving and cook for about 25 minutes, stirring occasionally.

Nutrition: Calories 389 Total Fat 18.2 g Saturated Fat 4.8 g Cholesterol 136 mg Total Carbs 4.3 g Sugar 2.4 g Fiber 0.7 g Sodium 149 mg Potassium 666 mg Protein 50.3 g

410) Beefwith Barley& Veggies

Ingredients:,

- ¾ cup filtered water
- ¼ cup pearl barley
- 2 teaspoons olive oil
- 7 ounces lean ground beef
- 1 cup fresh mushrooms, sliced,
- ¾ cup onion, chopped
- 2 cups frozen green beans
- ¼ cup low-sodium beef broth
- 2 tablespoon fresh parsley,chopped

Direction: Preparation Time: 15 minutes Cooking Time: 1hour 5 minutes Servings: 2

✓ In a pan, add water, barley anda pinch of salt and bring to a boil over medium heat.

✓ Now, reduce the heat to low and simmer, covered for about30-40 minutes or until all the liquid is absorbed.

✓ Remove from heat and setaside.

✓ In a skillet, heat oil over medium-high heat and cookbeef for about 8-10 minutes

✓ Add the mushroom and onionand cook for about 6-7 minutes.,Add the green beans and cookfor about 2-3 minutes. Stir in cooked barley and broth and cook for about 3-5 minutes more.

✓ Stir in the parsley and servehot.

Meal Prep Tip:

✓ Transfer the beef mixture intoa large bowl and set it aside tocool.

✓ Divide the mixture into 2 containers evenly. Cover the containers and refrigerate for1-2 days. Reheat in the microwave before serving.

Nutrition: Calories 374 Total Fat 11.4 g Saturated Fat 3.1 g Cholesterol 89 mg Total Carbs 32.7g Sugar 1.1 g Fiber 4.2 gSodium 136 mg Potassium 895 mg Protein 36.6 g

411) Beefwith Broccoli

Ingredients:

- 2 tablespoons olive oil, divided
- 2 garlic cloves, minced
- 1 pound beef sirloin steak, trimmed and sliced into thinstrips
- ¼ cup low-sodium chickenbroth
- 2 teaspoons fresh ginger,grated
- 1 tablespoon ground flax seeds
- ½ teaspoon red pepper flakes,crushed
- Salt and ground black pepper,as required
- 1 large carrot, peeled andsliced thinly
- 2 cups broccoli florets
- 1 medium scallion, slicedthinly

Direction: Preparation Time: 10 minutes Cooking Time: 14minutes Servings: 4

✓ In a large skillet, heat 1 tablespoon of oil over medium-high heat and sautéthe garlic for about 1 minute.

✓ Add the beef and cook for about 4-5 minutes or until browned. With a slotted spoon, transfer the beef into abowl.

✓ Remove the excess liquid fromthe skillet. In a bowl, add the broth, ginger, flax seeds, red

✓ pepper flakes, salt and blackpepper. In the same skillet, heat theremaining oil over mediumheat.

✓ Add the carrot, broccoli and ginger mixture and cook for about 3-4 minutes or until desired doneness. Stir in beefand scallion and cook for about 3-4 minutes.

Meal Prep Tip:

✓ Transfer the beef mixture intoa large bowl and set it aside tocool.

✓ Divide the mixture into 4 containers evenly. Cover the containers and refrigerate for

✓ 1-2 days. Reheat in the microwave before serving.

Nutrition: Calories 211 Total Fat 14.9 g Saturated Fat 3.9 g Cholesterol 101 mg Total Carbs 6.9 g Sugar 1.9 g Fiber 2.4 g Sodium 108 mg Potassium 706 mg Protein 36.5 g

412) Pan Grilled Steak

Ingredients:,

- 8 medium garlic cloves,crushed
- 1 (2-inch) piece fresh ginger,sliced thinly
- ¼ cup olive oil,Salt and ground black pepper,as required
- ½ pounds flank steak,trimmed

Direction: Preparation Time: 10 minutes Cooking Time: 16minutes Servings: 4

✓ *In a large sealable bag, mix together all ingredients exceptsteak.*

✓ *Add the steak and coat with marinade generously. Seal thebag and refrigerate to marinate for about 24 hours.*

✓ *Remove from refrigerator andkeep at room temperature forabout 15 minutes.*

✓ *Discard the excess marinadefrom the steak. Heat a lightlygreased grill pan over medium-high heat and cook the steak for about 6-8*

✓ *minutes per side.,Remove from grill pan and set aside for about 10 minutes before slicing.*

✓ *With a sharp knife cut intodesired slices and serve.*

Meal Prep Tip:

✓ *Transfer the steak slices onto awire rack to cool completely. With foil pieces, wrap the steak slices and refrigerate for about 1-2 days. Reheat in the microwave before serving.*

Nutrition: Calories 447 Total Fat 26.8 g Saturated Fat 7.7 gCholesterol 94 mg Total Carbs 2.1g Sugar 0.1 g Fiber 0.2 g Sodium 96 mg Potassium 601 mg Protein 47.7 g

413) *Lamb Stew Recipe 1*

Ingredients:,

- *1 teaspoon ground cumin*
- *1 teaspoon ground coriander*
- *½ teaspoon cayenne pepper*
- *½ teaspoon ground cinnamon*
- *2 tablespoons olive oil*
- *3 pounds lamb stew meat,trimmed and cubed*
- *Sea Salt and ground blackpepper, as required,*
- *1 onion, chopped*
- *2 garlic cloves, minced*
- *2¼ cups low-sodium chickenbroth*
- *2 cups tomatoes, choppedfinely*
- *1 medium head cauliflower,cut into 1-inch florets*

Direction: Preparation Time: 15 minutes Cooking Time: 2¼hours Servings: 8

✓ *Preheat the oven to 300degrees F.*

✓ *In a small bowl, mix togetherspices and set aside.*

✓ *In a large ovenproof pan, heatoil over medium heat and cook the lamb with a little saltand black pepper for about 10minutes or until browned from all sides.*

✓ *With a slotted spoon, transferthe lamb into a bowl.*

✓ *In the same pan, add onionand sauté for about 3-4,Add the cooked lamb, brothand tomatoes and bring to agentle boil.*

✓ *Immediately, cover the pan and transfer into oven—Bakefor about 1½ hours.*

✓ *Remove from oven and stir in cauliflower. Bake for*

about 30 minutes more or until cauliflower is done completely.Serve hot.

Meal Prep Tip:

✓ *Transfer the stew into a largebowl and set aside to cool.*

✓ *minutes. Add the garlic andspice mixture and sauté forabout 1 minute. Divide the stew into 8containers evenly.*

✓ *Cover the containers and refrigerate for 1-2 days. Reheatin the microwave before serving.*

Nutrition: Calories 375 Total Fat 16.2 g Saturated Fat 5 g Cholesterol 153 mg Total Carbs 5.6 g Sugar 2.6 g Fiber 1.8 g Sodium 162 mg Potassium 808 mg Protein 49.7 g

414) *Lamb Curry*

Ingredients:

For Spice Mixture:

- *2 teaspoons ground coriander*
- *2 teaspoons ground cumin*
- *1 teaspoon ground cinnamon*
- *½ teaspoon ground ginger*
- *1 tablespoon sweet paprika*
- *½ tablespoon cayenne pepper*
- *1 teaspoon red chili powder*
- *Salt and ground black pepper,as required*

For Curry:

- *1 tablespoon olive oil*
- *2 pounds boneless lamb,trimmed and cubed into*
- *1-inch size*
- *2 cups onions, chopped*
- *½ cup fat-free plain*
- *Greek yogurt, whipped*
- *1½ cups water*

Direction: Preparation Time: 15 minutes Cooking Time: 2¼hours Servings: 8

✓ *For spice mixture: in a bowl, add all spices and mix well. Setaside. In a large*

✓ *Dutch oven, heat the oil over medium-high heat and stir frythe lamb cubes for about 5 minutes.*

✓ *Add the onion and cook for about 4-5 minutes. Stir in thespice mixture and cook for about 1 minute.*

✓ *Add the yogurt and water andbring to a boil over high heat. Now, reduce the heat to low and simmer, covered for about1-2 hours or until the desired doneness of lamb. Uncover and simmer for about 3-4 minutes. Serve hot.*

Meal Prep Tip:

✓ *Transfer the curry into a largebowl and set it aside to cool.*

✓ *Divide the curry into 8containers evenly.*

✓ Cover the containers and refrigerate for 1-2 days. Reheat

✓ in the microwave beforeserving.

Nutrition: Calories 254 Total Fat 10.5 g Saturated Fat 3.3 gCholesterol 102 mg Total Carbs 4.7 g Sugar 1.9 g Fiber 1.4 g Sodium 99 mg Potassium 468 mg Protein 34 g

415) *Yummy Meatballs in Tomato Gravy*

Ingredients:

For Meatballs:

- 1 pound lean ground lamb
- 1 tablespoon homemadetomato paste
- ¼ cup fresh cilantro leaves,chopped
- 1 small onion, chopped finely
- 2 garlic cloves, minced
- ½ teaspoon ground cumin
- 1/8 teaspoon salt
- Ground black pepper, asrequired
- 1½ cups warm low-sodiumchicken broth

For Tomato Gravy:

- 3 tablespoons olive oil,divided
- 2 medium onions, choppedfinely
- 2 garlic cloves, minced
- ½ tablespoon fresh ginger,minced
- 1 teaspoon dried thyme,crushed
- 1 teaspoon dried oregano,crushed
- 3 large tomatoes, choppedfinely

Direction: Preparation Time: 20 minutes Cooking Time: 30minutes Servings: 6

For meatballs: in a large bowl,add all the ingredients and mix until well combined.

✓ Make small equal-sized balls from the mixture and set themaside.

For the gravy: in a large pan,heat 1 tablespoon of oil over medium heat.

✓ Add the meatballs and cook for about 4-5 minutes or until lightly browned from all sides.

✓ With a slotted spoon, transferthe meatballs onto a plate. In the same pan, heat the remaining oil over medium heat and sauté the onion for about 8-10 minutes.
Add the garlic, ginger and herbs and sauté for about 1minute.

✓ Add the tomatoes and cook forabout 3-4 minutes, crushing with the back of the spoon.

✓ Add the warm broth and bringto a boil. Carefully, place the meatballs and cook for 5 minutes, without stirring.

✓ Now, reduce the heat to low and cook partially covered forabout 15-20 minutes, stirringgently 2-3 times. Serve hot.

Meal Prep Tip:

✓ Transfer the meatballs mixture into a large bowl andset aside to cool. Divide the mixture into 6 containers evenly. Cover the containers and refrigerate for 1-2 days.

✓ Reheat in the microwavebefore serving.

Nutrition: Calories 248 Total Fat 12.9 g Saturated Fat 3 g Cholesterol 68 mg Total Carbs 10 g Sugar 4.8 g Fiber 2.5 g Sodium 138 mg Potassium 591 mg Protein 23.4 g

416) *Spiced Leg of Lamb*
Ingredients:

For Marinade:

- 2/3 cup fat-free plain Greekyogurt
- 1 tablespoon homemadetomato puree
- 1 tablespoon fresh lemon juice
- 3-4 garlic cloves, minced
- 2 tablespoons fresh rosemary,chopped 2 teaspoons ground coriander
- 1 teaspoon ground cumin
- 1 teaspoon ground cinnamon 1teaspoon red pepper flakes, crushed
- ¼ teaspoon sweet paprika
- Sea salt and freshly groundblack pepper, as required
- 1 (4½-pound) bone-in leg oflamb

Direction: Preparation Time: 15 minutes Cooking Time: 1hour 40 minutes Servings: 6

✓ In a large bowl, add yogurt, tomato puree, lemon juice, garlic, rosemary, and spices and mix until well combined.

✓ Add leg of lamb and coat with marinade generously. Cover and refrigerate to marinate for about 8-10 hours, flipping occasionally.

✓ Remove the marinated leg of lamb from the refrigerator andkeep it at room temperature for about 25-30 minutes before roasting.

✓ Preheat the oven to 425 ° F. Line a large roasting pan witha greased foil piece.

✓ Arrange the leg of lamb into aprepared roasting pan—roastfor 20 minutes.

✓ Remove the roasting pan from

✓ the oven and change the sideof the leg of lamb. Now, Now, reduce the temperature of oven to 325 °F.

✓ Roast for 40 minutes. Now loosely cover the roasting pan with a large piece of foil. Roastfor 40 minutes more. Remove from oven and place onto a cutting board for about 10-15 minutes before slicing.

✓ With a sharp knife cut the legof lamb in desired sized slicesand serve.

Meal Prep Tip:

✓ *Transfer the leg slices onto a wire rack to cool completely. With foil pieces, wrap the leg slices and refrigerate for about1-2 days. Reheat in the microwave before serving.*

Nutrition: Calories 478 Total Fat 15.5 g Saturated Fat 6.1 g Cholesterol 226 mg Total Carbs 3.3 g Sugar 1.3 g Fiber 0.9 g Sodium 226 mg Potassium 48 mg Protein 72.3 g

417) *Baked Lamb & Spinach*

Ingredients:

- *2 tablespoons olive oil*
- *2 pounds lamb necks,trimmed and cut into*
- *2-inch pieces crosswise*
- *Salt, as required*
- *2 medium onions, chopped*
- *3 tablespoons fresh ginger,minced*
- *4 garlic cloves, minced*
- *2 tablespoons groundcoriander*
- *1 tablespoon ground cumin*
- *1 teaspoon ground turmeric*
- *¼ cup fat-free plain Greekyogurt*
- *½ cup tomatoes, chopped 2cups boiling water*
- *30 ounces frozen spinach,thawed and squeezed*
- *1½ tablespoons garammasala*
- *1 tablespoon fresh lemon juice*
- *Ground black pepper, asrequired*

Direction: Preparation Time: 15 minutes Cooking Time: 2hours 55 minutes Servings: 6

✓ *Preheat the oven to 300degrees F. In a large*

✓ *Dutch oven, heat the oil over medium-high heat and stir frythe lamb necks with a little salt for about 4-5 minutes or until browned completely.*

✓ *With a slotted spoon, transferthe lamb onto a plate and Now, reduce the heat to medium.*

✓ *In the same pan, add the onion and sauté for about 10minutes.*

✓ *Add the ginger, garlic and spices and sauté for about 1minute.*

✓ *Add the yogurt and tomatoesand cook for about 3-4 minutes.*
With an immersion blender, blend the mixture until smooth. Add the lamb, boilingwater and salt and bring to a boil. Cover the pan and transfer into the oven.

✓ *Bake for about 2½ hours. Now, remove the pan from oven and place it over mediumheat. Stir in spinach and garam masala and cook for about 3-5 minutes. Stir in lemon juice, salt and black pepper and remove from heat.*

✓ *Serve hot.*

Meal Prep Tip:

✓ *Transfer the lamb mixture intoa large bowl and set aside to cool. Divide the mixture into 6containers evenly. Cover the containers and refrigerate for*

✓ *1-2 days. Reheat in the microwave before serving.*

Nutrition: Calories 469 Total Fat 32.4 g Saturated Fat 13.4 gCholesterol 0 mg Total Carbs 12.9 g Sugar 3.1 g Fiber 4.7 g Sodium 304 mg Potassium 957 mg Protein 34.1 g

418) *Pork Salad*

Ingredients:

- *1½ pounds pork tenderloin,trimmed and sliced thinly*
- *Salt and ground black pepper,as required*
- *3 tablespoon olive oil*
- *2 carrots, peeled and grated*
- *3 cups Napa cabbage,shredded*
- *2 scallions, chopped*
- *2 tablespoon fresh lime juice*
- *¼ cup fresh mint leaves,chopped*

Direction: Preparation Time: 15 minutes Cooking Time: 6minutes Servings: 5

✓ *Season the pork with salt andblack pepper lightly.*

✓ *In a large skillet, heat the oilover medium heat and cook the pork slices for about 2-3minutes per side or until cooked through.*

✓ *Remove from the heat and setaside to cool slightly. In a large bowl, add the pork and remaining ingredients except for mint leaves and tossto coat well. Serve with the garnishing of mint leaves.*

Meal Prep Tip:

✓ *In 5 containers, divide salad. Refrigerate the containers for*

✓ *about 1 day. Just before serving, stir the salad well*

Nutrition: Calories 292 Total Fat 13.3 g Saturated Fat 2.9 gCholesterol 99 mg Total Carbs 5.7 g Sugar 2.7 g Fiber 2.1 g Sodium 104 mg Potassium 760 mg Protein 36.6 g

419) *Porkwith Bell Peppers*

Ingredients:

- *1 tablespoon fresh ginger,chopped finely*
- *4 garlic cloves, chopped finely*
- *1 cup fresh cilantro, choppedand divided*
- *¼ cup plus*
- *1 tablespoon olive oil, divided*
- *1 pound tender pork, trimmed, sliced thinly*
- *2 onions, sliced thinly*
- *1 green bell pepper, seededand sliced thinly*
- *1 red bell pepper, seeded andsliced thinly*

- *1 tablespoon fresh lime juice*

Direction: Preparation Time: 15 minutes Cooking Time: 13minutes Servings: 4

✓ *In a large bowl, mix togetherginger, garlic, ½ cup of cilantro and ¼ cup of oil.*

✓ *Add the pork and coat withmixture generously.*

✓ *Refrigerate to marinate forabout 2 hours.*

✓ *Heat a large skillet over medium-high heat and stir frythe pork mixture for about 4-5minutes. Transfer the pork into a bowl. In the same skillet, heat remaining oil over medium heat and sauté the onion for about 3 minutes. Stir in the bell pepper and stir fry for about 3 minutes.*

✓ *Stir in the pork, lime juice andremaining cilantro and cook for about 2 minutes.*

✓ *Serve hot.*

Meal Prep Tip:

✓ *Transfer the pork mixture intoa large bowl and set aside to cool.*

✓ *Divide the mixture into 4containers evenly.*

✓ *Cover the containers andrefrigerate for 1-2 days. Reheat in the microwave*

✓ *before serving*

Nutrition: Calories 360 Total Fat 21.8 g Saturated Fat 3.9 gCholesterol 83 mg Total Carbs 11 g Sugar 5.4 g Fiber 2.2 g Sodium 71 mg Potassium 706 mg Protein 31.2 g

420) *Roasted Pork Shoulder*

Ingredients:

- *1 head garlic, peeled andcrushed*
- *¼ cup fresh rosemary, minced*
- *2 tablespoons fresh lemonjuice*
- *2 tablespoons balsamicvinegar*
- *1 (4-pound) pork shoulder,trimmed*

Direction: Preparation Time: 10 minutes Cooking Time: 6hours Servings: 12

✓ *In a bowl, add all the ingredients except pork shoulder and mix well.*

✓ *In a large roasting pan place pork shoulder and coat with marinade generously. With a large plastic wrap, cover the roasting pan and refrigerate tomarinate for at least 1-2 hours.*

✓ *Remove the roasting pan fromrefrigerator.*

✓ *Remove the plastic wrap from roasting pan and keep in roomtemperature for 1 hour. Preheat the oven to 275degrees F.*

✓ *Arrange the roasting pan inoven and roast for about 6 hours.*

✓ *Remove from the oven and setaside for about 15-20 minutes.With a sharp knife, cut the pork shoulder into desired slices and serve.*

Meal Prep Tip:

✓ *Transfer the pork slices onto awire rack to cool completely. With foil pieces, wrap the porkslices and refrigerate for about1-2 days. Reheat in the microwave before serving.*

Nutrition: Calories 450 Total Fat 32.6g Saturated Fat 12 g Cholesterol 136 mg Total Carbs 1.5 g Sugar 0.1 g Fiber 0.6 g Sodium 104 mg Potassium 522 mg Protein 35.4 g

421) *Pork Chops in Peach Glaze*

Ingredients:

- *2 (6-ounce) boneless porkchops, trimmed*
- *Sea Salt and ground blackpepper, as required*
- *½ of ripe yellow peach, peeled, pitted and chopped*
- *1 tablespoon olive oil*
- *2 tablespoons shallot, minced*
- *2 tablespoons garlic, minced*
- *2 tablespoons fresh ginger,minced*
- *4-6 drops liquid stevia*
- *1 tablespoon balsamic vinegar*
- *¼ teaspoon red pepper flakes,crushed*
- *¼ cup filtered water*

Direction: Preparation Time: 15 minutes Cooking Time: 16minutes Servings: 2

✓ *Season the pork chops with sea salt and black pepper generously. In a blender, addthe peach pieces and pulse until puree forms.*

✓ *Reserve the remaining peach pieces. In a skillet, heat the oilover medium heat and sauté the shallots for about 1-2 minutes.*

✓ *Add the garlic and ginger andsauté for about 1 minute. Stirin the remaining ingredients and bring to a boil.*

✓ *Now, reduce the heat to medium-low and simmer forabout 4-5 minutes or until a sticky glaze forms. Remove from the heat and reserve 1/3 of the glaze and setaside. Coat the chops with the remaining glaze.*

✓ *Heat a nonstick skillet over medium-high heat and sear the chops for about 4 minutesper side.*

✓ *Transfer the chops onto a plateand coat with the remaining glaze evenly. Serve immediately.*

Meal Prep Tip:

✓ *Transfer the pork chops into alarge bowl and set aside to cool.*

✓ *Divide the chops into 2containers evenly.*

✓ *Cover the containers and refrigerate for 1-2 days. Reheat*

✓ *in the microwave beforeserving.*

Nutrition: Calories 359 Total Fat 13.5 g Saturated Fat 3.2 g Total Carbs 12 g Sugar 3.8 g Protein 46.2 g

422) *Ground Pork with Spinach*

Ingredients:

- *1 tablespoon olive oil*
- *½ of white onion, chopped*
- *2 garlic cloves, chopped finely*
- *1 jalapeño pepper, choppedfinely*
- *1 pound lean ground pork*
- *1 teaspoon ground coriander*
- *1 teaspoon ground cumin*
- *½ teaspoon ground turmeric*
- *½ teaspoon ground cinnamon*
- *½ teaspoon ground fennelseeds*
- *Salt and ground black pepper,as required*
- *½ cup fresh cherry tomatoes,quartered*
- *1¼ pounds collard greens leaves stemmed and chopped*
- *1 teaspoon fresh lemon juice*

Direction: Preparation Time: 15 minutes Cooking Time: 15minutes Servings: 4

- ✓ *In a large skillet, heat the oil over medium heat and sauté the onion for about 4 minutes.*
- ✓ *Add the garlic and jalapeño pepper and sauté for about 1minute.*
- ✓ *Add the pork and spices andcook for about 6 minutes breaking into pieces with thespoon. Stir in the tomatoes and greens and cook, stirring gently for about 4 minutes. Stir in the lemon juice and remove from heat. Serve hot.*

Meal Prep Tip:

- ✓ *Transfer the pork mixture intoa large bowl and set it aside tocool. Divide the mixture into 4containers evenly. Cover the containers and refrigerate for*
- ✓ *1-2 days. Reheat in the microwave before serving.*

Nutrition: Calories 316 Total Fat 21.8 g Saturated Fat 0.5 gCholesterol 0 mg Total Carbs 11.4 g Sugar 1.4 g Fiber 5.7 g Sodium 27 mg Potassium 107 mg Protein 23 g

FISH AND SEA FOOD

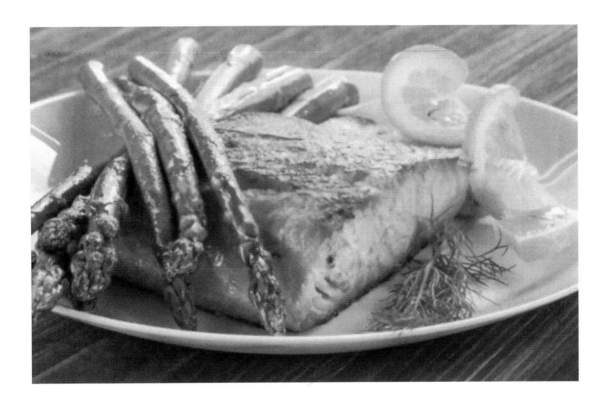

423)   Salmon Cakes in Air Fryer

Ingredients:

- 8 oz. Fresh salmon filled
- t 1 egg
- ⅛ tsp. salt
- ¼ tsp. garlic powder
- 1 sliced lemon

Direction: Preparation Time: 10 minutes Cooking Time: 10 minutes Servings: 2

✓ In the bowl, chop the salmon, add the egg and spices.

✓ Form tiny cakes.
  Let the Air fryer preheat to 390°F. On the bottom of the air fryer bowl lay sliced lemons—place cakes on top.

✓ Cook them for seven minutes. Based on your diet preferences, eat with your chosen dip.

Nutrition: Calories: 194 Fat: 9g Protein: 25g

424)   Coconut Shrimp

Ingredients:

- ½ cup pork rinds, crushed
- 4 cups. jumbo shrimp, deveined
- ½ cup coconut flakes preferably
- 2 eggs
- ½ cup coconut flour
- Any oil of your choice for frying at least half-inch in pan
- Freshly ground black pepper and kosher salt to taste

Dipping Sauce (Pina colada flavor):

- 2-3 tbsp. powdered Sugar as Substitute
- 3 tbsp. mayonnaise
- ½ cup our cream
- ¼ tsp. coconut extract or to taste
- 3 tbsp. coconut cream
- ¼ tsp. pineapple flavoring as much to taste
- 3 tbsp. coconut flakes preferably unsweetened this is optional

Direction: Preparation Time: 10 minutes Cooking Time: 30 minutes Servings: 4

✓ Pina Colada (Sauce):

✓ Mix all the ingredients into a tiny bowl for the Dipping sauce (Pina colada flavor). Combine well and put in the fridge until ready to serve.

✓ Shrimps:

✓ Whip all eggs in a deep bowl, and a small, shallow bowl, add the crushed pork rinds, coconut flour, sea salt, coconut flakes, and freshly ground black pepper.

✓ Put the shrimp one by one in the mixed eggs for dipping, then in the coconut flour blend. Put them on a clean plate or put them on your air fryer's basket.

✓ Place the shrimp battered in a single layer on your air fryer basket. Spritz the shrimp with oil and cook for 8–10 minutes at 360°F, flipping

✓ them through halfway.

✓ Enjoy hot with dipping sauce.

Nutrition: Calories: 340 Protein: 25g Fat 16g

425)   Crispy Fish Sticks in Air Fryer

Ingredients:

- lb. whitefish such as cod
- ¼ cup mayonnaise
- tbsp. Dijon mustard 2 tbsp. water
- 1 ½ cup pork rind
- ¾ tsp. cajun seasoning
- Kosher salt and pepper to taste

Direction: Preparation Time: 10 minutes Cooking Time: 15 minutes Servings: 4

✓ Spray non-stick cooking spray to the air fryer rack.

✓ Pat the fish dry and cut into sticks about 1 inch by 2 inches' broad

✓ Stir together the mayo, mustard, and water in a tiny small dish. Mix the pork rinds and Cajun seasoning into another small container.

✓ Adding kosher salt and pepper to taste (both pork rinds and seasoning can have a decent amount of kosher salt, so you can dip a finger to see how salty it is).
  Working for 1 slice of fish at a time, dip to cover in the mayo, mix and then tap off the excess. Dip into the mixture of pork rind, then flip to cover. Place on the rack of an air fryer.

✓ Set at 400°F to Air Fry and bake for 5 minutes, then turn the fish with tongs and bake for another 5 minutes. Serve.

Nutrition: Calories: 263 Fat: 16g Protein: 26.4g

426)   Honey-Glazed Salmon

Ingredients:

- 6 tsp. gluten-free soy Sauce
- 2 pcs. salmon Fillets
- 3 tsp. sweet rice wine
- 1 tsp. water
- 6 tbsp. Honey

Direction: Preparation Time: 10 minutes Cooking

Time: 15 minutes Servings: 2

✓ In a bowl, mix sweet rice wine, soy sauce, honey, and water.

✓ Set half of it aside.

✓ In half of it, marinate the fish and let it rest for 2 hours.

✓ Let the air fryer preheat to 180°C. Cook the fish for 8 minutes, flip halfway through and cook for another 5 minutes.

✓ Baste the salmon with marinade mixture after 3 or 4 minutes.

✓ The half of marinade, pour in a saucepan reduce to half, serve with a sauce.

Nutrition: Calories: 254 Protein: 20g Fat: 12g

427) Basil-Parmesan Crusted Salmon

Ingredients:

- 3 tbsp. grated parmesan
- 4 salmon fillets, skinless
- ¼ tsp. salt
- Freshly ground black pepper
- 3 tbsp. low-fat mayonnaise Basil leaves, chopped
- Half lemon

Direction: Preparation Time: 5 minutes Cooking Time: 15 minutes Servings: 4

✓ Let the air fryer preheat to 400°F. Spray the basket with olive oil.

✓ With salt, pepper, and lemon juice, season the salmon.

✓ In a bowl, mix 2 tbsp—Parmesan cheese with mayonnaise and basil leaves.

✓ Add this mix and more parmesan on top of salmon and cook for seven minutes or until fully cooked. Serve hot.

Nutrition: Calories: 289 Protein: 30g Fat: 18.5g

428) Cajun Shrimp in Air Fryer

Ingredients:

- 24 extra-jumbo shrimp, peeled
- 2 tbsp. olive oil
- 1 tbsp. cajun seasoning
- 1 zucchini, thick slices (half-moons)
- ¼ cup cooked Turkey
- Yellow squash, sliced half-moons
- ¼ tsp. kosher salt

Direction: Preparation Time: 10 minutes Cooking Time: 21 minutes Servings: 4

✓ In a bowl, mix the shrimp with Cajun seasoning.

✓ In another bowl, add zucchini, turkey, salt, squash,

and coat with oil.

✓ Let the air fryer preheat to 400°F

✓ Move the shrimp and vegetable mix to the fryer basket and cook for 3 minutes.

✓ Serve hot.

Nutrition: Calories: 284 Protein: 31g Fat: 14g

429) Crispy Air Fryer Fish

Ingredients:

- 2 tsp. old bay
- 4-6, cut in half, Whiting Fish fillets
- ¾ cup fine cornmeal
- ¼ cup flour
- 1 tsp. paprika
- ½ tsp. garlic powder 1 ½ tsp. salt
- ½ tsp. freshly ground black pepper

Direction: Preparation Time: 10 minutes Cooking Time: 17 minutes Servings: 4

✓ In a Ziploc bag, add all ingredients and coat the fish fillets with it.

✓ Spray oil on the basket of the air fryer and put the fish in it.

✓ Cook for ten minutes at 400°F. flip fish if necessary and coat with oil spray and cook for another seven-minute.

✓ Serve with salad green.

Nutrition: Calories: 254 Fat: 12.7g Protein: 17.5g

430) Air Fryer Lemon Cod

Ingredients:

- 1 cod fillet
- Dried parsley
- Kosher salt and pepper to taste
- Garlic powder
- 1 lemon

Direction: Preparation Time: 5 minutes Cooking Time: 10 minutes Servings: 1

✓ In a bowl, mix all ingredients and coat the fish fillet with spices.

✓ Slice the lemon and lay it at the bottom of the air fryer basket.

✓ Put spiced fish on top. Cover the fish with lemon slices.

✓ Cook for ten minutes at 375°F, the internal temperature of the fish should be 145°F.

✓ Serve with a micro green salad.

Nutrition: Calories: 101 Protein: 16g Fat: 1g

431) *Air Fryer Salmon Fillets*

Ingredients:

- ¼ cup low-fat Greek yogurt 2 salmon fillets
- 1 tbsp. fresh dill, chopped
- 1 lemon and lemon juice
- ½ tsp. garlic powder
- Kosher salt and pepper

Direction: Preparation Time: 5 minutes Cooking Time: 15 minutes Servings: 2

- ✓ Cut the lemon into slices and lay it at the bottom of the air fryer basket.
- ✓ Season the salmon with kosher salt and pepper. Put salmon on top of lemons.
- ✓ Let it cook at 330°F for 15 minutes. In the meantime, mix garlic powder, lemon juice, salt, pepper with yogurt and dill.
- ✓ Serve the fish with sauce.

Nutrition: Calories: 194 Protein: 25g Fat: 7g

432) *Air Fryer Fish & Chips*

Ingredients:

- 4 cups any fish fillet
- ¼ cup flour
- 1 cup whole-wheat breadcrumbs
- 1 egg
- 2 tbsp. oil
- Potatoes
- 1 tsp. salt

Direction: Preparation Time: 10 minutes Cooking Time: 35 minutes Servings: 4

- ✓ Cut the potatoes in fries. Then coat with oil and salt.
- ✓ Cook in the air fryer for 20 minutes at 400°F, toss the fries halfway through.
- ✓ In the meantime, coat fish in flour, then in the whisked egg, and finally in breadcrumbs mix. Place the fish in the air fryer and let it cook at 330°F for 15 minutes.
- ✓ Flip it halfway through, if needed.
- ✓ Serve with tartar sauce and salad green.

Nutrition: Calories: 409 Protein: 30g Fat: 11g

433) *Grilled Salmon with Lemon*

Ingredients:

- 2 tbsp. olive oil
- 2 Salmon fillets
- Lemon juice
- ¹/3 cup water
- ¹/3 cup gluten-free light soy sauce

- ¹/3 cup Honey Scallion slices
- Cherry tomato
- Freshly ground black pepper, garlic powder, Kosher salt to taste

Direction: Preparation Time: 10 minutes Cooking Time: 21 minutes Servings: 4

- ✓ Season salmon with pepper and salt
- ✓ In a bowl, mix honey, soy sauce, lemon juice, water, oil. Add salmon to this marinade and let it rest for at least 2 hours.
- ✓ Let the air fryer preheat at 180°C Place fish in the air fryer and cook for 8 minutes.
- ✓ Move to a dish and top with scallion slices.

Nutrition: Calories: 211 Protein: 15g Fat: 9g

434) *Air-Fried Fish Nuggets*

Ingredients:

- 2 cups fish fillets in cubes, skinless 1 egg, beaten
- 5 tbsp. flour
- 5 tbsp. water
- Kosher salt and pepper to taste
- Breadcrumbs mix
- 1 tbsp. Smoked paprika
- ¼ cup whole wheat breadcrumbs 1 tbsp. garlic powder

Direction: Preparation Time: 15 minutes Cooking Time: 10 minutes Servings: 4

- ✓ Season the fish cubes with kosher salt and pepper.
- ✓ In a bowl, add flour and gradually add water, mixing as you add.
- ✓ Then mix in the egg. And keep mixing but do not over mix.
- ✓ Coat the cubes in batter, then in the breadcrumb mix. Coat well
- ✓ Place the cubes in a baking tray and spray with oil.
- ✓ Let the air fryer preheat to 200°C.
- ✓ Place cubes in the air fryer and cook for 12 minutes or until well cooked and golden brown.
- ✓ Serve with salad greens.

Nutrition: Calories: 184 Protein: 19g Fat: 3.3g

435) *Garlic Rosemary Grilled Prawns*

Ingredients:

- ½ tbsp. melted butter
- Green capsicum, sliced
- 8 prawns
- Rosemary leaves
- Kosher salt and freshly ground black pepper

- *3–4 cloves of minced garlic*

Direction: Preparation Time: 6 minutes Cooking Time: 11 minutes Servings: 2

✓ *In a bowl, mix all the ingredients and marinate the prawns in it for at least 60 minutes or more*

✓ *Add 2 prawns and 2 slices of capsicum on each skewer.*

✓ *Let the air fryer preheat to 180°C. Cook for 5–6 minutes. Then change the temperature to 200°C and cook for another minute.*

✓ *Serve with lemon wedges.*

Nutrition: Calories: 194 Fat: 10g Carbohydrates: 12g

436) *Air-Fried Crumbed Fish*

Ingredients:

- *4 fish fillets*
- *4 tbsp. olive oil*
- *1 egg beaten*
- *¼ cup whole wheat breadcrumbs*

Direction: Preparation Time: 10 minutes Cooking Time: 13 minutes Servings: 2

✓ *Let the air fryer preheat to 180°C.*

✓ *In a bowl, mix breadcrumbs with oil. Mix well*

✓ *First, coat the fish in the egg mix (egg mix with water) then in the breadcrumb mix. Coat well Place in the air fryer, let it cook for 10–12 minutes.*

✓ *Serve hot with salad green and lemon.*

Nutrition: Calories: 254 Fat 12.7g Protein: 15.5g

437) *Parmesan Garlic Crusted Salmon*

Ingredients:

- *¼ cup whole wheat breadcrumbs*
- *4 cups salmon*
- *2 tbsp. butter melted*
- *¼ tsp. freshly ground black pepper*
- *¼ cup parmesan cheese, grated*
- *2 tsp. garlic, minced*
- *½ tsp. Italian seasoning*

Direction: Preparation Time: 5 minutes Cooking Time: 15 minutes Servings: 2

✓ *Let the air fryer preheat to 400°F, spray the oil over the air fryer basket.*

✓ *Pat dries the salmon. In a bowl, mix Parmesan cheese, Italian seasoning, and breadcrumbs. In another pan, mix melted butter with garlic and add to the breadcrumbs mix. Mix well*

✓ *Add kosher salt and freshly ground black pepper to salmon. On top of every salmon piece, add the crust*

mix and press gently.

✓ *Let the air fryer preheat to 400°F and add salmon to it. Cook until done to your liking.*

✓ *Serve hot with vegetable side dishes.*

Nutrition: Calories: 330 Fat 19g Protein: 31g

438) *Air Fryer Salmon with Maple Soy Glaze*

Ingredients:

- *3 tbsp. pure maple syrup*
- *3 tbsp. gluten-free soy sauce*
- *1 tbsp. sriracha hot sauce*
- *1 clove of minced garlic*
- *4 fillets salmon, skinless*

Direction: Preparation Time: 6 minutes Cooking Time: 8 minutes Servings: 4

✓ *In a Ziploc bag, mix sriracha, maple syrup, garlic, and soy sauce with salmon.*

✓ *Mix well and let it marinate for at least half an hour.*

✓ *Let the air fryer preheat to 400°F with oil spray the basket*

✓ *Take fish out from the marinade, pat dry.*

✓

Put the salmon in the air fryer, cook for 7 to 8 minutes, or longer.

✓ *In the meantime, in a saucepan, add the marinade, let it simmer until reduced to half.*

✓ *Add glaze over salmon and serve.*

Nutrition: Calories: 292 Protein: 35g Fat: 11g

439) *Air Fried Cajun Salmon*

Ingredients:

- *1-piece fresh salmon*
- *2tbsp. cajun seasoning*
- *Lemon juice*

Direction: Preparation Time: 10 minutes Cooking Time: 21 minutes Servings: 1

✓ *Let the air fryer preheat to 180°C.*

✓ *Pat dries the salmon fillet. Rub lemon juice and Cajun seasoning over the fish fillet. Place in the air fryer, cook for 7 minutes. Serve with salad greens and lime wedges.*

Nutrition: Calories: 216 Fat 19g Protein: 19.2g

440) *Air Fryer Shrimp Scampi*

Ingredients:

- *4 cups raw Shrimp*

- 1 tbsp. lemon juice
- Chopped fresh basil
- 2 tsp. red pepper flakes
- 2.5 tbsp. butter
- Chopped chives
- tbsp. chicken stock
- 1 tbsp. minced garlic

Direction: Preparation Time: 5 minutes Cooking Time: 11 minutes Servings: 2

✓ Let the air fryer preheat with a metal pan to 330°F

✓ In the hot pan, add garlic, red pepper flakes, and half of the butter. Let it cook for 2 minutes.

✓ Add the butter, shrimp, chicken stock, minced garlic, chives, lemon juice, basil to the pan. Let it cook for 5 minutes. Bathe the shrimp in melted butter.

✓ Take out from the air fryer and let it rest for 1 minute.

✓ Add fresh basil leaves and chives and serve.

Nutrition: Calories: 287 Fat 5.5g Protein: 18g

441) *Sesame Seeds Fish Fillet*

Ingredients:

- 3 tbsp. plain flour
- 1 egg, beaten
- 5 frozen fish fillets

For Coating:

- 2 tbsp. oil
- ½ cup sesame seeds Rosemary herbs
- 5–6 biscuit's crumbs
- Kosher salt and pepper to taste

Direction: Preparation Time: 10 minutes Cooking Time: 22 minutes Servings: 2

✓ For 2 minutes, sauté the sesame seeds in a pan, without oil. Brown them and set it aside.

✓ On a plate, mix all coating ingredients

✓ Place the aluminum foil on the air fryer basket and let it preheat at 200°C.
First, coat the fish in flour. Then in egg, then in the coating mix.

✓ Place in the Air fryer. If fillets are frozen, cook for ten minutes, then turn the fillet and cook for another 4 minutes.

✓ If not frozen, then cook for eight minutes and 2 minutes.

Nutrition: Calories: 250 Fat: 8g Protein: 20g

442) *Mixed Chowder*

Ingredients:

- 1 lb. fish stew mix

- 2 cups white sauce
  3 tbsp. old bay seasoning

Direction: Preparation Time: 16 minutes Cooking Time: 35 minutes Servings: 2

✓ Mix all the ingredients in your Instant Pot.

✓ Cook on Stew for 35 minutes.

✓ Release the pressure naturally.

Nutrition: Calories: 320 Fat: 16g Protein: 41g

443) *Lemon Pepper Shrimp in Air Fryer*

Ingredients:

- 1 ½ cup peeled raw shrimp, deveined
- ½ tbsp. olive oil
- ¼ tsp. garlic powder
- 1 tsp. lemon pepper
- ¼ tsp. paprika
- 1 lemon, juiced

Direction: Preparation Time: 6 minutes Cooking Time: 11 minutes Servings: 2

✓ Let the air fryer preheat to 400°F

✓ In a bowl, mix lemon pepper, olive oil, paprika, garlic powder, and lemon juice. Mix well. Add shrimps and coat well
Add shrimps in the air fryer, cook for 8 minutes and top with lemon slices and serve.

Nutrition: Calories: 237 Fat: 6g Protein: 36g

444) *Monk-Fish Curry*

Ingredients:

- ½ lb. monk-fish
- 1 thinly sliced sweet yellow onion
- ½ cup chopped tomato
- 3 tbsp. strong curry paste
- 1 tbsp. oil or ghee

Direction: Preparation Time: 15 minutes Cooking Time: 21 minutes Servings: 2

✓ Set the Instant Pot to sauté and add the onion, oil, and curry paste.

✓ When the onion is soft, add the remaining ingredients and seal.

✓ Cook on Stew for 20 minutes.

✓ Release the pressure naturally.

Nutrition: Calories: 270 Protein: 45g Fat: 11g

445) *Salmon Bake*

Ingredients:

- 1 lb. salmon

- *1 lb. chopped Mediterranean vegetables*
- *1 cup low sodium fish broth*
- *Half a lemon, juiced*
- *Sea salt as desired*

Direction: Preparation Time: 15 minutes Cooking Time: 15 minutes Servings: 2

✓ *Mix all the ingredients except the broth in a foil pouch.*
✓ *Place the pouch in the steamer basket of your Instant Pot.*
✓ *Pour the broth into your Instant Pot. Cook on Steam for 15 minutes.*
✓ *Release the pressure naturally.*

Nutrition: Calories: 260 Protein: 36g Fat: 12g

446) *Trout Bake*

Ingredients:

- *1 lb. trout fillets, boneless*
- *1 lb. chopped winter vegetables*
- *1 cup low sodium fish broth*
- *1 tbsp. mixed herbs*
- *Sea salt as desired*

Direction: Preparation Time: 10 minutes Cooking Time: 38 minutes Servings: 2

✓ *Mix all the ingredients except the broth in a foil pouch.*
✓ *Place the pouch in the steamer basket in your Instant Pot.*
✓ *Pour the broth into the Instant Pot.*
✓ *Cook on Steam for 35 minutes.*
✓ *Release the pressure naturally.*

Nutrition: Calories: 310 Fat: 12g Protein: 40g

447) *Tuna Sweetcorn Casserole*

Ingredients:

- *3 small tins of tuna*
- *½ lb. sweetcorn kernels*
- *1 lb. chopped vegetables*
- *1 cup low sodium vegetable broth*
- *2 tbsp. spicy seasoning*

Direction: Preparation Time: 16 minutes Cooking Time: 35 minutes Servings: 2

✓ *Mix all the ingredients in your Instant Pot.*
✓ *Cook on Stew for 35 minutes.*
✓ *Release the pressure naturally.*

Nutrition: Calories: 300 Fat: 9g Protein: 43g

448) *Swordfish Steak*

Ingredients:

- *1 lb. swordfish steak, whole*
- *1lb. chopped Mediterranean vegetables*
- *1 cup low sodium fish broth*
- *tbsp. soy sauce*

Direction: Preparation Time: 16 minutes Cooking Time: 35 minutes Servings: 2

✓ *Mix all the ingredients except the broth in a foil pouch.*
✓ *Place the pouch in the steamer basket for your Instant Pot.*
✓ *Pour the broth into the Instant Pot. Lower the steamer basket into the Instant Pot. Cook on Steam for 35 minutes.*
✓ *Release the pressure naturally.*

Nutrition: Calories: 270 Fat: 10g Protein: 48g

449) *Shrimp Coconut Curry*

Ingredients:

- *½ lb. cooked shrimp*
- *1 thinly sliced onion*
- *1 cup coconut yogurt 3 tbsp. curry paste*
- *1 tbsp. oil or ghee*

Direction: Preparation Time: 14 minutes Cooking Time: 25 minutes Servings: 2

✓ *Set the Instant Pot to sauté and add the onion, oil, and curry paste.*
✓ *When the onion is soft, add the remaining ingredients and seal.*
✓ *Cook on Stew for 20 minutes.*
✓ *Release the pressure naturally.*

Nutrition: Calories: 380 Fat: 22g Protein: 40g

450) *Tuna and Cheddar*

Ingredients:

- *3 small cans of tuna*
- *1 lb. finely chopped vegetables 1 cup low sodium vegetable broth*
- *½ cup shredded cheddar*

Direction: Preparation Time: 20 minutes Cooking Time: 31 minutes Servings: 2

✓ *Mix all the ingredients in your Instant Pot.*
✓ *Cook on Stew for 35 minutes.*
✓ *Release the pressure naturally.*

Nutrition: Calories: 320 Fat: 11g Protein: 37g

451)   *Chili Shrimp*

Ingredients:

- 1 ½ lb. cooked shrimp
- 1 lb. stir fry vegetables
- 1 cup ready-mixed fish sauce
- 2 tbsp. chili flakes

Direction: Preparation Time: 16 minutes Cooking Time: 35 minutes Servings: 2

✓ Mix all the ingredients in your Instant Pot.

✓ Cook on Stew for 35 minutes.

✓ Release the pressure naturally.

Nutrition: Calories: 270 Fat: 8g Protein: 51g

452)   *Sardine Curry*

Ingredients:

- 5 tins of sardines in tomato
- 1 lb. chopped vegetables
- 1 cup low sodium fish broth
- 3 tbsp. curry paste

Direction: Preparation Time: 15 minutes Cooking Time: 35 minutes Servings: 2

✓ Mix all the ingredients in your Instant Pot.

✓ Cook on Stew for 35 minutes
   Release the pressure naturally.

Nutrition: Calories: 320 Fat: 16g Protein: 42g

453)   *Mussels and Spaghetti Squash*

Ingredients:

- 1 lb. cooked, shelled mussels
- ½ a spaghetti squash, to fit the Instant Pot
- 1 cup low sodium fish broth
- 3 tbsp. crushed garlic
- sea salt to taste

Direction: Preparation Time: 14 minutes Cooking Time: 35 minutes Servings: 2

✓ Mix the mussels with garlic and salt.

✓ Place the mussels inside the squash.

✓ Lower the squash into your Instant Pot.

✓ Pour the broth around it.
   Cook on Stew for 35 minutes.

✓ Release the pressure naturally.

✓ Shred the squash, mixing the "spaghetti" with the mussels.

Nutrition: Calories: 265 Fat: 9g Protein: 48g

454)   *Cod in WhiteSource*

Ingredients:

- 1 lb. cod fillets
- 1 lb. chopped swede and carrots
- 2 cups white sauce
- 1 cup peas
- 3 tbsp. black pepper

Direction: Preparation Time: 16 minutes Cooking Time: 5 minutes Servings: 2

✓ Mix all the ingredients in your Instant Pot.

✓ Cook on Stew for 5 minutes.
   Release the pressure naturally.

Nutrition: Calories: 390 Fat: 26g Protein: 41g

455)   *Cod in Parsley Sauce*

Ingredients:

- 1 lb. boneless, skinless cod fillets
- ½ lb green peas
- 1 cup white sauce
- A lemon, juiced
- 2 tbsp. dry parsley

Direction: Preparation Time: 17 minutes Cooking Time: 5 minutes Servings: 2

✓ Mix all the ingredients in your Instant Pot.

✓ Cook on Stew for 35 minutes.
   Release the pressure naturally.

Nutrition: Calories: 330 Fat: 19g Protein: 40g

456)   *Shrimp with Tomatoes and Feta*

Ingredients:

- 3 tomatoes, coarsely chopped
- ½ cup chopped sun-dried tomatoes
- 2 tsp. minced garlic
- 2 tsp. extra-virgin olive oil
- 1tsp. chopped fresh oregano
   Freshly ground black pepper
- 1½ pounds (16–20 count) shrimp, peeled, deveined, tails removed
- 4 tsp. freshly squeezed lemon juice
- ½ cup low-sodium feta cheese, crumbled

Direction: Preparation Time: 10 minutes Cooking Time: 30 minutes Servings: 4

✓ Heat the oven to 450°F.

✓ In a medium bowl, toss the tomatoes, sun-dried tomatoes, garlic, oil, and oregano until well combined.

✓ Season the mixture lightly with pepper.

✓ Transfer the tomato mixture to a 9-by-13-inch glass baking dish.
Bake until softened, about 15 minutes.

✓ Stir the shrimp and lemon juice into the hot tomato mixture and top evenly with the feta.

✓ Bake until the shrimp are cooked through, about 15 minutes more.

Nutrition: Calories: 306 Fat: 11g Protein: 39g

457)   *Orange-Infused Scallops*

Ingredients:

- lb. sea scallops Sea salt
- Freshly ground black pepper
- 2 tbsp. extra-virgin olive oil
- 1 tbsp. minced garlic
- ¼ cup freshly squeezed orange juice
- 1 tsp. orange zest
- 2 tsp. chopped fresh thyme, for garnish

Direction: Preparation Time: 10 minutes Cooking Time: 12 minutes Servings: 4

✓ Clean the scallops and pat them dry with paper towels, then season them lightly with salt and

✓ pepper.

✓ Place a large skillet over medium-high heat and add the olive oil.

✓ Sauté the garlic until it is softened and translucent, about 3 minutes.

✓ Add the scallops to the skillet and cook until they are lightly seared and just cooked through, turning once, about 4 minutes per side.

✓ Transfer the scallops to a plate, cover them to keep warm, and set them aside.

✓ Add the orange juice and zest to the skillet and stir to scrape up any cooked bits.

✓ Spoon the sauce over the scallops and serve, garnished with the thyme.

Nutrition: Calories: 267 Fat: 8g Protein: 38g

458)   *Crab Cakes with Honeydew Melon Salsa*

Ingredients:

For The Salsa:
- 1 cup finely chopped honeydew melon
- 1 scallion, white and green parts, finely chopped
- 1 red bell pepper, seeded, finely chopped
- 1 tsp. chopped fresh thyme Pinch sea salt
- Pinch freshly ground black pepper

For The Crab Cakes:
- 1 lb. lump crabmeat, drained and picked over
- ¼ cup finely chopped red onion
- ¼ cup panko bread crumbs
- 1 tbsp. chopped fresh parsley
- 1 tsp. lemon zest
- 1 egg
- ¼ cup whole-wheat flour Nonstick cooking spray

Direction: Preparation Time: 90 minutes Cooking Time: 13 minutes Servings: 4

✓ For The Salsa:

✓ In a small bowl, stir together the melon, scallion, bell pepper, and thyme.

✓ Season the salsa with salt and pepper and set aside.

✓ For The Crab Cakes:

✓ In a medium bowl, mix together the crab, onion, bread crumbs, parsley,

✓ lemon zest, and egg until very well combined.

✓ Divide the crab mixture into 8 equal portions and form them into patties about ¾-inch thick.

✓ Chill the crab cakes in the refrigerator for at least 1 hour to firm them up.

✓ Dredge the chilled crab cakes in the flour until lightly coated, shaking off any excess flour.

✓ Place a large skillet over medium heat and lightly coat it with cooking spray.

✓ Cook the crab cakes until they are golden brown, turning once, about 5 minutes per side.

✓ Serve warm with the salsa.

Nutrition: Calories: 232 Fat: 3g Protein: 32g

459)   *Seafood Stew*

Ingredients:

- tbsp. extra-virgin olive oil
- 1 sweet onion, chopped
- 2 tsp. minced garlic
- 3 celery stalks, chopped
- 2 carrots, peeled and chopped
- (28 oz.) can sodium-free diced tomatoes, undrained
- 3 cups low-sodium chicken broth
- ½ cup clam juice
- ¼ cup dry white wine
- 2 tsp. chopped fresh basil
- 2 tsp. chopped fresh oregano
- 2 (4 oz.) haddock fillets, cut into 1-inch chunks
- 1 lb. mussels, scrubbed, debearded
- 8 oz. (16–20 count) shrimp, peeled, deveined, quartered
- Sea salt
- Freshly ground black pepper

- *2 tbsp. chopped fresh parsley*

Direction: Preparation Time: 20 minutes Cooking Time: 31 minutes Servings: 6

✓ *Place a large saucepan over medium-high heat and add the olive oil.*

✓ *Sauté the onion and garlic until softened and translucent, about 3 minutes.*

✓ *Stir in the celery and carrots and sauté for 4 minutes.*

✓ *Stir in the tomatoes, chicken broth, clam juice, white wine, basil, and oregano.*

✓ *Bring the sauce to a boil, then reduce the heat to low. Simmer for 15 minutes.*

✓ *Add the fish and mussels, cover, and cook until the mussels open, about 5 minutes.*

✓ *Discard any unopened mussels.*

✓ *Add the shrimp to the pan and cook until the shrimp are opaque, about 2 minutes.*

✓ *Season with salt and pepper.*

✓ *Serve garnished with the chopped parsley.*

Nutrition: Calories: 248 Fat: 7g Protein: 28g

460) *Sole Piccata*

Ingredients:

- *1 tsp. extra-virgin olive oil*
- *4 (5 oz.) sole fillets, patted dry*
- *3 tbsp. butter*
- *2 tsp. minced garlic*
  2 tbsp. all-purpose flour
- *2 cups low-sodium chicken broth*
- *½ lemon, juiced and zested 2 tbsp. capers*

Direction: Preparation Time: 10 minutes Cooking Time: 22 minutes Servings: 4

✓ *Place a large skillet over medium-high heat and add the olive oil.*

✓ *Pat the sole fillets dry with paper towels then pan-sear them until the fish flakes easily when tested with a fork, about 4 minutes on each side. Transfer the fish to a plate and set it aside.*

✓ *Return the skillet to the stove and add the butter.*

✓ *Sauté the garlic until translucent, about 3 minutes.*

✓ *Whisk in the flour to make a thick paste and cook, stirring constantly, until the mixture is golden brown, about 2 minutes.*

✓ *Whisk in the chicken broth, lemon juice, and lemon zest.*

✓ *Cook until the sauce has thickened, about 4 minutes.*

✓ *Stir in the capers and serve the sauce over the fish.*

Nutrition: Calories: 271 Fat: 13g Protein: 30g

461) *Spicy Citrus Sole*

Ingredients:

- *1 tsp. chili powder 1 tsp. garlic powder*
- *½ tsp. lime zest*
- *½ tsp. lemon zest*
- *¼ tsp. freshly ground black pepper*
- *¼ tsp. smoked paprika Pinch sea salt*
- *4 (6 oz.) sole fillets, patted dry*
- *1 tbsp. extra-virgin olive oil*
- *2 tsp. freshly squeezed lime juice*

Direction: Preparation Time: 10 minutes Cooking Time: 12 minutes Servings: 4

✓ *Preheat the oven to 450°F.*

✓ *Line a baking sheet with aluminum foil and set it aside.*

✓ *In a small bowl, stir together the chili powder, garlic powder, lime zest, lemon zest, pepper, paprika, and salt until well mixed.*

✓ *Pat the fish fillets dry with paper towels, place them on the baking sheet, and rub them lightly all over with the spice mixture.*

✓ *Drizzle the olive oil and lime juice on the top of the fish.*

✓ *Bake until the fish flakes when pressed lightly with a fork, about 8 minutes. Serve immediately.*

Nutrition: Calories: 184 Fat: 5g Protein: 32g

462) *Haddock with Creamy Cucumber Sauce*

Ingredients:

- *¼ cup 2 percent plain Greek yogurt*
- *½ English cucumber, grated, liquid squeezed out*
- *½ scallion, white and green parts, finely chopped*
- *2 tsp. chopped fresh mint*
- *1 tsp. honey*
- *Sea salt*
- *4 (5 oz.) haddock fillets*
- *Freshly ground black pepper*
- *Nonstick cooking spray*

Direction: Preparation Time: 10 minutes Cooking Time: 13 minutes Servings: 4

✓ *In a small bowl, stir together the yogurt, cucumber, scallion, mint, honey, and a pinch of salt. Set it aside.*

✓ *Pat the fish fillets dry with paper towels and season them lightly with salt and pepper.*

✓ *Place a large skillet over medium-high heat and spray lightly with cooking spray.*

✓ Cook the haddock, turning once, until it is just cooked through, about 5 minutes per side.

✓ Remove the fish from the heat and transfer to plates.

✓ Serve topped with the cucumber sauce.

Nutrition: Calories: 164 Fat: 2g Protein: 27g

463)   *Herb-Crusted Halibut*

Ingredients:

- 4 (5 oz.) halibut fillets
- Extra-virgin olive oil, for brushing
- ½ cup coarsely ground unsalted pistachios
- 1 tbsp. chopped fresh parsley
- 1 tsp. chopped fresh thyme
- 1 tsp. chopped fresh basil Pinch sea salt
- Pinch freshly ground black pepper

Direction: Preparation Time: 10 minutes Cooking Time: 21 minutes Servings: 4

✓ Preheat the oven to 350°F.

✓ Line a baking sheet with parchment paper.

✓ Pat the halibut fillets dry with a paper towel and place them on the baking sheet.

✓ Brush the halibut generously with olive oil.

✓ In a small bowl, stir together the pistachios, parsley, thyme, basil, salt, and pepper.

✓ Spoon the nut and herb mixture evenly on the fish, spreading it out so the tops of the fillets are covered.

✓ Bake the halibut until it flakes when pressed with a fork, about 20 minutes.

✓ Serve immediately.

Nutrition: Calories: 262 Fat: 11g Protein: 32g

464)   *Salmon Florentine*

Ingredients:

- 1 tsp. extra-virgin olive oil
- ½ sweet onion, finely chopped 1 tsp. minced garlic
- 3 cups baby spinach
- 1 cup kale, tough stems removed, torn into 3-inch pieces
- Sea salt
- Freshly ground black pepper
- 4 (5 oz.) salmon fillets
- Lemon wedges, for serving

Direction: Preparation Time: 10 minutes Cooking Time: 32 minutes Servings: 4

✓ Preheat the oven to 350°F.

✓ Place a large skillet over medium-high heat and add the oil.

✓ Sauté the onion and garlic until softened and translucent, about 3 minutes.

✓ Add the spinach and kale and sauté until the greens wilt, about 5 minutes.

✓ Remove the skillet from the heat and season the greens with salt and pepper.

✓ Place the salmon fillets so they are nestled in the greens and partially covered by them. Bake the salmon until it is opaque, about 20 minutes.

✓ Serve immediately with a squeeze of fresh lemon.

Nutrition: Calories: 281 Fat: 16g Protein: 29g

465)   *Baked Salmon with Lemon Sauce*

Ingredients:

- 4 (5 oz.) salmon fillets Sea salt
- Freshly ground black pepper
- 1 tbsp. extra-virgin olive oil
- ½ cup low-sodium vegetable broth
- 1 lemon, juiced and zested 1 tsp. chopped fresh thyme
- ½ cup fat-free sour cream
- 1 tsp. honey
- 1 tbsp. chopped fresh chives

Direction: Preparation Time: 10 minutes Cooking Time: 15 minutes Servings: 4

✓ Preheat the oven to 400°F.

✓ Season the salmon lightly on both sides with salt and pepper.

✓ Place a large ovenproof skillet over medium-high heat and add the olive oil.

✓ Sear the salmon fillets on both sides until golden, about 3 minutes per side.

✓ Transfer the salmon to a baking dish and bake until it is just cooked through, about 10 minutes.

✓ While the salmon is baking, whisk together the vegetable broth, lemon juice, zest, and thyme in a small saucepan over medium-high heat until the liquid reduces by about ¼, about 5 minutes.

✓ Whisk in the sour cream and honey.

✓ Stir in the chives and serve the sauce over the salmon.

Nutrition: Calories: 310 Fat: 18g Protein: 29g

466)   *Tomato Tuna Melts*

Ingredients:

- 1 (5 oz.) can chunk light tuna packed in water, drained
- 2 tbsp. plain nonfat Greek yogurt

- 2 tsp. freshly squeezed lemon juice
- 2 tbsp. finely chopped celery
- 1 tbsp. finely chopped red onion
- Pinch cayenne pepper
- large tomato, cut into ¾-inch-thick rounds
- ½ cup shredded cheddar cheese

Direction: Preparation Time: 6 minutes Cooking Time: 5 minutes Servings: 2

✓ Preheat the broiler to high.

✓ In a medium bowl, combine the tuna, yogurt, lemon juice, celery, red onion, and cayenne pepper. Stir well.

✓ Arrange the tomato slices on a baking sheet. Top each with some tuna salad and cheddar cheese.

✓ Broil for 3 to 4 minutes until the cheese is melted and bubbly. Serve.

Nutrition: Calories: 243 Fat: 10g Protein: 30g

467) *Peppercorn-Crusted Baked Salmon*

Ingredients:

- Nonstick cooking spray
- ½ tsp. freshly ground black pepper
- ¼ tsp. salt
- ½ lemon zested and juiced
- ¼ tsp. dried thyme
- 1 lb. salmon fillet

Direction: Preparation Time: 6 minutes Cooking Time: 22 minutes Servings: 4

✓ Preheat the oven to 425°F. Spray a baking sheet with nonstick cooking spray.

✓ In a small bowl, combine the pepper, salt, lemon zest and juice, and thyme. Stir to combine.

✓ Place the salmon on the prepared baking sheet, skin-side down. Spread the seasoning mixture evenly over the fillet.

✓ Bake for 15 to 20 minutes, depending on the thickness of the fillet, until the flesh flakes easily.

Nutrition: Calories: 163 Fat: 7g Protein: 23g

468) *Roasted Salmon with Honey-Mustard Sauce*

Ingredients:

- Nonstick cooking spray
- 2 tbsp. wholegrain mustard
- 1 tbsp. honey
- 2 garlic cloves, minced
- ¼ tsp. salt
- ¼ tsp. freshly ground black pepper
- 1 lb. salmon fillet

Direction: Preparation Time: 6 minutes Cooking Time: 21 minutes Servings: 4

✓ Preheat the oven to 425°F. Spray a baking sheet with nonstick cooking spray.

✓ In a small bowl, whisk together the mustard, honey, garlic, salt, and pepper.

✓ Place the salmon fillet on the prepared baking sheet, skin-side down. Spoon the sauce onto the salmon and spread evenly.

✓ Roast for 15 to 20 minutes, depending on the thickness of the fillet, until the flesh flakes easily.

Nutrition: Calories: 186 Protein: 23g Fat: 7g

469) *Ginger-Glazed Salmon and Broccoli*

Ingredients:

- Nonstick cooking spray
- 1 tbsp. low-sodium tamari or gluten-free soy sauce
- 1 lemon, juiced
- 1 tbsp. honey
- 1 (1-inch) piece fresh ginger, grated
- 1 garlic clove, minced
- 1 lb. salmon fillet
- ¼ tsp. Salt, divided
- ⅛ tsp. freshly ground black pepper
- 2 broccoli heads, cut into florets
- 1 tbsp. extra-virgin olive oil

Direction: Preparation Time: 10 minutes Cooking Time: 15 minutes Servings: 4

✓ Preheat the oven to 400°F. Spray a baking sheet with nonstick cooking spray.

✓ In a small bowl, mix the tamari, lemon juice, honey, ginger, and garlic. Set aside.

✓ Place the salmon skin-side down on the prepared baking sheet. Season with ⅛ tsp. of salt and pepper.

✓ In a large mixing bowl, toss the broccoli and olive oil. Season with the remaining ⅛ tsp. of salt. Arrange in a single layer on the baking sheet next to the salmon. Bake for 15 to 20 minutes until the salmon flakes easily with a fork and the broccoli is fork-tender.

✓ In a small pan over medium heat, bring the tamari ginger mixture to a simmer and cook for 1 to 2 minutes until it just begins to thicken.

✓ Drizzle the sauce over the salmon and serve.

Nutrition: Calories: 238 Fat: 11g Protein: 25g

470) *Roasted Salmon with Salsa Verde*

Ingredients:

- Nonstick cooking spray

- *8 oz. tomatillos, husks removed*
- *½ onion, quartered*
- *1 jalapeño or serrano pepper, seeded*
- *1 garlic clove, unpeeled*
- *1 tsp. extra-virgin olive oil*
- *½ tsp. salt, divided*
- *4 (4 oz.) wild-caught salmon fillets*
- *¼ tsp. freshly ground black pepper*
- *¼ cup chopped fresh cilantro*
- *1 lime, juiced*

Direction: Preparation Time: 6 minutes Cooking Time: 25 minutes Servings: 4

✓ *Preheat the oven to 425°F. Spray a baking sheet with nonstick cooking spray.*

✓ *In a large bowl, toss the tomatillos, onion, jalapeño, garlic, olive oil, and ¼ tsp. of salt to coat. Arrange in a single layer on the prepared baking sheet, and roast for about 10 minutes until just softened. Transfer to a dish or plate and set aside.*

✓ *Place the salmon fillets skin side down on the same baking sheet and season with the remaining salt and pepper. Bake for 12–15 min. until the fish is firm and flakes easily.*
Meanwhile, peel the roasted garlic and place it and the roasted vegetables in a blender or food processor. Add a scant ¼ cup water to the jar, and process until smooth.

✓ *Add the cilantro and lime juice and process until smooth. Serve the salmon topped with the salsa verde.*

Nutrition: Calories: 199 Fat: 9g Protein: 23g

471) *Baked Salmon with Garlic Parmesan Topping*

Ingredients:

- *¼ cup light mayonnaise*
- *2-3 cloves garlic, diced*
- *2 tbsp. parsley*
- *Salt and pepper*

Direction: Preparation time: 5 minutes, Cooking time: 20 minutes, Servings: 4

✓ *Reduce heat to low and add remaining ingredients. Stir until everything is melted and combined.*

✓ *Spread evenly over salmon and bake 15 minutes for thawed fish or 20 for frozen. Salmon is done when it flakes easily with a fork. Serve.*

Nutrition: Calories 408; Total Carbs 4g; Protein 41g; Fat 24g; Sugar 1g; Fiber 0g

472) *Blackened Shrimp*

Ingredients:

- *1 1/2 lbs. shrimp, peel & devein*
- *4 lime wedges*
- *4 tbsp. cilantro, chopped*

What you'll need from the store cupboard:

- *4 cloves garlic, diced*
- *1 tbsp. chili powder*
- *1 tbsp. paprika*
- *1 tbsp. olive oil*
- *2 tsp. Splenda brown sugar*
- *1 tsp. cumin*
- *1 tsp. oregano*
- *1 tsp. garlic powder*
- *1 tsp. salt*
- *1/2tsp. pepper*

Direction: Preparation time: 5 minutes Cooking time: 5 minutes Servings: 4

✓ *In a small bowl combine seasonings and Splenda brown sugar.*

✓ *Heat oil in a skillet over med-high heat. Add shrimp, in a single layer, and cook 1-2 minutes per side.*
Add seasonings, and cook, stirring, 30 seconds.

✓ *Serve garnished with cilantro and a lime wedge.*

Nutrition: Calories 252; Total Carbs 7g; Net Carbs 6g; Protein 39g; Fat 7g; Sugar 2g; Fiber 1g

473) *Cajun Catfish*

Ingredients:

- *4 (8 oz.) catfish fillets*
- *What you'll need from the store cupboard:*
- *2 tbsp. olive oil*
- *2 tsp. garlic salt*
- *2 tsp. thyme*
- *2 tsp. paprika*
- *1/2tsp. cayenne pepper*
- *1/2tsp. red hot sauce*
- *¼ tsp. black pepper*
- *Nonstick cooking spray*

Direction: Preparation time: 5 minutes Cooking time: 15 minutes Servings: 4

✓ *Heat oven to 450 degrees. Spray a 9x13-inch baking dish with cooking spray.*

✓ *In a small bowl whisk together everything but catfish. Brush both sides of fillets, using all the spice mix.*

✓ *Bake 10-13 minutes or until fish flakes easily with a*

fork. Serve.

Nutrition: Calories 366; Total Carbs 0g; Protein 35g; Fat 24g; Sugar 0g; Fiber 0g

474)   *Cajun Flounder & Tomatoes*

Ingredients:

- *4 flounder fillets*
- *2 1/2 cups tomatoes, diced*
- *¾ cup onion, diced*
- *¾ cup green bell pepper, diced*

What you'll need from the store cupboard:

- *2 cloves garlic, diced fine*
- *1 tbsp. Cajun seasoning*
- *1 tsp. olive oil*

Direction: Preparation time: 10 minutes Cooking time: 15 minutes Servings: 4

✓ *Heat oil in a large skillet over med-high heat. Add onion and garlic and cook 2 minutes, or until soft. Add tomatoes, peppers and spices, and cook 2-3 minutes until tomatoes soften.*
Lay fish over the top. Cover, reduce heat to medium and cook, 5-8 minutes, or until fish flakes easily with a fork. Transfer fish to serving plates and top with sauce.

Nutrition: Calories 194; Total Carbs 8g; Net Carbs 6g; Protein 32g; Fat 3g; Sugar 5g; Fiber 2g

475)   *Cajun Shrimp & Roasted Vegetables*

Ingredients:

- *1 lb. large shrimp, peeled and deveined*
- *2 zucchinis, sliced*
- *2 yellow squash, sliced*
- *1/2 bunch asparagus, cut into thirds*
- *2 red bell pepper, cut into chunks*

What you'll need from store cupboard:

- *2 tbsp. olive oil*
- *2 tbsp. Cajun Seasoning*
- *Salt & pepper, to taste*

Direction: Preparation time: 5 minutes Cooking time: 15 minutes Servings: 4

✓ *Heat oven to 400 degrees.*

✓ *Combine shrimp and vegetables in a large bowl. Add oil and seasoning and toss to coat.*
Spread evenly in a large baking sheet and bake 15-20 minutes, or until vegetables are tender. Serve.

Nutrition: Calories 251; Total Carbs 13g; Net Carbs 9g; Protein 30g; Fat 9g; Sugar 6g; Fiber 4g

476)   *Cilantro Lime Grilled Shrimp*

Ingredients:

- *1 1/2 lbs. large shrimp raw, peeled, deveined with tails on*
- *Juice and zest of 1 lime*
- *2 tbsp. fresh cilantro chopped*

What you'll need from store cupboard:

- *¼ cup olive oil*
- *2 cloves garlic, diced fine*
- *1 tsp. smoked paprika*
- *¼ tsp. cumin*
- *1/2 teaspoon salt*
- *¼ tsp. cayenne pepper*

Direction: Preparation time: 5 minutes, Cooking time: 5 minutes, Servings: 6

✓ *Place the shrimp in a large Ziploc bag.*

✓ *Mix remaining ingredients in a small bowl and pour over shrimp. Let marinate 20-30 minutes. Heat up the grill. Skewer the shrimp and cook 2-3 minutes, per side, just until they turn to pick. Be careful not to overcook them. Serve garnished with cilantro.*

Nutrition: Calories 317; Total Carbs 4g; Protein 39g; Fat 15g; Sugar 0g; Fiber 0g

477)   *Crab Frittata*

Ingredients:

- *4 eggs*
- *2 cups lump crabmeat*
- *1 cup half-n-half*
- *1 cup green onions, diced*

What you'll need from store cupboard:

- *1 cup reduced-fat parmesan cheese, grated*
- *1 tsp. salt*
- *1 tsp. pepper*
- *1 tsp. smoked paprika*
- *1 tsp. Italian seasoning*
- *Nonstick cooking spray*

Direction: Preparation time: 10 minutes Cooking time: 50 minutes Servings: 4

✓ *Heat oven to 350 degrees. Spray an 8-inch springform pan, or pie plate with cooking spray.*

✓ *In a large bowl, whisk together the eggs and half-n-half. Add seasonings and parmesan cheese, stir to mix.*

✓ *Stir in the onions and crab meat. Pour into prepared pan and bake 35-40 minutes, or eggs are set and top is lightly browned.*

✓ *Let cool 10 minutes, then slice and serve warm or*

at room temperature.

Nutrition: Calories 276; Net Carbs 4g; Protein 25g; Fat 17g

478) Crunchy Lemon Shrimp

Ingredients:

- *1 lb. raw shrimp, peeled and deveined*
- *2 tbsp. Italian parsley, roughly chopped*
- *2 tbsp. lemon juice, divided*

What you'll need from the store cupboard:

- *2/3 cup panko bread crumbs*
- *21/2 tbsp. olive oil, divided*
- *Salt and pepper, to taste*

Direction: Preparation time: 5 minutes Cooking time: 10 minutes, Servings: 4

- ✓ *Heat oven to 400 degrees.*
- ✓ *Place the shrimp evenly in a baking dish and sprinkle with salt and pepper.*
- ✓ *Drizzle on 1 tablespoon lemon juice and 1 tablespoon of olive oil. Set aside.*
  In a medium bowl, combine parsley, remaining lemon juice, bread crumbs, remaining olive oil, and ¼ tsp. each of salt and pepper. Layer the panko mixture evenly on top of the shrimp.
- ✓ *Bake 8-10 minutes or until shrimp are cooked through and the panko is golden brown.*

Nutrition: Calories 283; Total Carbs 15g; Net Carbs 14g; Protein 28g; Fat 12g; Sugar 1g; Fiber 1g

479) Grilled Tuna Steaks

Ingredients:

- *6 6 oz. tuna steaks*
- *3 tbsp. fresh basil, diced*

What you'll need from the store cupboard:

- *4 1/2tsp. olive oil*
- *¾ tsp. salt*
- *¼ tsp. pepper*
- *Nonstick cooking spray*

Direction: Preparation time: 5 minutes Cooking time: 10 minutes, Servings: 6

- ✓ *Heat grill to medium heat. Spray rack with cooking spray.*
- ✓ *Drizzle both sides of the tuna with oil. Sprinkle with basil, salt and pepper.*
  Place on grill and cook 5 minutes per side, tuna should be slightly pink in the center. Serve.

Nutrition: Calories 343; Total Carbs 0g; Protein 51g; Fat 14g; Sugar 0g; Fiber 0g

480) Red Clam Sauce & Pasta

Ingredients:

- *1 onion, diced*
- *¼ cup fresh parsley, diced*
- *What you'll need from the store cupboard:*
- *2 6 1/2 oz. cans clams, chopped, undrained*
- *14 1/2 oz. tomatoes, diced, undrained*
- *6 oz. tomato paste*
- *2 cloves garlic, diced*
  1 bay leaf
- *1 tbsp. sunflower oil*
- *1 tsp. Splenda*
- *1 tsp. basil*
- *1/2tsp. thyme*
- *1/2 Homemade Pasta, cook & drain*

Direction: Preparation time: 10 minutes, Cooking time: 3 hours, Servings: 4

- ✓ *Heat oil in a small skillet over med-high heat. Add onion and cook until tender,*
- ✓ *Add garlic and cook 1 minute more. Transfer to crockpot.*
  Add remaining ingredients, except pasta, cover and cook on low 3-4 hours.
- ✓ *Discard bay leaf and serve over cooked pasta.*

Nutrition: Calories 223; Total Carbs 32g; Net Carbs 27g; Protein 12g; Fat 6g; Sugar 15g Fiber 5g

481) Salmon Milano

Ingredients:

- *2 1/2 lb. salmon filet*
- *2 tomatoes, sliced*
- *1/2 cup margarine*
  What you'll need from store cupboard:
- *1/2 cup basil pesto*

Direction: Preparation time: 10 minutes,

Cooking time: 20 minutes, Servings: 6

- ✓ *Heat the oven to 400 degrees. Line a 9x15-inch baking sheet with foil, making sure it covers the sides. Place another large piece of foil onto the baking sheet and place the salmon filet on top of it.*
- ✓ *Place the pesto and margarine in a blender or food processor and pulse until smooth. Spread evenly over salmon.*
- ✓ *Place tomato slices on top.*
  Wrap the foil around the salmon, tenting around the top to prevent foil from touching the salmon as much as possible.
- ✓ *Bake 15-25 minutes, or salmon flakes easily with a fork. Serve.*

Nutrition: Calories 444; Total Carbs 2g; Protein 55g; Fat 24g; Sugar 1g; Fiber 0g

482)   *Shrimp & Artichoke Skillet*

Ingredients:

- 1 1/2 cups shrimp, peel & devein
- 2 shallots, diced
- 1 tbsp. margarine

What you'll need from the store cupboard

- 2 12 oz. jars artichoke hearts, drain & rinse
- 2 cups white wine
- 2 cloves garlic, diced fine

Direction: Preparation time: 5 minutes Cooking time: 10 minutes Servings: 4

✓ *Melt margarine in a large skillet over med-high heat. Add shallot and garlic and cook until they start to brown, stirring frequently.*
Add artichokes and cook 5 minutes. Reduce heat and add wine. Cook 3 minutes, stirring occasionally.

✓ *Add the shrimp and cook just until they turn pink. Serve.*

Nutrition: Calories 487; Total Carbs 26g; Net Carbs 17g; Protein 64g; Fat 5; Sugar 3g; Fiber 9g

483)   *Tuna Carbonara*

Ingredients:

- 1/2 lb. tuna fillet, cut in pieces
- 2 eggs
- 4 tbsp. fresh parsley, diced

What you'll need from the store cupboard:

- 1/2 Homemade Pasta, cook & drain,
- 1/2 cup reduced-fat parmesan cheese
- 2 cloves garlic, peeled
- 2 tbsp. extra virgin olive oil
- Salt & pepper, to taste

Direction: Preparation time: 5 minutes Cooking time: 25 minutes Servings: 4

✓ *In a small bowl, beat the eggs, parmesan and a dash of pepper.*

✓ *Heat the oil in a large skillet over med-high heat.*

✓ *Add garlic and cook until browned. Add the tuna and cook 2-3 minutes, or until tuna is almost cooked through. Discard the garlic.*
Add the pasta and reduce heat. Stir in egg mixture and cook, constantly stirring, 2 minutes if the sauce is too thick, thin with water, a little bit at a time, until it has a creamy texture.

✓ *Salt and pepper to taste and serve garnished with parsley.*

Nutrition: Calories 409; Total Carbs 7g; Net Carbs 6g; Protein 25g; Fat 30g; Sugar 3g; Fiber 1g

484)   *Mediterranean Fish Fillets*

Ingredients:

- 4 cod fillets
- 1 lb. grape tomatoes, halved
- 1 cup olives, pitted and sliced
- 2 tbsp. capers
- 1 tsp. dried thyme
- 2 tbsp. olive oil
- 1 tsp. garlic, minced
- Pepper
- Salt

Direction: Preparation Time: 10 minutes Cooking Time: 3 minutes Servings: 4

✓ *Pour 1 cup of water into the instant pot then place the steamer rack in the pot.*

✓ *Spray heat-safe baking dish with cooking spray.*

✓ *Add half grape tomatoes into the dish and season with pepper and salt.*

✓ *Arrange fish fillets on top of cherry tomatoes. Drizzle with oil and season with garlic, thyme, capers, pepper, and salt.*
Spread olives and remaining grape tomatoes on top of fish fillets.

✓ *Place dish on top of steamer rack in the pot.*

✓ *Seal pot with a lid and select manual and cook on high for 3 minutes.*

✓ *Once done, release pressure using quick release. Remove lid.*

✓ *Serve and enjoy.*

Nutrition: Calories 212; Fat 11.9 g; Carbs 7.1 g; Sugar 3 g; Protein 21.4 g; Cholesterol 55 mg

485)   *Lemony Salmon*

Ingredients:

- 1 pound salmon fillet, cut into 3 pieces
- 3 teaspoons fresh dill, chopped
- 5 tablespoons fresh lemon juice, divided
- Salt and ground black pepper, as required

Direction: Preparation Time: 10 minutesCooking Time: 3 Minutes Servings: 3

✓ *Arrange a steamer trivet in Instant Pot and pour ¼ cup of lemon juice.*

✓ *Season the salmon with salt and black pepper evenly.*

✓ *Place the salmon pieces on top of the trivet, skin side down and drizzle with remaining lemon juice.*

✓ *Now, sprinkle the salmon pieces with dill evenly. Close the lid and place the pressure valve to the "Seal" position.*

✓ *Press "Steam" and use the default time of 3 minutes.*

✓ Press "Cancel" and allow a "Natural" release.

✓ Open the lid and serve hot.

Nutrition: Calories 20 Fats 9.6g, Carbs 1.1g, Sugar 0.5g, Proteins 29.7g, Sodium 74mg

486) Shrimp with Green Beans

Ingredients:

- ¾ pound fresh green beans, trimmed
- 1 pound medium frozen shrimp, peeled and deveined
- 2 tablespoons fresh lemon juice
- 2 tablespoons olive oil
- Salt and ground black pepper, as required

Direction: Preparation Time: 10 minutesCooking Time: 2 Minutes Servings: 4

✓ Arrange a steamer trivet in the Instant Pot and pour a cup of water.

✓ Arrange the green beans on top of trivet in a single layer and top with shrimp.

✓ Drizzle with oil and lemon juice.

✓ Sprinkle with salt and black pepper.
Close the lid and place the pressure valve in the "Seal" position.

✓ Press "Steam" and just use the default time of 2 minutes.

✓ Press "Cancel" and allow a "Natural" release.

✓ Open the lid and serve.

Nutrition: Calories 223, Fats 1g, Carbs 7.9g, Sugar 1.4g, Proteins 27.4g, Sodium 322mg

487) Crab Curry

Ingredients:

- 0.5lb chopped crab
- 1 thinly sliced red onion
- 0.5 cup chopped tomato
- 3tbsp curry paste
- 1tbsp oil or ghee

Direction: Preparation Time: 10 minutesCooking Time: 20 Minutes Servings: 2

✓ Set the Instant Pot to sauté and add the onion, oil, and curry paste.

✓ When the onion is soft, add the remaining ingredients and seal.
Cook on Stew for 20 minutes.

✓ Release the pressure naturally.

Nutrition: Calories 2; Carbs 11; Sugar 4; Fat 10; Protein 24; GL 9

488) Mixed Chowder

Ingredients:

- 1lb fish stew mix
- 2 cups white sauce
- 3tbsp old bay seasoning

Direction: Preparation Time: 10 minutesCooking Time: 35 Minutes Servings: 2

✓ Mix all the ingredients in your Instant Pot.

✓ Cook on Stew for 35 minutes.
Release the pressure naturally.

Nutrition: : Calories 320; Carbs 9; Sugar 2; Fat 16; Protein GL 4

489) Mussels in Tomato Sauce

Ingredients:

- 2 tomatoes, seeded and chopped finely
- 2 pounds mussels, scrubbed and de-bearded
- 1 cup low-sodium chicken broth
- 1 tablespoon fresh lemon juice
- 2 garlic cloves, minced

Direction: Preparation Time: 10 minutes

Cooking Time: 3 Minutes Servings: 4

✓ In the pot of Instant Pot, place tomatoes, garlic, wine and bay leaf and stir to combine.

✓ Arrange the mussels on top.

✓ Close the lid and place the pressure valve in the "Seal" position.
Press "Manual" and cook under "High Pressure" for about 3 minutes.

✓ Press "Cancel" and carefully allow a "Quick" release.

✓ Open the lid and serve hot.

Nutrition: Calories 213, Fats 25.2g, Carbs 11g, Sugar 1. Proteins 28.2g, Sodium 670mg

490) Citrus Salmon

Ingredients:

- 4 (4-ounce) salmon fillets
- 1 cup low-sodium chicken broth
- 1 teaspoon fresh ginger, minced
- 2 teaspoons fresh orange zest, grated finely
- 3 tablespoons fresh orange juice
- 1 tablespoon olive oil
- Ground black pepper, as required

Direction: Preparation Time: 10 minutesCooking Time: 7 Minutes Servings: 4

✓ In Instant Pot, add all ingredients and mix.

✓ *Close the lid and place the pressure valve to the "Seal" position.*

✓ *Press "Manual" and cook under "High Pressure" for about 7 minutes.*
Press "Cancel" and allow a "Natural" release.

✓ *Open the lid and serve the salmon fillets with the topping of cooking sauce.*

Nutrition: Calories 190, Fats 10.5g, Carbs 1.8g, Sugar 1g, Proteins 22. Sodium 68mg

491) *Herbed Salmon*

Ingredients:

- *4 (4-ounce) salmon fillets*
- *¼ cup olive oil*
- *2 tablespoons fresh lemon juice*
- *1 garlic clove, minced*
- *¼ teaspoon dried oregano*
- *Salt and ground black pepper, as required*
- *4 fresh rosemary sprigs*
- *4 lemon slices*

Direction: Preparation Time: 10 minutes Cooking Time: 3 Minutes Servings: 4

✓ *For the dressing: in a large bowl, add oil, lemon juice, garlic, oregano, salt and black pepper and beat until well co combined.*

✓ *Arrange a steamer trivet in the Instant Pot and pour 11/2 cups of water in Instant Pot.*

✓ *Place the salmon fillets on top of trivet in a single layer and top with dressing.*

✓ *Arrange 1 rosemary sprig and 1 lemon slice over each fillet.*
Close the lid and place the pressure valve in "Seal" position.

✓ *Press "Steam" and just use the default time of 3 minutes.*

✓ *Press "Cancel" and carefully allow a "Quick" release.*

✓ *Open the lid and serve hot.*

Nutrition: Calories 262, Fats 17g, Carbs 0.7g, Sugar 0.2g, Proteins 22.1g, Sodium 91mg

492) *Salmon in Green Sauce*

Ingredients:

- *4 (6-ounce) salmon fillets*
- *1 avocado, peeled, pitted and chopped*
- *1/2 cup fresh basil, chopped*
- *3 garlic cloves, chopped*
- *1 tablespoon fresh lemon zest, grated finely*

Direction: Preparation Time: 10 minutesCooking Time: 12 Minutes Servings: 4

✓ *Grease a large piece of foil.*

✓ *In a large bowl, add all ingredients except salmon and water and with a fork, mash completely.*

✓ *Place fillets in the center of foil and top with the avocado mixture evenly.*

✓ *Fold the foil around fillets to seal them.*

✓ *Arrange a steamer trivet in the Instant Pot and pour 1/2 cup of water.*

✓ *Place the foil packet on top of the trivet.*

✓ *Close the lid and place the pressure valve to the "Seal" position.*
Press "Manual" and cook under "High Pressure" for about minutes.

✓ *Meanwhile, preheat the oven to the broiler.*

✓ *Press "Cancel" and allow a "Natural" release.*

✓ *Open the lid and transfer the salmon fillets onto a broiler pan.*

✓ *Broil for about 3-4 minutes.*

✓ *Serve warm.*

Nutrition: Calories 333, Fats 20.3g, Carbs 5.5g, Sugar 0.4g, Proteins 34.2g, Sodium 79mg

493) *Braised Shrimp*

Ingredients:

- *1 pound frozen large shrimp, peeled and deveined*
- *2 shallots, chopped*
- *¾ cup low-sodium chicken broth*
- *2 tablespoons fresh lemon juice*
- *2 tablespoons olive oil*
- *1 tablespoon garlic, crushed*
- *Ground black pepper, as required*

Direction: Preparation Time: 10 minutes Cooking Time: 4 Minutes Servings: 4

✓ *In the Instant Pot, place oil and press "Sauté." Now add the shallots and cook for about 2 minutes.*

✓ *Add the garlic and cook for about 1 minute.*

✓ *Press "Cancel" and stir in the shrimp, broth, lemon juice and black pepper.*

✓ *Close the lid and place the pressure valve to the "Seal" position.*
Press "Manual" and cook under "High Pressure" for about 1 minute.

✓ *Press "Cancel" and carefully allow a "Quick" release.*

✓ *Open the lid and serve hot.*

Nutrition: Calories 209, Fats 9g, Carbs 4.3g, Sugar 0.2g, Proteins 26.6g, Sodium 293mg

494) *Shrimp Coconut Curry*

Ingredients:

- *0.5lb cooked shrimp*
- *1 thinly sliced onion*
- *1 cup coconut yogurt*
- *3tbsp curry paste*
- *1tbsp oil or ghee*

Direction: Preparation Time: 10 minutes

Cooking Time: 20 Minutes Servings: 2

✓ *Set the Instant Pot to sauté and add the onion, oil, and curry paste.*

✓ *When the onion is soft, add the remaining ingredients and seal.*

✓ *Cook on Stew for 20 minutes.*

✓ *Release the pressure naturally.*

Nutrition: Calories: 380 Carbs 13; Sugar 4; Fat 22; Protein 40; GL 14

495) *Trout Bake*

Ingredients:

- *1lb trout fillets, boneless*
- *1lb chopped winter vegetables*
- *1 cup low sodium fish broth*
- *1tbsp mixed herbs*
- *sea salt as desired*

Direction: Preparation Time: 10 minutes Cooking Time: 35 Minutes Servings: 2

✓ *Mix all the ingredients except the broth in a foil pouch.*

✓ *Place the pouch in the steamer basket your Instant Pot.*

✓ *Pour the broth into the Instant Pot.*

✓ *Cook on Steam for 35 minutes.*

✓ *Release the pressure naturally.*

Nutrition: : Calories 310; Carbs 14; Sugar 2; Fat 12; Protein 40; GL 5

496) *Sardine Curry*

Ingredients:

- *5 tins of sardines in tomato*
- *1lb chopped vegetables*
- *1 cup low sodium fish broth*
- *3tbsp curry paste*

Direction: Preparation Time: 10 minutes

Cooking Time: 35 Minutes Servings: 2

✓ *Mix all the ingredients in your Instant Pot.*

✓ *Cook on Stew for 35 minutes.*

Release the pressure naturally.

Nutrition: Calories 320; Carbs 8; Sugar 2; Fat 16; Protein GL 3

497) *Swordfish Steak*

Ingredients:

- *1lb swordfish steak, whole*
- *1lb chopped Mediterranean vegetables*
- *1 cup low sodium fish broth*
- *2tbsp soy sauce*

Direction: Preparation Time: 10 minutes

Cooking Time: 35 Minutes Servings: 2

✓ *Mix all the ingredients except the broth in a foil pouch.*

✓ *Place the pouch in the steamer basket for your Instant Pot.*

✓ *Pour the broth into the Instant Pot. Lower the steamer basket into the Instant Pot. Cook on Steam for 35 minutes.*

✓ *Release the pressure naturally.*

Nutrition: Calories 270; Carbs 5; Sugar 1; Fat 10; Protein 48; GL 1

498) *Lemon Sole*

Ingredients:

- *1lb sole fillets, boned and skinned*
- *1 cup low sodium fish broth*
- *2 shredded sweet onions*
- *juice of half a lemon*
- *2tbsp dried cilantro*

Direction: Preparation Time: 10 minutes

Cooking Time: 5 Minutes Servings: 2

✓ *Mix all the ingredients in your Instant Pot.*

✓ *Cook on Stew for 5 minutes. Release the pressure naturally.*

Nutrition: Calories 230; Carbs Sugar 1; Fat 6; Protein 46; GL 1

499) *Tuna Sweet corn Casserole*

Ingredients:

- *3 small tins of tuna*
- *0.5lb sweet corn kernels*
- *1lb chopped vegetables*
- *1 cup low sodium vegetable broth*
- *2tbsp spicy seasoning*

Direction: Preparation Time: 10 minutes Cooking Time: 35 Minutes Servings: 2

✓ *Mix all the ingredients in your Instant Pot.*

✓ Cook on Stew for 35 minutes.

✓ Release the pressure naturally.

Nutrition: Calories: 300;Carbs: 6 ;Sugar: 1 ;Fat: 9 ;Protein: ;GL: 2

500) *Lemon Pepper Salmon*

Ingredients:

- 3 tbsps. ghee or avocado oil
- 1 lb. skin-on salmon filet
- 1 julienned red bell pepper
- 1 julienned green zucchini
- 1 julienned carrot
- ¾ cup water
- A few sprigs of parsley, tarragon, dill, basil or a combination
- 1/2 sliced lemon
- 1/2 tsp. black pepper
- ¼ tsp. sea salt

Direction: Preparation Time: 10 minutesCooking Time: 10 Minutes Servings: 4

✓ Add the water and the herbs into the bottom of the Instant Pot and put in a wire steamer rack making sure the handles extend upwards.

✓ Place the salmon filet onto the wire rack, with the skin side facing down.

✓ Drizzle the salmon with ghee, season with black pepper and salt, and top with the lemon slices.

✓ Close and seal the Instant Pot, making sure the vent is turned to "Sealing."

✓ Select the "Steam" setting and cook for 3 minutes.

✓ While the salmon cooks, julienne the vegetables and set them aside.
Once done, quickly release the pressure, and then press the "Keep Warm/Cancel" button.

✓ Uncover and wearing oven mitts, carefully remove the steamer rack with the salmon.

✓ Remove the herbs and discard them.

✓ Add the vegetables to the pot and put the lid back on.

✓ Select the "Sauté" function and cook for 1-2 minutes.

✓ Serve the vegetables with salmon and add the remaining fat to the pot.

✓ Pour a little of the sauce over the fish and vegetables if desired.

Nutrition: Cal 296, Carbs 8g, Fat 15 g, Protein 31 g,

501) *Almond Crusted Baked Chili Mahi Mahi*

Ingredients:

- 4 mahimahi fillets 1 lime

- 2 teaspoons olive oil Salt and pepper to taste
- ½ cup almonds
- ¼ teaspoon paprika
- ¼ teaspoon onion powder
- ¾ teaspoon chili powder
- ½ cup red bell pepper, chopped
- ¼ cup onion, chopped
- ¼ cup fresh cilantro, chopped

Direction: Preparation Time: 20 minutes Cooking Time: 15 minutes Servings: 4

✓ Preheat your oven to 325 degrees F. Line your baking pan with parchment paper. Squeeze juice from the lime.

✓ Grate zest from the peel. Put juice and zest in a bowl. Add the oil, salt and pepper. In another bowl, add the almonds, paprika, onion powder and chili powder.

✓ Put the almond mixture in a food processor. Pulse until powdery.
Dip each fillet in the oil mixture.

✓ Dredge with the almond and chili mixture.

✓ Arrange on a single layer in the oven—Bake for 12 to 15 minutes or until fully cooked.

✓ Serve with red bell pepper, onion and cilantro.

Nutrition: Calories 322 Total Fat 12 g Saturated Fat 2 g Cholesterol 83 mg Sodium 328 mg Total Carbohydrate 28 g Dietary Fiber 4 g Total Sugars 10 g Protein 28 g Potassium 829 mg

502) *Salmon & Asparagus*

Ingredients:

- 2 salmon fillets
- 8 spears asparagus, trimmed
- 2 tablespoons balsamic vinegar
- 1 teaspoon olive oil
- 1 teaspoon dried dill
- Salt and pepper to taste

Direction: Preparation Time: 15 minutes Cooking Time: 10 minutes Servings: 2

✓ Preheat your oven to 325 degrees F.

✓ Dry salmon with paper towels.

✓ Arrange the asparagus around the salmon fillets on a baking pan. In a bowl, mix the rest of the ingredients.

✓ Pour mixture over the salmon and vegetables.

✓ Bake in the oven for 10 minutes or until the fish is fully cooked.

Nutrition: Calories 328 Total Fat 15 g Saturated Fat 3 g Cholesterol 67 mg Sodium 365 mg Total Carbohydrate 6 g Dietary Fiber 4 g Total Sugars 5 g Protein 28 g Potassium 258 mg

503) Halibut with Spicy Apricot Sauce

Ingredients:

- 4 fresh apricots, pitted
- ⅓ cup apricot preserves
- ½ cup apricot nectar
- ½ teaspoon dried oregano
- 3 tablespoons scallion, sliced
- 1 teaspoon hot pepper sauce Salt to taste
- 4 halibut steaks
- 1 tablespoon olive oil

Direction: Preparation Time: 15 minutes Cooking Time: 17 minutes Servings: 4

✓ Put the apricots, preserves, nectar, oregano, scallion, hot pepper sauce and salt in a saucepan.

✓ Bring to a boil and then simmer for 8 minutes. Set aside.

✓ Brush the halibut steaks with olive oil. Grill for 7 to 9 minutes or until the fish is flaky

✓ Brush one tablespoon of the sauce on both sides of the fish. Serve with the reserved sauce.

Nutrition:: Calories 304 Total Fat 8 g Saturated Fat 1 g Cholesterol 73 mg Sodium 260 mg Total Carbohydrate 27 g Dietary Fiber 2 g Total Sugars 16 g Protein 29 g Potassium 637 mg

504) Popcorn Shrimp

Ingredients:

- Cooking spray
- ½ cup all-purpose flour
- 2 eggs, beaten
- 2 tablespoons water
- 1 ½ cups panko breadcrumbs
- 1 tablespoon garlic powder
- ½ cup ketchup
- 2 tablespoons fresh cilantro, chopped
- 2 tablespoons lime juice Salt to taste
- 1 tablespoon ground cumin
- 1 lb. shrimp, peeled and deveined

Direction: Preparation Time: 15 minutes Cooking Time: 8 minutes Servings: 4

✓ Coat the air fryer basket with cooking spray

✓ Put the flour in a dish. In the second dish, beat the eggs and water.

✓ In the third dish, mix the breadcrumbs, garlic powder and cumin.

✓ Dip each shrimp in each of the three dishes, first in the dish with flour, then the egg and then the breadcrumb mixture. Place the shrimp in the air fryer basket.

✓ Cook at 360 degrees F for 8 minutes, flipping once halfway through.

✓ Combine the rest of the ingredients as dipping sauce for the shrimp.

Nutrition:Calories 297 Total Fat 4 g Saturated Fat 1 g Cholesterol 276 mg Sodium 291 mg Total Carbohydrate 35 g

505) Shrimp Lemon Kebab

Ingredients:

- 1 ½ lb. shrimp, peeled and deveined but with tails intact
- ⅓ cup olive oil
- ¼ cup lemon juice
- 2 teaspoons lemon zest
- 1 tablespoon fresh parsley, chopped
- 8 cherry tomatoes, quartered
- 2 scallions, sliced

Direction: Preparation Time: 10 minutes Cooking Time: 5 minutes Servings: 4

✓ Mix the olive oil, lemon juice, lemon zest and parsley in a bowl.

✓ Marinate the shrimp in this mixture for 15 minutes. Thread each shrimp into the skewers.

✓ Grill for 4 to 5 minutes, turning once halfway through.

✓ Serve with tomatoes and scallions.

Nutrition: Calories 271 Total Fat 12 g Saturated Fat 2 g Cholesterol 259 mg Sodium 255 mg Total Carbohydrate 4 g Dietary Fiber 1 g Total Sugars 1 g Protein 25 g Potassium 429 mg

506) Grilled Herbed Salmon with Raspberry Sauce & Cucumber Dill Dip

Ingredients:

- 3 salmon fillets
- 1 tablespoon olive oil
- Salt and pepper to taste
- 1 teaspoon fresh sage, chopped
- 1 tablespoon fresh parsley, chopped
- 2 tablespoons apple juice
- 1 cup raspberries
- 1 teaspoon Worcestershire sauce
- 1 cup cucumber, chopped
- 2 tablespoons light mayonnaise
- ½ teaspoon dried dill

Direction: Preparation Time: 15 minutes Cooking Time: 30 minutes Servings: 4

✓ Coat the salmon fillets with oil—season with salt, pepper, sage and parsley.

✓ Cover the salmon with foil.

✓ *Grill for 20 minutes or until the fish is flaky. While waiting, mix the apple juice, raspberries and Worcestershire sauce.*

✓ *Pour the mixture into a saucepan over medium heat. Bring to a boil and then simmer for 8 minutes.*

✓ *In another bowl, mix the rest of the ingredients.*

✓ *Serve salmon with raspberry sauce and cucumber dip.*

Nutrition: Calories 256 Total Fat 15 g Saturated Fat 3 g Cholesterol 68 mg Sodium 176 mg Total Carbohydrate 6 g Dietary Fiber 1 g Total Sugars 5 g Protein 23 g Potassium 359 mg

507) *Tarragon Scallops*

Ingredients:

- *1 cup water*
- *1 lb. asparagus spears, trimmed*
- *2 lemons*
- *1 ¼ lb. scallops*
- *Salt and pepper to taste*
- *1 tablespoon olive oil*
- *1 tablespoon fresh tarragon, chopped*

Direction: Preparation Time: 10 minutes Cooking Time: 15 minutes Servings: 4

✓ *Pour water into a pot. Bring to a boil. Add asparagus spears. Cover and cook for 5 minutes.*

✓ *Drain and transfer to a plate. Slice one lemon into wedges.*

✓ *Squeeze juice and shred zest from the remaining lemon.*

✓ *Season the scallops with salt and pepper. Put a pan over medium heat.*

✓ *Add oil to the pan.*

✓ *Cook the scallops until golden brown.*

✓ *Transfer to the same plate, putting scallops beside the asparagus.*

✓ *Add lemon zest, juice and tarragon to the pan. Cook for 1 minute.*

✓ *Drizzle tarragon sauce over the scallops and asparagus.*

Nutrition: Calories 253 Total Fat 12 g Saturated Fat 2 g Cholesterol 47 mg Sodium 436 mg Total Carbohydrate 14 g Dietary Fiber 5 g Total Sugars 3 g Protein 27 g Potassium 773 mg

508) *Garlic Shrimp & Spinach*

Ingredients:

- *3 tablespoons olive oil, divided*
- *6 clove garlic, sliced and divided*
- *1 lb. spinach Salt to taste*
  1 tablespoon lemon juice

- *1 lb. shrimp, peeled and deveined*
- *¼ teaspoon red pepper, crushed*
- *1 tablespoon parsley, chopped*
- *1 teaspoon lemon zest*

Direction: Preparation Time: 10 minutes Cooking Time: 10 minutes Servings: 4

✓ *Pour 1 tablespoon olive oil in a pot over medium heat.*

✓ *Cook the garlic for 1 minute.*

✓ *Add the spinach and season with salt.*

✓ *Cook for 3 minutes. Stir in lemon juice. Transfer to a bowl. Pour the remaining oil.*

✓ *Add the shrimp. Season with salt and add red pepper.*

✓ *Cook for 5 minutes.*

✓ *Sprinkle parsley and lemon zest over the shrimp before serving*

Nutrition: Calories 226 Total Fat 12 g Saturated Fat 2 g Cholesterol 183 mg Sodium 444 mg Total Carbohydrate 6 g Dietary Fiber 3 g Total Sugars 1 g Protein 26 g Potassium 963 mg

509) *Herring & Veggies Soup*

Ingredients:

- *2 tablespoons olive oil*
- *1 shallot, chopped*
- *2 small garlic cloves, minced*
- *1 jalapeño pepper, chopped*
- *1 head cabbage, chopped*
- *1 small red bell pepper, seeded and chopped finely*
- *1 small yellow bell pepper, seeded and chopped finely*
- *5 cups low-sodium chicken broth*
- *2 (4-ounce) boneless herring fillets, cubed*
- *¼ cup fresh cilantro, minced*
- *2 tablespoons fresh lemon juice*
- *Ground black pepper, as required*
- *2 scallions, chopped*

Direction: Preparation Time: 15 minutes Cooking Time: 25 minutes Servings: 5

✓ *In a large soup pan, heat the oil over medium heat and sauté shallot and garlic for 2-3 minutes.*

✓ *Add the cabbage and bell peppers and sauté for about 3-4 minutes.*

✓ *Add the broth and bring to a boil over high heat.*

✓ *Now, reduce the heat to medium-low and simmer for about 10 minutes.*
  Add the herring cubes and cook for about 5-6 minutes.

✓ Stir in the cilantro, lemon juice, salt and black pepper and cook for about 1-2 minutes.

✓ Serve hot with the topping of scallion.

✓ **Meal Prep Tip:**

✓ Transfer the soup into a large bowl and set it aside to cool. Divide the soup into 5 containers evenly. Cover the containers and refrigerate for 1-2 days. Reheat in the microwave before serving.

Nutrition: Calories 215 Total Fat 11.2g Saturated Fat 2.1 g Cholesterol 35 mg Total Carbs 14.7 g Sugar 7 g Fiber 4.5 g Sodium 152 mg Potassium 574 mg Protein 15.1 g

510)   Salmon Soup

Ingredients:

- 1 tablespoon olive oil
- 1 yellow onion, chopped
- 1 garlic clove, minced
- 4 cups low-sodium chicken broth
- 1 pound boneless salmon, cubed
- 2 tablespoon fresh cilantro, chopped
- Ground black pepper, as required
- 1 tablespoon fresh lime juice

Direction: Preparation Time: 15 minutes Cooking Time: 20 minutes Servings: 4

✓ In a large pan heat the oil over medium heat and sauté the onion for about 5 minutes.

✓ Add the garlic and sauté for about 1 minute.

✓ Stir in the broth and bring to a boil over high heat. Now, reduce the heat to low and simmer for about 10 minutes.
Add the salmon and soy sauce and cook for about 3-4 minutes. Stir in black pepper, lime juice, and cilantro and serve hot.

Meal Prep Tip:

✓ Transfer the soup into a large bowl and set it aside to cool.

✓ Divide the soup into 4 containers evenly.

✓ Cover the containers and refrigerate for 1-2 days. Reheat in the microwave before serving.

Nutrition: Calories 208 Total Fat 10.5 g Saturated Fat 1.5 g Cholesterol 50 mg Total Carbs 3.9 g Sugar 1.2 g Fiber 0.6 g Sodium 121 mg Potassium 331 mg Protein 24.4 g

511)   Salmon Curry

Ingredients:

- 6 (4-ounce) salmon fillets
- 1 teaspoon ground turmeric, divided Salt, as required
- 3 tablespoon olive oil, divided

- 1 yellow onion, chopped finely
- 1 teaspoon garlic paste
- 1 teaspoon fresh ginger paste
- 3-4 green chilies, halved
- 1 teaspoon red chili powder
- ½ teaspoon ground cumin
- ½ teaspoon ground cinnamon
- ¾ cup fat-free plain Greek yogurt, whipped
- ¾ cup filtered water 3 tablespoon fresh cilantro, chopped

Direction: Preparation Time: 15 minutes Cooking Time: 30 minutes Servings: 6

✓ Season each salmon fillet with ½ teaspoon of turmeric and salt.

✓ In a large skillet, melt 1 tablespoon of the butter over medium heat and cook the salmon fillets for about 2 minutes per side.

✓ Transfer the salmon onto a plate. In the same skillet, melt the remaining butter over medium heat and sauté the onion for about 4-5 minutes.

✓ Add the garlic paste, ginger paste, green chilies, remaining turmeric and spices and sauté for about 1 minute.
Now, reduce the heat to medium-low. Slowly add the yogurt and water, stirring continuously until smooth.

✓ Cover the skillet and simmer for about 10-15 minutes or until the desired doneness of the sauce.

✓ Carefully, add the salmon fillets and simmer for about 5 minutes. Serve hot with the garnishing of cilantro.

✓ **Meal Prep Tip:**

✓ Transfer the curry into a large bowl and set it aside to cool. Divide the curry into 6 containers evenly.

✓ Cover the containers and refrigerate for 1-2 days. Reheat in the microwave before serving.

Nutrition: Calories 242 Total Fat 14.3 g Saturated Fat 2 g Cholesterol 51 mg Total Carbs 4.1 g Sugar 2 g Fiber 0.8 g Sodium 98 mg Potassium 493 mg Protein 25.4 g

512)   Salmon with Bell Peppers

Ingredients:

- 6 (3-ounce) salmon fillets Pinch of salt
- Ground black pepper, as required
- 1 yellow bell pepper, seeded and cubed
- 1 red bell pepper, seeded and cubed, 4 plum tomatoes, cubed
- 1 small onion, sliced thinly
- ½ cup fresh parsley, chopped
- ¼ cup olive oil
- 2 tablespoons fresh lemon juice

Direction: Preparation Time: 15 minutes Cooking Time: 20 minutes Servings: 6

✓ Preheat the oven to 400 degrees F. Season each salmon fillet with salt and black pepper lightly. In a bowl, mix together the bell peppers, tomato and onion.

✓ Arrange 6 foil pieces onto a smooth surface. Place 1 salmon fillet over each foil paper and sprinkle with salt and black pepper.

✓ Place veggie mixture over each fillet evenly and top with parsley and capers evenly.
Drizzle with oil and lemon juice. Fold each foil around the salmon mixture to seal it. Arrange the foil packets onto a large baking sheet in a single layer.

✓ Bake for about 20 minutes. Serve hot.

✓ Transfer the salmon mixture into a large bowl and set aside to cool. Divide the salmon mixture into 6 containers evenly.

✓ Cover the containers and refrigerate for 1 day. Reheat in the microwave before serving.

Nutrition: Calories 220 Total Fat 14 g Saturated Fat 2 g Cholesterol 38 mg Total Carbs 7.7 g Sugar 4.8 g Fiber 2 g Sodium 74 mg Potassium 647 mg Protein 17.9 g

513) *Shrimp Salad*

Ingredients:

* For Salad: 1 pound shrimp, peeled and deveined
* Salt and ground black pepper, as required
* 1 teaspoon olive oil
* 1½ cups carrots, peeled and julienned
* 1½ cups red cabbage, shredded1
* ½ cup cucumber, julienned
* 5 cups fresh baby arugula
* ¼ cup fresh basil, chopped
* ¼ cup fresh cilantro, chopped
* 4 cups lettuce, torn
* ¼ cup almonds, chopped

For Dressing:
* 2 tablespoons natural almond butter
* 1 garlic clove, crushed
* 1 tablespoon fresh cilantro, chopped
* 1 tablespoon fresh lime juice
* 1 tablespoon unsweetened applesauce
* 2 teaspoons balsamic vinegar
* ½ teaspoon cayenne pepper Salt, as required
* 1 tablespoon water
* 1/3 cup olive oil

Direction: Preparation Time: 20 minutes Cooking Time: 4 minutes Servings: 6

✓ Slowly add the oil, beating continuously until

smooth. For the salad: in a bowl, add shrimp, salt, black pepper and oil and toss to coat well. Heat a skillet over medium-high heat and cook the shrimp for about 2 minutes per side.

✓ Remove from the heat and set aside to cool. In a large bowl, add the shrimp, vegetables and mix well. For the dressing: in a bowl, add all ingredients except oil and beat until well combined. Place the dressing over shrimp mixture and gently toss to coat well. Serve immediately.

✓ **Meal Prep Tip:**

✓ Divide dressing into 6 large mason jars evenly. Place the remaining ingredients in the layers of carrots, followed by cabbage, cucumber, arugula, basil, cilantro, shrimp, lettuce and almonds.

✓ Cover each jar with the lid tightly and refrigerate for about 1 day. Shake the jars well just before serving.

Nutrition: Calories 274 Total Fat 17.7 g Saturated Fat 2.4 g Cholesterol 159 mg Total Carbs 10 g Sugar 3.8 g Fiber 2.9 g Sodium 242 mg Potassium 481 mg Protein 20.5 g

514) *Shrimp & Veggies Curry*

Ingredients:

* 2 teaspoons olive oil
* 1½ medium white onions, sliced
* 2 medium green bell peppers, seeded and sliced
* 3 medium carrots, peeled and sliced thinly
* 3 garlic cloves, chopped finely
* 1 tablespoon fresh ginger, chopped finely
* 2½ teaspoons curry powder
* 1½ pounds shrimp, peeled and deveined
* 1 cup filtered water
* 2 tablespoons fresh lime juice
* Salt and ground black pepper, as required
* 2 tablespoons fresh cilantro, chopped

Direction: Preparation Time: 20 minutes Cooking Time: 20 minutes Servings: 6

✓ In a large skillet, heat oil over medium-high heat and sauté the onion for about 4-5 minutes.

✓ Add the bell peppers and carrot and sauté for about 3-4 minutes. Add the garlic, ginger and curry powder and sauté for about 1 minute.

✓ Add the shrimp and sauté for about 1 minute. Stir in the water and cook for about 4-6 minutes, stirring occasionally.
Stir in lime juice and remove from heat. Serve hot with the garnishing of cilantro.

Meal Prep Tip:

✓ Transfer the curry into a large bowl and set it aside to cool. Divide the curry into 6 containers evenly.

✓ Cover the containers and refrigerate for 1-2 days.

Reheat in the microwave before serving.

Nutrition: Calories 193 Total Fat 3.8 g Saturated Fat 0.9 g Cholesterol 239 mg Total Carbs 12 g Sugar 4.7 g Fiber 2.3 g Sodium 328 mg Potassium 437 mg Protein 27.1 g

515)   *Shrimp with Zucchini*

Ingredients:

- *3 tablespoons olive oil*
- *1 pound medium shrimp, peeled and deveined*
- *1 shallot, minced 4 garlic cloves, minced*
- *¼ teaspoon red pepper flakes, crushed*
- *Salt and ground black pepper, as required*
- *¼ cup low-sodium chicken broth*
- *2 tablespoons fresh lemon juice*
- *1 teaspoon fresh lemon zest, grated finely*
- *½ pound zucchini, spiralized with Blade C*

Direction: Preparation Time: 20 minutes Cooking Time: 8 minutes Servings: 4

- ✓ *In a large skillet, heat the oil and butter over medium-high heat and cook the shrimp, shallot, garlic, red pepper flakes, salt and black pepper for about 2 minutes, stirring occasionally.*
- ✓ *Stir in the broth, lemon juice and lemon zest and bring to a gentle boil.*
- ✓ *Stir in zucchini noodles and cook for about 1-2 minutes.*
  Serve hot.

Meal Prep Tip:

- ✓ *Transfer the shrimp mixture into a large bowl and set it aside to cool.*
- ✓ *Divide the shrimp mixture into 4 containers. Cover the containers and refrigerate for about 1-2 days.*
- ✓ *Reheat in microwave before serving.*

Nutrition: Calories 245 Total Fat 12.6 g Saturated Fat 2.2 g Cholesterol 239 mg Total Carbs 5.8 g Sugar 1.2 g Fiber 08 g Sodium 289 mg Potassium 381 mg Protein 27 g

516)   *Shrimp with Broccoli*

Ingredients:

- *2 tablespoons olive oil, divided*
- *4 cups broccoli, chopped*
- *2-3 tablespoons filtered water*
- *1½ pounds large shrimp, peeled and deveined*
- *2 garlic cloves, minced*
- *1 (1-inch) piece fresh ginger, minced*
- *Salt and ground black pepper, as required*

Direction: Preparation Time: 15 minutes Cooking Time: 12 minutes Servings: 6

- ✓ *: In a large skillet, heat 1 tablespoon of oil over*

medium-high heat and cook the broccoli for about 1-2 minutes stirring continuously.

- ✓ *Stir in the water and cook, covered for about 3-4 minutes, stirring occasionally.*
- ✓ *With a spoon, push the broccoli to the side of the pan. Add the remaining oil and let it heat.*
- ✓ *Add the shrimp and cook for about 1-2 minutes, tossing occasionally.*
  Add the remaining ingredients and sauté for about 2-3 minutes. Serve hot.
- ✓ **Meal Prep Tip:**
- ✓ *Transfer the shrimp mixture into a large bowl and set it aside to cool.*
- ✓ *Divide the shrimp mixture into 6 containers evenly.*
- ✓ *Cover the containers and refrigerate for 1 day. Reheat in the microwave before serving.*

Nutrition: Calories 197 Total Fat 6.8 g Saturated Fat 1.3 g Cholesterol 239 mg Total Carbs 6.1 g Sugar 1.1 g Fiber 1.6 g Sodium 324 mg Potassium 389 mg Protein 27.6 g

517)   *Grilled Salmon with Ginger Sauce*

Ingredients:

- *1 tablespoon toasted sesame oil*
- *1 tablespoon fresh cilantro, chopped*
- *1 tablespoon lime juice*
- *1 teaspoon fish sauce*
- *1 clove garlic, mashed*
- *1 teaspoon fresh ginger, grated*
- *1 teaspoon jalapeño pepper, minced*
- *4 salmon fillets*
- *1 tablespoon olive oil*
- *Salt and pepper to taste*

Direction: Preparation Time: 15 minutes Cooking Time: 8 minutes Servings: 4

- ✓ *In a bowl, mix the sesame oil, cilantro, lime juice, fish sauce, garlic, ginger and jalapeño pepper.*
- ✓ *Preheat your grill.*
- ✓ *Brush oil on salmon. Season both sides with salt and pepper.*
  Grill salmon for 6 to 8 minutes, turning once or twice.
- ✓ *Take 1 tablespoon from the oil mixture.*
- ✓ *Brush this on the salmon while grilling.*
- ✓ *Serve grilled salmon with the remaining sauce.*

Nutrition: Calories 204 Total Fat 11 g Saturated Fat 2 g Cholesterol 53 mg Total Carbs 2 g Protein 23 g

518)   *Swordfish with Tomato Salsa*

Ingredients:

- *1 cup tomato, chopped*

- ¼ cup tomatillo, chopped
- 2 tablespoons fresh cilantro, chopped
- ¼ cup avocado, chopped
- 1 clove garlic, minced
- 1 jalapeño pepper, chopped
- 1 tablespoon lime juice
- Salt and pepper to taste
- 4 swordfish steaks
- 1 clove garlic, sliced in half
- 2 tablespoons lemon juice
- ½ teaspoon ground cumin

Direction: Preparation Time: 20 minutes Cooking Time: 12 minutes Servings: 4

✓ Preheat your grill. In a bowl, mix the tomato, tomatillo, cilantro, avocado, garlic, jalapeño, lime juice, salt and pepper.

✓ Cover the bowl with foil and put it in the refrigerator.
Rub each swordfish steak with sliced garlic—drizzle lemon juice on both sides.

✓ Season with salt, pepper and cumin.

✓ Grill for 12 minutes or until the fish is fully cooked. Serve with salsa.

Nutrition: Calories 190 Total Fat 8 g Saturated Fat 2 g Cholesterol 43 mg Sodium 254 mg Total Carbohydrate 6 g Dietary Fiber 3 g Total Sugars 1 g Protein 24 g Potassium 453 mg

519) *Grilled Herbed Salmon with Raspberry Sauce & Cucumber Dill Dip*

Ingredients:

- 3 salmon fillets
- 1 tablespoon olive oil Salt and pepper to taste
- 1 teaspoon fresh sage, chopped
- 1 tablespoon fresh parsley, chopped
- 2 tablespoons apple juice
- 1 cup raspberries 1 teaspoon Worcestershire sauce
- 1 cup cucumber, chopped
- 2 tablespoons light mayonnaise
- ½ teaspoon dried dill

Direction: Preparation Time: 15 minutes Cooking Time: 30 minutes Servings: 4

✓ Coat the salmon fillets with oil. Season with salt, pepper, sage and parsley.

✓ Cover the salmon with foil. Grill for 20 minutes or until fish is flaky.

✓ While waiting, mix the apple juice, raspberries and Worcestershire sauce.
Pour the mixture into a saucepan over medium heat.

✓ Bring to a boil and then simmer for 8 minutes.

✓ In another bowl, mix the rest of the ingredients.

✓ Serve salmon with raspberry sauce and cucumber dip.

Nutrition: Calories 256 Total Fat 15 g Saturated Fat 3 g Cholesterol 68 mg Sodium 176 mg Total Carbohydrate 6 g Dietary Fiber 1 g Protein 23 g

520) *Salmon & Shrimp Stew*

Ingredients:

- 2 tablespoons olive oil
- 1/2 cup onion, chopped finely
- 2 garlic cloves, minced
- 1 Serrano pepper, chopped
- 1 teaspoon smoked paprika
- 4 cups fresh tomatoes, chopped
- 4 cups low-sodium chicken broth
  1 pound salmon fillets, cubed
- 1 pound shrimp, peeled and deveined
- 2 tablespoons fresh lime juice
- ¼ cup fresh basil, chopped
- ¼ cup fresh parsley, chopped
- Ground black pepper, as required
- 2 scallions, chopped

Direction: Preparation Time: 20 minutes Cooking Time: 21 minutes Servings: 6

✓ In a large soup pan, melt coconut oil over medium-high heat and sauté the onion for about 5-6 minutes.

✓ Add the garlic, Serrano pepper and smoked paprika and sauté for about 1 minute.

✓ Add the tomatoes and broth and bring to a gentle simmer over medium heat.

✓ Simmer for about 5 minutes.
Add the salmon and simmer for about 3-4 minutes.

✓ Stir in the remaining seafood and cook for about 4-5 minutes.

✓ Stir in the lemon juice, basil, parsley, sea salt and black pepper and remove from heat.

✓ Serve hot with the garnishing of scallion.

Nutrition: Calories 271; Total Fat 11 g; Saturated Fat 1.8 g; Total Carbs 8.6 g; Protein 34.7 g

SIDE DISH

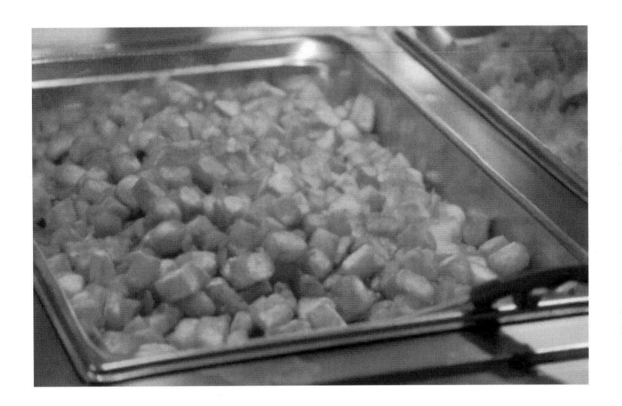

521)   *Lemon Garlic Green Beans*

Ingredients:

- 1 1/2 pounds green beans, trimmed
- 2 tablespoons olive oil
- 1 tablespoon fresh lemon juice
- 2 cloves minced garlic
- Salt and pepper

Direction: Preparation time: 5 minutesCooking Time: 10 minutes Servings: 6

- ✓ Fill a large bowl with ice water and set it aside.
- ✓ Bring a pot of salted water to boil then add the green beans.
- ✓ Cook for 3 minutes then drain and immediately place in the ice water.
  Cool the beans completely then drain them well.
- ✓ Heat the oil in a large skillet over medium-high heat.
- ✓ Add the green beans, tossing to coat, then add the lemon juice, garlic, salt, and pepper.
- ✓ Sauté for 3 minutes until the beans are tender-crisp then serve hot.

Nutrition: Calories 75, Total Fat 4.8g, Saturated Fat 0.7g, Total Carbs 8.5g, Net Carbs 4.6g, Protein 2.1g, Sugar 1.7g, Fiber 3.9g, Sodium 7mg

522)   *Brown Rice & Lentil Salad*

Ingredients:

- 1 cup water
- 1/2 cup instant brown rice
- 2 tablespoons olive oil
- 2 tablespoons red wine vinegar
- 1 tablespoon Dijon mustard
- 1 tablespoon minced onion
- 1/2 teaspoon paprika
- Salt and pepper
- 1 (15-ounce) can brown lentils, rinsed and drained
- 1 medium carrot, shredded
- 2 tablespoons fresh chopped parsley

Direction: Preparation time: 10 minutes Cooking Time: 10 minutes Servings: 4

- ✓ Stir together the water and instant brown rice in a medium saucepan.
- ✓ Bring to a boil then simmer for 10 minutes, covered.
- ✓ Remove from heat and set aside while you prepare the salad.
  Whisk together the olive oil, vinegar, Dijon mustard, onion, paprika, salt, and pepper in a medium bowl.

- ✓ Toss in the cooked rice, lentils, carrots, and parsley.
- ✓ Adjust seasoning to taste then stir well and serve warm.

Nutrition: Calories 145, Total Fat 7.7g, Saturated Fat 1g, Total Carbs 13.1g, Net Carbs 10.9g, Protein 6g, Sugar 1g, Fiber 2.2g, Sodium 57mg

523)   *Mashed Butternut Squash*

Ingredients:

- 3 pounds whole butternut squash (about 2 medium)
- 2 tablespoons olive oil
- Salt and pepper

Direction: Preparation time: 5 minutesCooking Time: 25 minutes Servings: 6

- ✓ Preheat the oven to 400F and line a baking sheet with parchment.
- ✓ Cut the squash in half and remove the seeds.
- ✓ Cut the squash into cubes and toss with oil then spread on the baking sheet.
  Roast for 25 minutes until tender then places in a food processor.
- ✓ Blend smooth then season with salt and pepper to taste.

Nutrition: Calories 90, Total Fat 4.8g, Saturated Fat 0.7g, Total Carbs 12.3g, Net Carbs 10.2g, Protein 1.1g, Sugar 2.3g, Fiber 2.1g, Sodium 4mg

524)   *Cilantro Lime Quinoa*

Ingredients:

- 1 cup uncooked quinoa
- 1 tablespoon olive oil
- 1 medium yellow onion, diced
- 2 cloves minced garlic
- 1 (4-ounce) can diced green chiles, drained
- 1 1/2 cups fat-free chicken broth
- ¾ cup fresh chopped cilantro
- 1/2 cup sliced green onion
- 2 tablespoons lime juice
- Salt and pepper

Direction: Preparation time: 5 minutes Cooking Time: 25 minutes Servings: 6

- ✓ Rinse the quinoa thoroughly in cool water using a fine mesh sieve.
- ✓ Heat the oil in a large saucepan over medium heat.
- ✓ Add the onion and sauté for 2 minutes then stir in the chile and garlic.
- ✓ Cook for 1 minute then stir in the quinoa and chicken broth.
  Bring to a boil then reduce heat and simmer, covered, until the quinoa absorbs the liquid – about

20 to 25 minutes.

✓ Remove from heat then stir in the cilantro, green onions, and lime juice.

✓ Season with salt and pepper to taste and serve hot.

Nutrition: Calories 150, Total Fat 4.1g, Saturated Fat 0.5g, Total Carbs 22.5g, Net Carbs 19.8g, Protein 6g, Sugar 1.7g, Fiber 2.7g, Sodium 179mg

525)   Oven-Roasted Veggies

Ingredients:

- 1 pound cauliflower florets
- 1/2 pound broccoli florets
- 1 large yellow onion, cut into chunks
- 1 large red pepper, cored and chopped
- 2 medium carrots, peeled and sliced
- 2 tablespoons olive oil
- 2 tablespoons apple cider vinegar
- Salt and pepper

Direction: Preparation time: 5 minutes

Cooking Time: 25 minutes Servings: 6

✓ Preheat the oven to 425F and line a large rimmed baking sheet with parchment.

✓ Spread the veggies on the baking sheet and drizzle with oil and vinegar.

✓ Toss well and season with salt and pepper. Spread the veggies in a single layer then roast for 20 to 25 minutes, stirring every 10 minutes, until tender.

✓ Adjust seasoning to taste and serve hot.

Nutrition: Calories 100, Total Fat 5g, Saturated Fat 0.7g, Total Carbs 12.4g, Net Carbs 8.2g, Protein 3.2g, Sugar 5.5g, Fiber 4.2g, Sodium 51mg

526)   Vegetable Rice Pilaf

Ingredients:

- 1 tablespoon olive oil
- 1/2 medium yellow onion, diced
- 1 cup uncooked long-grain brown rice
- 2 cloves minced garlic
- 1/2 teaspoon dried basil
- Salt and pepper
- 2 cups fat-free chicken broth
- 1 cup frozen mixed veggies

Direction: Preparation time: 5 minutesCooking Time: 25 minutes Servings: 6

✓ Heat the oil in a large skillet over medium heat.

✓ Add the onion and sauté for 3 minutes until translucent.

✓ Stir in the rice and cook until lightly toasted.

✓ Add the garlic, basil, salt, and pepper then stir to combine.
Stir in the chicken broth then bring to a boil.

✓ Reduce heat and simmer, covered, for 10 minutes.

✓ Stir in the frozen veggies then cover and cook for another 10 minutes until heated through. Serve hot.

Nutrition: Calories 90, Total Fat 2.7g, Saturated Fat 0.4g, Total Carbs 12.6g, Net Carbs 10.4g, Protein 3.9g, Sugar 1.5g, Fiber 2.2g, Sodium 143mg

527)   Curry Roasted Cauliflower Florets

Ingredients:

- 8 cups cauliflower florets
- 2 tablespoons olive oil
- 1 teaspoon curry powder
- 1/2 teaspoon garlic powder
- Salt and pepper

Direction: Preparation time: 5 minutes

Cooking Time: 25 minutes Servings: 6

✓ Preheat the oven to 425F and line a baking sheet with foil.

✓ Toss the cauliflower with olive oil and spread it on the baking sheet.
Sprinkle with curry powder, garlic powder, salt, and pepper.

✓ Roast for 25 minutes or until just tender. Serve hot.

Nutrition: Calories 75, Total Fat 4.9g, Saturated Fat 0.7g, Total Carbs 7.4g, Net Carbs 3.9g, Protein 2.7g, Sugar 3.3g,

528)   Mushroom Barley Risotto

Ingredients:

- 4 cups fat-free beef broth
- 2 tablespoons olive oil
- 1 small onion, diced well
- 2 cloves minced garlic
- 8 ounces thinly sliced mushrooms
- ¼ tsp. dried thyme
- Salt and pepper
- 1 cup pearled barley
- 1/2 cup dry white wine

Direction: Preparation time: 5 minutesCooking Time: 25 minutes Servings: 8

✓ Heat the beef broth in a medium saucepan and keep it warm.

✓ Heat the oil in a large, deep skillet over medium heat.

✓ Add the onions and garlic and sauté for 2 minutes then stir in the mushrooms and thyme.

✓ *Season with salt and pepper and sauté for 2 minutes more.*

✓ *Add the barley and sauté for 1 minute then pour in the wine.*
Ladle about 1/2 cup of beef broth into the skillet and stir well to combine.

✓ *Cook until most of the broth has been absorbed then add another ladle.*

✓ *Repeat until you have used all of the broth and the barley is cooked to al dente.*

✓ *Adjust seasoning to taste with salt and pepper and serve hot.*

Nutrition: Calories 155, Total Fat 4.4g, Saturated Fat 0.6g, Total Carbs 21.9g, Net Carbs 17.5g, Protein 5.5g, Sugar 1.2g,

529) *Braised Summer Squash*

Ingredients:

- *3 tablespoons olive oil*
- *3 cloves minced garlic*
- *¼ teaspoon crushed red pepper flakes*
- *1 pound summer squash, sliced*
- *1 pound zucchini, sliced*
- *1 teaspoon dried oregano*
- *Salt and pepper*

Direction: Preparation time: 10 minutes

Cooking Time: 20 minutes Servings: 6

✓ *Heat the oil in a large skillet over medium heat.*

✓ *Add the garlic and crushed red pepper and cook for 2 minutes.*
Add the summer squash and zucchini and cook for 15 minutes, often stirring, until just tender.

✓ *Stir in the oregano then season with salt and pepper to taste. Serve hot.*

Nutrition: Calories 90, Total Fat 7.4g, Saturated Fat 1.1g, Total Carbs 6.2g, Net Carbs 4.4g, Protein 1.8g, Sugar 4g, Fiber 1.8g, Sodium 10mg

530) *Parsley Tabbouleh*

Ingredients:

- *1 cup water*
- *1/2 cup bulgur*
- *¼ cup fresh lemon juice*
- *2 tablespoons olive oil*
- *2 cloves minced garlic*
- *Salt and pepper*
- *2 cups fresh chopped parsley*
- *2 medium tomatoes died*
- *1 small cucumber, diced*
- *¼ cup fresh chopped mint*

Direction: Preparation time: 5 minutes Cooking Time: 25 minutes Servings: 6

✓ *Bring the water and bulgur to a boil in a small saucepan then remove from heat.*

✓ *Cover and let stand until the water is fully absorbed, about 25 minutes.*

✓ *Meanwhile, whisk together the lemon juice, olive oil, garlic, salt, and pepper in a medium bowl. Toss in the cooked bulgur along with the parsley, tomatoes, cucumber, and mint.*

✓ *Season with salt and pepper to taste and serve.*

Nutrition: Calories 110, Total Fat 5.3g, Saturated Fat 0.9g, Total Carbs 14.4g, Net Carbs 10.5g, Protein 3g, Sugar 2.4g, Fiber 3.9g, Sodium 21mg

531) *Chicken Salad in Cucumber Cups*

Ingredients:

- *½ chicken breast, skinless, boiled, and shredded*
- *2 long cucumbers, cut into 8 thick rounds each, scooped out (won't use in a).*
- *1 tsp. ginger, minced*
- *1 tsp. lime zest, grated*
- *4 tsp. olive oil*
- *1 tsp. Sesame oil 1 tsp. lime juice*
- *Salt and pepper to taste*

Direction: Preparation Time: 5 minutes Cooking Time: 15 minutes Servings: 4

✓ *In a bowl combine lime zest, juice, olive, and sesame oils, ginger, and season with salt.*

✓ *Toss the chicken with the dressing and fill the cucumber cups with the salad.*

Nutrition: Carbohydrates: 4g Protein: 12g Calories: 116g

532) *French Lentils*

Ingredients:

- *2 tablespoons olive oil*
- *1 medium onion, diced*
- *1 medium carrot, peeled and diced*
- *2 cloves minced garlic*
- *5 1/2 cups water*
- *2 ¼ cups French lentils, rinsed and drained*
- *1 teaspoon dried thyme*
- *2 small bay leaves*
- *Salt and pepper*

Direction: Preparation time: 5 minutes Cooking Time: 25 minutes Servings: 10

✓ *Heat the oil in a large saucepan over medium heat.*

✓ *Add the onions, carrot, and garlic and sauté for 3*

minutes.

✓ *Stir in the water, lentils, thyme, and bay leaves – season with salt.*
Bring to a boil then reduce to a simmer and cook until tender, about 20 minutes.

✓ *Drain any excess water and adjust seasoning to taste. Serve hot.*

Nutrition: Calories 185, Total Fat 3.3g, Saturated Fat 0.5g, Total Carbs 27.9g, Net Carbs 14.2g, Protein 11.4g, Sugar 1.7g, Fiber 13.7g, Sodium 11mg

533) *Grain-Free Berry Cobbler*

Ingredients:

- *4 cups fresh mixed berries*
- *1/2 cup ground flaxseed*
- *¼ cup almond meal*
- *¼ cup unsweetened shredded coconut*
- *1/2 tablespoon baking powder*
- *1 teaspoon ground cinnamon*
- *¼ teaspoon salt*
- *Powdered stevia, to taste*
- *6 tablespoons coconut oil*

Direction: Preparation time: 5 minutes Cooking Time: 25 minutes Servings: 10

✓ *Preheat the oven to 375F and lightly grease a 10-inch cast-iron skillet.*

✓ *Spread the berries on the bottom of the skillet.*

✓ *Whisk together the dry ingredients in a mixing bowl.*
Cut in the coconut oil using a fork to create a crumbled mixture.

✓ *Spread the crumble over the berries and bake for 25 minutes until hot and bubbling.*

✓ *Cool the cobbler for 5 to 10 minutes before serving.*

Nutrition: Calories 215 Total Fat 16.8g, Saturated Fat 10.4g, Total Carbs 13.1g, Net Carbs 6.7g, Protein 3.7g, Sugar 5.3g, Fiber 6.4g, Sodium 61mg

534) *Spicy Spinach*

Ingredients:

- *1 tablespoon olive oil*
- *1 red onion, chopped finely*
- *6 garlic cloves, minced*
- *1 (1-inch) piece fresh ginger, minced*
- *1 teaspoon garam masala*
- *1 teaspoon ground coriander*
- *½ teaspoon ground cumin*
- *¼ teaspoon ground turmeric*
- *6 cups fresh spinach, chopped*
- *Salt and ground black pepper, as required*
- *1-2 tablespoons water*

Direction: Preparation Time: 10 minutes Cooking Time: 20 minutes Servings: 3

✓ *Heat the olive oil in a large nonstick skillet over medium heat and sauté the onion for about 6-7 minutes.*

✓ *Add the garlic, ginger and spices and sauté for about 1 minute.*

✓ *Add the spinach, salt and black pepper and water and cook, covered for about 10 minutes.*
Uncover and stir fry for about 2 minutes. Serve hot.

✓ ***Meal Prep Tip:***

✓ *Transfer the spinach mixture into a large bowl and set aside to cool completely. Divide the mixture into 3 containers evenly.*

✓ *Cover the containers and refrigerate for about 1-2 days. Reheat in the microwave before serving.*

Nutrition: Calories 80 Total Fat 5.1 g Saturated Fat 0.7 g Cholesterol 0 mg Total Carbs 8 g Sugar 1.9 g Fiber 2.3 g Sodium 52 mg Potassium 331 mg Protein 2.6 g

535) *Herbed Asparagus*

Ingredients:

- *2 tablespoons olive oil*
- *2 tablespoons fresh lemon juice*
- *1 tablespoon balsamic vinegar*
- *1 teaspoon garlic, minced*
- *1 tablespoon fresh parsley, chopped*
- *1 teaspoon dried oregano*
- *Salt and ground black pepper, as required*
- *1 pound fresh asparagus, ends removed*

Direction: Preparation Time: 10 minutes Cooking Time: 10 minutes Servings: 4

✓ *Preheat oven to 400 degrees F and lightly grease a rimmed baking sheet.*

✓ *Place the oil, lemon juice, vinegar, garlic, herbs, salt and black pepper in a bowl and beat until well combined.*

✓ *Arrange the asparagus onto the prepared baking sheet in a single layer. Top with half of the herb mixture and toss to coat.*

✓ *Roast for about 8-10 minutes. Remove from the oven and transfer the asparagus onto a platter. Drizzle with the remaining herb mixture and serve.*

✓ ***Meal Prep Tip:***

✓ *Transfer the asparagus into a large bowl and set it aside to cool completely.*

✓ *Divide the asparagus into 4 containers evenly. Cover the containers and refrigerate for about 1-2 days. Reheat in the microwave before serving.*

Nutrition: Calories 88 Total Fat 7.3 g Saturated Fat 1.1 g Total Carbs 5.1 g Sugar 2.4 g Protein 2.7 g

536) *Lemony Brussels Sprout*

Ingredients:

- ½ pound Brussels sprouts, halved
- 1 tablespoon olive oil
- 1 garlic clove, minced
- ½ teaspoon red pepper flakes, crushed
- Salt and ground black pepper, as required
- 1 tablespoon fresh lemon juice

Direction: Preparation Time: 10 minutes Cooking Time: 7 minutes Servings: 2

✓ Heat the olive oil in a large skillet over medium heat and cook the garlic and red pepper flakes for about 1 minute, stirring continuously.

✓ Stir in the Brussels sprouts, salt and black pepper and sauté for about 4-5 minutes.

✓ Stir in lemon juice and sauté for about 1 minute more. Serve hot.

Meal Prep Tip:

✓ Transfer the Brussels sprouts into a large bowl and set them aside to cool completely.

✓ Divide the Brussels sprouts into 2 containers evenly. Cover the containers and refrigerate for about 1-2 days.

✓ Reheat in the microwave before serving.

Nutrition: Calories 114 Total Fat 7.5 g Saturated Fat 1.2 g Cholesterol 0 mg Total Carbs 11.2 g Sugar 2.7 g Fiber 4.4 g Sodium 108 mg Potassium 465 mg Protein 4.1 g

537) *Gingered Cauliflower*

Ingredients:

- 2 cups cauliflower, cut into
- 1-inch florets Salt, as required
- 2 tablespoons olive oil
- 1 teaspoon fresh ginger root, sliced thinly
- 2 fresh thyme sprigs

Direction: Preparation Time: 0 minutes Cooking Time: 0 minutes Servings: 2

✓ In a pan of water, add the cauliflower and salt over medium heat and bring to a boil.

✓ Cover and cook for about 10-12 minutes.

✓ Drain the cauliflower well and transfer it onto a serving platter.

✓ Meanwhile, in a small skillet, melt the coconut oil over medium-low heat.

✓ Add the ginger and thyme sprigs and swirl the pan occasionally for about 2-3 minutes. Discard the ginger and thyme sprigs.

✓ Pour the oil over cauliflower and serve immediately.

Meal Prep Tip:

✓ Transfer the cauliflower into a large bowl and set it aside to cool completely.

✓ Divide the cauliflower into 2 containers evenly.

✓ Cover the containers and refrigerate for about 1-2 days. Reheat in the microwave before serving.

Nutrition: Calories 147 Total Fat 14.2 g Saturated Fat 2 g Cholesterol 0 mg Total Carbs 5.7 g Sugar 2.4 g Fiber 2.7 g Sodium 108 mg Potassium 310 mg Protein 2 g

538) *Roasted Broccoli*

Ingredients:

- 2 cups fresh broccoli florets
- 1 small yellow onion, cut into wedges
- ¼ teaspoon garlic powder
- 1/8 teaspoon paprika
- 1/8 teaspoon freshly ground black pepper
- 2 tablespoons olive oil

Direction: Preparation Time: 10 minutes Cooking Time: 15 minutes Servings: 2

✓ Preheat the grill to medium heat. In a large bowl, add all the ingredients and toss to coat well.

✓ Transfer the broccoli mixture over a double thickness of foil paper.

✓ Fold the foil paper around the broccoli mixture to seal it.
Grill for about 10-15 minutes. Serve hot.

Meal Prep Tip:

✓ Transfer the broccoli mixture into a large bowl and set aside to cool completely.

✓ Divide the broccoli mixture into 2 containers evenly.

✓ Cover the containers and refrigerate for about 1-2 days. Reheat in the microwave before serving.

Nutrition: Calories 167 Total Fat 14.4 g Saturated Fat 2 g Cholesterol 0 mg Total Carbs 9.7 g Sugar 3.1 g Fiber 3.2 g Sodium 32 mg Protein 3 g

539) *Garlicky Cabbage*

Ingredients:

- 1 tablespoon olive oil
- 2 garlic cloves, minced
- 1 pound cabbage, shredded
- 2-3 tablespoons filtered water
- 1½ tablespoons fresh lemon juice
- Salt and ground black pepper, as required

Direction: Preparation Time: 10 minutes Cooking Time: 10 minutes Servings: 4

✓ In a large skillet, heat the oil over medium heat and sauté the garlic for about 1 minute.

✓ Stir in the cabbage and cook, covered for about 2-3 minutes.

✓ Stir in the water and cook for about 2-3 minutes, stirring continuously.

✓ Increase the heat to high and stir in the lemon juice, salt and black pepper.
Cook for about 2-3 minutes, stirring continuously.
Serve hot.

Meal Prep Tip:

✓ Transfer the cabbage mixture into a large bowl and set aside to cool completely. Divide the cabbage mixture into 2 containers evenly. Cover the containers and refrigerate for about 1-2 days. Reheat in the microwave before serving.

Nutrition: Calories 62 Total Fat 3.7 g Saturated Fat 0.6 g Cholesterol 0 mg Total Carbs 7.2 g Sugar 3.8 g Fiber 2.9 g Sodium 168 mg Potassium 206 mg Protein 1.6 g

540)   Stir Fried Zucchini

Ingredients:

- 1 tablespoon olive oil
- ½ cup yellow onion, sliced
- 4 cups zucchini, sliced
- 1½ teaspoons garlic, minced
- ¼ cup water
- Salt and ground black pepper, as required

Direction: Preparation Time: 10 minutes Cooking Time: 10 minutes Servings: 4

✓ In a large skillet, heat the oil over medium-high heat and sauté the onion and zucchini for about 4-5 minutes.

✓ Add the garlic and sauté for about 1 minute.

✓ Add the remaining ingredients and stir to combine.

✓ Now, reduce the heat to medium and cook for about 3-4 minutes, stirring occasionally.
Serve hot.

Meal Prep Tip:

Transfer the zucchini mixture into a large bowl and set it aside to cool completely.

✓ Divide the zucchini mixture into 4 containers evenly.

✓ Cover the containers and refrigerate for about 1-2 days. Reheat in the microwave before serving.

Nutrition: Calories 55 Total Fat 3.7 g Saturated Fat 0.5 g Cholesterol 0 mg Total Carbs 5.5 g Sugar 2.6 g Fiber 1.6 g Sodium 51 mg Potassium 321 mg Protein 1.6 g

541)   Green Beans with Tomatoes

Ingredients:

- ¼ teaspoon fresh lemon peel, grated finely
- 2 teaspoons olive oil
- Salt and freshly ground white pepper, as required
- 4 cups grape tomatoes
- 1½ pounds fresh green beans, trimmed

Direction: Preparation Time: 15 minutes Cooking Time: 40 minutes Servings: 8

✓ Preheat the oven to 350 degrees F. In a large bowl, mix together lemon peel, oil, salt and white pepper.

✓ Add the cherry tomatoes and toss to coat well.

✓ Transfer the tomato mixture into a roasting pan.

✓ Roast for about 35-40 minutes, stirring once in a middle way.

✓ Meanwhile, in a pan of boiling water, arrange a steamer basket.
Place the green beans in a steamer basket and steam, covered for about 7-8 minutes.

✓ Drain the green beans well.

✓ Divide the green beans and tomatoes onto serving plates and serve.

Meal Prep Tip:

✓ Transfer the green beans and tomatoes into a large bowl and set aside to cool completely.

✓ Divide the green beans and tomatoes into 8 containers evenly.

✓ Cover the containers and refrigerate for about 1-2 days. Reheat in the microwave before serving.

Nutrition: Calories 53 Total Fat 1.5 g Saturated Fat 0.2 g Cholesterol 0 mg Total Carbs 9.6 g Sugar 3.6 g Fiber 4 g Sodium 29 mg Potassium 391 mg Protein 2.3 g

SOUPS AND STEWS

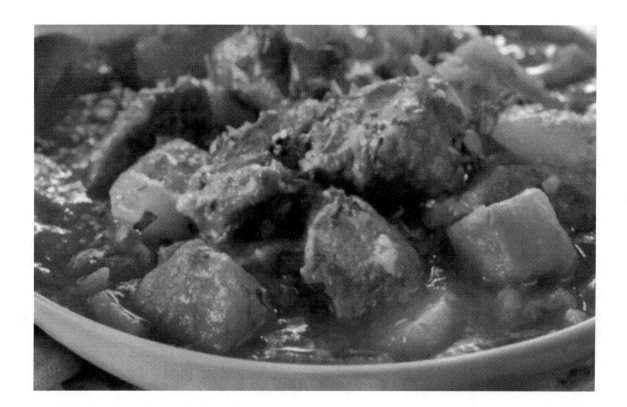

542) *Mexican Beef Stew*

Ingredients:

- *1 cup onion, diced*
- *1 ½ lb. Beef round steak, sliced into ½-inch pieces*
- *1 ¾ cups tomatoes, diced*
- *1 cup carrots, diced*
- *¼ cup sweet red pepper, diced*
- *2 tbsp. cilantro, diced*
- *1 jalapeno, seeded and diced*
- *2 tbsp. flour*
- *tbsp. water*
- *1 ¾ cups low-sodium beef broth*
- *1 garlic clove, diced*
- *½ tsp. sea salt*
- *1 ½ tbsp. chili powder*
- *1 tbsp. vegetable oil*

Direction: Preparation Time: 15 minutes Cooking Time: 90 minutes Servings: 6

✓ *Heat your oil in a pot over medium-high heat. Add the steak and cook until brown.*

✓ *Add the broth, onion, carrots, red pepper, jalapeno, garlic, and seasonings, and bring to a boil. Reduce your heat to low and cover, then simmer for 45 minutes.*

✓ *Stir stew occasionally.*

✓ *Add your tomatoes and continue to cook for 15 minutes.*

✓ *Stir the flour and water together in a bowl until smooth.*

✓ *Add to your stew with the cilantro, then continue to cook for an additional 30 minutes; or until the stew has thickened.*

✓ *Serve!*

Nutrition: Calories: 312 Fat: 13g Protein: 39g

543) *Italian Veggie Soup*

Ingredients:

- *4 cups cabbage, chopped*
- *1 cup green beans, sliced into 1-inch pieces*
- *2 cups fresh spinach, chopped*
- *small onion, diced*
- *green bell peppers, diced*
- *2 celery stalks, diced*
- *28 oz. can tomato, low-sodium, diced*
- *6 cups low-sodium vegetable broth*
- *1 tbsp. parsley*
- *2 tbsp. tomato paste*
- *½ tsp. Italian seasoning*
- *2 bay leaves*
- *garlic cloves, fine diced*
- *1 tbsp. basil*
- *pepper to taste*

Direction: Preparation Time: 16 minutes Cooking Time: 4 hours Servings: 8

✓ *Add your vegetables to a crockpot.*

✓ *Add the canned tomatoes, tomato paste, broth, bay leaves, Italian seasoning, and pepper and stir to combine.*

✓ *Cover with a pot lid and cook on high for 5 hours. Add the basil, spinach, and parsley and cook for another additional 5 minutes.*

Nutrition: Calories: 85 Fats: 1g Protein: 3g

544) *Korean Beef Soup*

Ingredients:

- *1-gallon water 1 tbsp. oil*
- *3 tbsp. soy sauce*
- *1 tbsp. sesame seeds, toasted*
- *2 garlic cloves, diced fine*
- *1 tsp. sea salt*
- *1 tsp. black ground pepper*
- *1 lb. Beef, cubed*
- *1 Korean white radish, peeled and diced 1 cup green onions, diced*

Direction: Preparation Time: 16 minutes Cooking Time: 4 hours Servings: 8

✓ *Set the crockpot to high and add the water.*

✓ *In a mixing bowl, mix the soy sauce, green onions, sesame seeds, oil, sea salt, and pepper. Divide evenly between 2 Ziploc bags.*

✓ *Place the meat in 1 bag and the radish in the other and allow to sit for 1 hour.*

✓ *Turn the crockpot down to low and add the contents of the meat bag. Let cook for an hour, then add the contents of the radish bag. Cook for another 3–4 hours.*

Nutrition: Calories: 120 Fats: 4g Protein: 19g

545) *Italian Sausage Soup*

Ingredients:

- *1 lb. Ground pork*
- *1 large onion, chopped*
- *2 cups kale, fresh chopped*
- *¾ lb. tiny red new potatoes, cut into pieces*
- *4 cups low-sodium chicken broth*
- *1 tsp. oregano*

- *2 tbsp. cornstarch*
- *1 (12 oz.) fat-free evaporated milk*
- *2 garlic cloves, fine diced*
- *¼ tsp. sea salt*
- *¼ to ½ tsp. crushed red pepper*

Direction: Preparation Time: 10 minutes Cooking Time: 7 hours Servings: 6

✓ *Place skillet over medium-high heat; prepare your pork, garlic, and onion until the meat is browned. Drain the fat from the pan.*

✓ *Return your meat to the skillet and add the seasonings—Cook for another minute or so.*

✓ *Transfer to your crockpot. Add the potatoes and broth. Cover, then cook the dish on low for 6–8 hours or on high for 3–4 hours.*

✓ *Whisk your cornstarch and milk in a small bowl until smooth. Add to the crockpot along with kale. Cook for about 60 minutes or until the soup begins to bubble around the edges. Serve topped with red pepper flakes, and enjoy!*

Nutrition: Calories: 209 Fats: 3g Protein: 27g

546)   *Bell Pepper Stew*

Ingredients:

- *3 cups onion, diced*
- *3 cups green pepper, diced*
- *1 lb. Hot Italian sausage, chopped*
- *3 ½ cups tomatoes, diced*
- *1 cup cauliflower, grated*
- *1 lb. Lean ground sirloin*
- *4 cups low-sodium beef broth*
- *4 garlic cloves, fine diced*
- *2 tbsp. olive oil*
- *1 cup tomato sauce*
- *½ tsp. oregano*
- *1 tsp. basil*

Direction: Preparation Time: 20 minutes Cooking Time: 4 hours Servings: 8

✓ *Heat your oil in a large skillet over medium-high heat.*

✓ *Add your onions and peppers to the pan and cook until tender.*

✓ *Add your Italian chopped sausage to the pan and continue to cook for about 5 minutes or until the sausage is cooked.*

✓ *Add remaining ingredients to crockpot, along with cooked sausage, onion, and peppers—cook on high for 4 hours. Serve hot and enjoy!*

Nutrition: Calories: 212 Fats: 6g Protein: 28g

547)   *Seafood Chowder*

Ingredients:

- *3 celery stalks, diced*
- *1 ½ lb. Frozen mixed seafood, thawed and cut into bite-sized pieces*
- *1 ½ cups onion, diced*
- *5 tbsp. dill, fresh chopped*
- *½ cup half-n-half*
- *½ cups white wine*
- *2½ cups low-sodium chicken broth*
- *1 ½ tbsp. olive oil*
- *1 ½ tbsp. cold water*
- *½ tsp. garlic, fine diced*
- *sea salt and black pepper to taste*

Direction: Preparation Time: 5 minutes Cooking Time: 25 minutes Servings: 4

✓ *Heat your oil in a soup pot over medium heat. Add the celery and onion to the pot and cook until softened, for about 7 minutes. Stir in your garlic and cook for an additional 30 seconds.*

✓ *Add the wine to the pot and bring to a low boil, cooking until most of the liquid has disappeared.*

✓ *Combine cornstarch along with water in a bowl, stirring until dissolved. Add the cornstarch mixture to your chicken broth. Simmer the dish for 10 minutes or until broth thickens.*

✓ *Season your soup to taste with salt and pepper, then add the seafood and dill to the soup pot. Simmer for 7 minutes or until the seafood is cooked through. Stir in the half-n-half and cook until heated through. Serve soup using dill for garnish, and enjoy!*

Nutrition: Calories: 353 Fats: 10g Protein: 27g

548)   *Creamy Chicken & Cauliflower Rice Soup*

Ingredients:

- *2 stalks celery, peeled and diced*
- *2 carrots, peeled and diced*
- *2 cups skim milk*
- *½ onion, diced*
- *2 cups cauliflower, riced*
- *1 cup chicken, cooked and shredded*
- *½ tsp. Rosemary*
- *5 garlic cloves, diced*
- *4 cups low-sodium chicken broth*
- *3 tbsp. margarine*
- *1 bay leaf*
- *½ tsp. parsley*
- *½ tsp. thyme*

Direction: Preparation Time: 20 minutes Cooking Time: 5 hours Servings: 6

✓ Melt your margarine in a large skillet over medium heat. Add your onion, garlic, and carrots. Cook, while often stirring, for about 5 minutes. Place into a crockpot.

✓ Add the chicken broth and seasonings, then cover and cook for 4 hours.
Add the chicken, milk, and cauliflower rice. Cook for 60 minutes or until the cauliflower is tender. Discard the bay leaf before serving and enjoy!

Nutrition: Calories: 151 Fats: 6g Protein: 12g

549) *Chunky Chicken Noodle Soup*

Ingredients:

- lb. Chicken thighs, boneless and skinless
- 2 celery stalks, sliced
- 2 carrots, sliced
- 2 tsp. fresh ginger, grated
- 8 cups low-sodium chicken broth
- 2 cups homemade pasta
- tbsp. garlic, fine diced
- 1 tbsp. chicken bouillon
- Salt and black pepper to taste

Direction: Preparation Time: 10 minutes Cooking Time: 35 minutes Servings: 8

✓ Add the chicken and 1 cup broth in a large soup pot over medium heat. Bring to a simmer and cook the chicken until done, for about 20 minutes. Transfer the chicken to a bowl and, using 2 forks, shred the chicken.

✓ Add the celery, garlic, ginger, carrots, and bouillon to the soup pot and stir to mix. Add in the remaining broth and bring it back to a boil. Reduce the heat to a simmer until the vegetables are tender, for about 15 minutes.

✓ Add your pasta and cook for an additional 5 minutes. Add the chicken to the soup along with salt and pepper. Serve and enjoy!

Nutrition: Calories: 210 Fats: 7g Protein: 23g

550) *Cheesy Ham & Broccoli Soup*

Ingredients:

- cups cheddar cheese, grated 2 cups broccoli florets
- 8 cups low-sodium vegetable broth 1 ½ cups ham, slice into small cubes 1 onion, diced
- 2 stalks celery, peeled and diced 1 bay leaf
- tbsp. olive oil
- sea salt and black pepper to taste

Direction: Preparation Time: 10 minutes Cooking Time: 6 hours Servings: 8

✓ Heat your oil in a skillet over medium-high heat. Add the celery and onion, cooking for 5 minutes and stirring often.

✓ Add the ham, broth, seasoning, and celery mixture to the crockpot. Cook on low for 3–4 hours.

✓ Add your broccoli and continue to cook for an additional 2 hours or until the broccoli starts to become tender. Stir in the cheese and cook until melted. Discard the bay leaf. Serve soup and enjoy!

Nutrition: Calories: 214 Fats: 15g Protein: 12g

551) *Potlikker Soup*

Ingredients:

- 3 cups chicken broth or store-bought low-sodium chicken broth, divided
- 1 medium onion, chopped
- 3 garlic cloves, minced
- 1 bunch collard greens or mustard greens including stems, roughly chopped
- 1 fresh ham bone
- 5 carrots, peeled and cut into 1-inch rounds 2 fresh thyme sprigs
- 3 bay leaves
- Freshly ground black pepper

Direction: Preparation Time: 16 minutes Cooking Time: 25 minutes Servings: 6

✓ Select the Sauté setting on an electric pressure cooker, and combine ½ cup chicken broth, the onion, and garlic and cook for 3 to 5 minutes, or until the onion and garlic are translucent.

✓ Add the collard greens, ham bone, carrots, remaining 2½ cups broth, thyme, and bay leaves.

✓ Close and lock the lid and set the pressure valve to sealing.

✓ Change to the Manual/Pressure Cook setting, and cook for 15 minutes.

✓ Once cooking is complete, quick-release the pressure, carefully remove the lid. Discard the bay leaves.

✓ Serve with Skillet Bivalves.

Nutrition: Calories: 99 Fats: 4g Protein: 6g

552) *Burgoo*

Ingredients:

- 2 pounds' pork butt, chopped into 1-inch pieces
- 2 pounds beef stew meat, chopped into 1-inch pieces
- 1 lb. boneless, skinless chicken thighs, chopped into 1-inch pieces

- *1 tsp. cayenne pepper*
- *1 tsp. Not Old Bay Seasoning*
- *3 cups chicken broth or store-bought low-sodium chicken broth 2 pounds' potatoes, cut into 1-inch cubes*
- *3 onions, chopped*
- *2 green bell peppers, chopped*
- *4 carrots, peeled and chopped*
- *2 cups frozen corn*
- *1 lb. okra, cut into 1-inch rounds*
- *2 celery stalks, roughly chopped*
- *1 cup frozen lima beans*
- *2 large tomatoes, chopped*
- *2 tbsp. tomato paste*
- *¼ large cabbage, roughly chopped*

Direction: Preparation Time: 16 minutes Cooking Time: 60 minutes Servings: 16

✓ *In an electric pressure cooker, combine the pork, beef, chicken, cayenne, and seasoning.*

✓ *Cover with the broth, close and lock the lid, and set the pressure valve to sealing.*

✓ *Select the Manual/Pressure Cook setting, and cook for 20 minutes.*

✓ *Once cooking is complete, allow the pressure to release naturally. Carefully remove the lid.*

✓ *Remove the meat, and shred with 2 forks. Select the Manual/Pressure Cook setting, and cook for 10 minutes.*

✓ *Once cooking is complete, allow the pressure to release naturally. Carefully remove the lid.*

✓ *Return the meat to the pressure cooker, change to the Sauté setting, and cook for 5 minutes, uncovered, or until the flavors meld.*

Nutrition: Calories: 354 Fat: 12g Protein: 36g

553)   *She-Crab Soup*

Ingredients:

- *2 cups Seafood Broth (here)*
- *1 shallot, chopped*
- *2 celery stalks, chopped*
- *1 garlic clove, minced*
- *1 tsp. Not Old Bay Seasoning*
- *1 cup fat-free milk*
- *½ cup half-and-half*
- *1 tsp. hot sauce*
- *1 tsp. Worcestershire sauce*
- *1 ⅛ pound backfin lump crab meat*
- *1 bunch chives, chopped*
- *Freshly ground black pepper*
- *Lemon wedges*

Direction: Preparation Time: 16 minutes Cooking Time: 25 minutes Servings: 6

✓ *In a heavy-bottomed stockpot, bring the broth to a simmer.*

✓ *Add the shallot, celery, garlic, and seasoning and cook for 3 to 5 minutes, or until softened.*

✓ *Reduce the heat to low, and whisk in the milk, half-and-half, hot sauce, and Worcestershire sauce. Simmer for 10 minutes.*

✓ *Add the crab and cook for 5 to 7 minutes, or until the flavors come together.*

✓ *Serve with chives, pepper, and lemon wedges.*

Nutrition: Calories: 116 Fat: 4g Protein: 16g

554)   *Sweet Potato and Pumpkin Soup with Peanuts*

Ingredients:

- *3 cups Vegetable Broth (here) or store-bought low-sodium vegetable broth, divided*
- *1 celery stalk, roughly chopped*
- *1 cup roughly chopped tomato*
- *1 red bell pepper, chopped*
- *1 large sweet potato, peeled and cut into 2-inch cubes*
- *1 small pumpkin, peeled and cut into 2-inch cubes*
- *1 bay leaf*
- *tsp. paprika*
- *2 cups roasted unsalted peanuts*
- *Baby sage leaves (optional)*

Direction: Preparation Time: 10 minutes Cooking Time: 45 minutes Servings: 8

✓ *In a large Dutch oven, bring 1 cup broth to a simmer over medium heat.*

✓ *Add the celery, tomato, and bell pepper and cook for 5 to 7 minutes, or until softened.*

✓ *Add the sweet potato, pumpkin, bay leaf, paprika, and the remaining 2 cups broth. Cover and cook for 30 minutes, or until the sweet potato and pumpkin are soft.*

✓ *Add the peanuts and cook for 5 minutes, or until the peanuts become less crunchy. Discard the bay leaf.*

✓ *Transfer to a heat-safe blender, and pulse until the soup has a batter-like consistency.*

✓ *Serve with Grilled Hearts of Romaine with Buttermilk Dressing and protein of your choice. If using, garnish with baby sage leaves.*

Nutrition: Calories: 266 Fat: 18g Protein: 12g

555) *Spicy Chicken Stew*

Ingredients:

- *3 cups chicken broth or store-bought low-sodium chicken broth*
- *6 boneless, skinless chicken breasts*
- *1 tbsp. Blackened Rub*
- *2 carrots, peeled and cut into 1-inch rounds*
- *1 onion, roughly chopped*
- *2 celery stalks, roughly chopped*
- *1 medium sweet potato, cut into 1-inch chunks*
- *2 cups fresh peas*
- *cups roughly chopped green beans*
- *2 garlic cloves, minced*
- *1 cup chopped tomatoes*
- *1 tbsp. tomato paste*

Direction: Preparation Time: 16 minutes Cooking Time: 21 minutes Servings: 8

✓ *Select the Sauté setting on an electric pressure cooker, and combine the broth, chicken, and rub. Cook for 5 minutes, or until the exterior of the chicken is lightly browned.*

✓ *Add the carrots, onion, celery, sweet potato, peas, green beans, garlic, tomatoes, and tomato paste.*

✓ *Close and lock the lid and set the pressure valve to sealing.*

✓ *Change to the Manual/Pressure Cook setting, and cook for 15 minutes at high pressure.*

✓ *Once cooking is complete, quick-release the pressure, carefully remove the lid, and serve.*

Nutrition: Calories: 145 Fat: 1g Protein: 22g

556) *Tomato-Based Stew*

Ingredients:

- *5 cups chicken broth or store-bought low-sodium chicken broth, divided*
- *1 medium onion, roughly chopped*
- *2 garlic cloves, minced*
- *4 boneless, skinless chicken thighs, roughly cut into chunks*
- *3 sun-dried tomatoes, drained and*
- *2 cups fresh lima beans*
- *1 cup fresh corn kernels*
- *1 zucchini, cut into 1-inch chunks*
- *1 cup Barbecue Sauce*
- *1 tbsp. Worcestershire sauce*
- *½ tsp. Not Old Bay Seasoning*

Direction: Preparation Time: 16 minutes Cooking Time: 61 minutes Servings: 8

✓ *Select the Sauté setting on an electric pressure cooker, and combine 1 cup broth, the onion, and*

garlic and cook for 1 to 2 minutes, or until the onion and garlic are translucent.

✓ *Add the chicken, sun-dried tomatoes, lima beans, corn, zucchini, barbecue sauce, remaining 4 cups broth, the Worcestershire sauce, and seasoning.*

✓ *Close and lock the lid and set the pressure valve to sealing.*

✓ *Change to the Manual/Pressure Cook setting, and cook for 1 hour at high pressure.*

✓ *Once cooking is complete, quick-release the pressure, carefully remove the lid, and serve.*

Nutrition: Calories: 262 Fat: 4g Protein: 22g

557) *Down South Corn Soup*

Ingredients:

- *1 tbsp. extra-virgin olive oil*
- *½ Vidalia onion, minced*
- *2 garlic cloves, minced*
- *3 cups chopped cabbage*
- *1 small cauliflower, broken into florets, or 1 (10 oz.) bag frozen cauliflower*
- *1 (10 oz.) bag frozen corn*
- *1 cup Vegetable Broth (here) or store-bought low-sodium vegetable broth*
- *1 tsp. smoked paprika 1 tsp. ground cumin*
- *1 tsp. dried dill*
- *½ tsp. freshly ground black pepper*
- *1 cup plain unsweetened cashew milk*

Direction: Preparation Time: 10 minutes Cooking Time: 35 minutes Servings: 8

✓ *In a large stockpot, heat the oil over medium heat.*

✓ *Add the onion and garlic, and sauté, stirring to prevent the garlic from scorching, for 3 to 5 minutes, or until translucent.*

✓ *Add the cabbage and a splash of water, cover, and cook for 5 minutes, or until tender.*

✓ *Add the cauliflower, corn, broth, paprika, cumin, dill, and pepper. Cover and cook for 20 minutes, or until tender.*

✓ *Add the cashew milk and stir well. Cover and cook for 5 minutes, letting the flavors come together.*

✓ *Serve with a heaping plate of greens and seafood of your choice.*

Nutrition: Calories: 120 Fat: 4g Protein: 3g

558) *Carrot Soup*

Ingredients:

- *4 cups Vegetable Broth (here) or store-bought low-sodium vegetable broth, divided*
- *2 celery stalks, halved*

- 1 small yellow onion, roughly chopped
- ½ fennel bulb, cored and roughly chopped
- 1 (1-inch) piece fresh ginger, peeled and chopped
- 1 lb. carrots, peeled and halved
- tsp. ground cumin 1 garlic clove, peeled
- 1 tbsp. almond butter

Direction: Preparation Time: 16 minutes Cooking Time: 25 minutes Servings: 6

✓ Select the Sauté setting on an electric pressure cooker, and combine ½ cup broth, the celery, onion, fennel, and ginger. Cook for 5 minutes, or until the vegetables are tender.

✓ Add the carrots, cumin, garlic, remaining 3½ cups broth, and the almond butter.

✓ Close and lock the lid, and set the pressure valve to sealing.

✓ Change to the Manual/Pressure Cook setting, and cook for 15 minutes.

✓ Once cooking is complete, quick-release the pressure. Carefully remove the lid, and let cool for 5 minutes.

✓ Using a stand mixer or an immersion blender, carefully purée the soup. Serve with a heaping plate of greens.

Nutrition: Calories: 82 Fat: 2g Protein: 3g

559) *Bean Field Stew*

Ingredients:

- 6 cups Vegetable Broth (here) or store-bought low-sodium vegetable broth
- 1 cup dried lima beans 1 cup dried black beans
- 1 cup dried pinto beans
- 1 cup dried kidney beans
- 1 cup roughly chopped tomato
- 2 carrots, peeled and roughly chopped
- 1 zucchini, chopped
- ½ cup chopped white onion
- 1 celery stalk, roughly chopped
- 2 garlic cloves, minced
- 1tsp. dried oregano
- 1 tsp. dried thyme
- ¼ tsp. freshly ground black pepper

Direction: Preparation Time: 20 minutes Cooking Time: 41 minutes Servings: 8

✓ In an electric pressure cooker, combine the broth, lima beans, black beans, pinto beans, kidney beans, tomato, carrots, zucchini, onion, celery, garlic, oregano, thyme, and pepper.

✓ Close and lock the lid, and set the pressure valve to sealing.

✓ Select the Manual/Pressure Cook setting, and cook

for 40 minutes.

✓ Once cooking is complete, quick-release the pressure. Carefully remove the lid.

✓ Serve with Barbecue Chicken.

Nutrition: Calories: 298 Fat: 1g Protein: 19g

560) *Pumpkin Soup*

Ingredients:

- 2 cups Seafood Broth (here), divided
- 1 bunch collard greens, stemmed and cut into ribbons
- 1 tomato, chopped
- 1 garlic clove, minced
- 1 butternut squash or other winter squash, peeled and cut into 1-inch cubes
- 1tsp. paprika
- 1 tsp. dried dill
- (5 oz.) cans boneless, skinless salmon in water, rinsed

Direction: Preparation Time: 14 minutes Cooking Time: 31 minutes Servings: 6

✓ In a heavy-bottomed large stockpot, bring ½ cup broth to a simmer over medium heat.

✓ Add the collard greens, tomato, and garlic and cook for 5 minutes, or until the greens are wilted and the garlic is softened.

✓ Add the squash, paprika, dill, and remaining 1½ cups broth. Cover and cook for 20 minutes, or until the squash is tender.

✓ Add the salmon and cook for 3 minutes, or just enough for the flavors to come together.

Nutrition: Calories: 152 Fat: 2g Protein: 14g

561) *Low Country Boil*

Ingredients:

- 2 pounds small new potatoes
- 1-pound low-sodium chicken sausage, cut into 2-inch pieces
- 1 lb. shell-on medium shrimp, deveined
- ½ cup Not Old Bay Seasoning
- 2 small onions, quartered
- 1 garlic bulb
- celery stalk including leaves, halved
- 2 bay leaves
- 2 cups water
- 4 ears fresh corn, halved
- Lemons, cut into eighths, for serving

Direction: Preparation Time: 15 minutes Cooking Time: 10 minutes Servings: 8

✓ *In an electric pressure cooker, combine the potatoes, sausage, shrimp, seasoning, onions, garlic, celery, and bay leaves. Cover with the water, and top with the corn.*

✓ *Close and lock the lid, and set the pressure valve to sealing.*

✓ *Select the Manual/Pressure Cook setting, and cook for 7 minutes.*

✓ *Once cooking is complete, quick-release the pressure. Carefully remove the lid.*

✓ *Drain the liquid and discard the bay leaves. Transfer the shrimp, sausage, and vegetables to a bowl and serve immediately. Garnish each portion with a lemon wedge (if using).*

Nutrition: Calories: 294 Fat: 6g Protein: 25g

562)   *North Carolina Fish Stew*

Ingredients:

- *½ cup Seafood Broth (here)*
- *2 large white onions, chopped*
- *4 garlic cloves, minced*
- *¼ cup tomato paste*
- *1 tsp. red pepper flakes*
- *2 tsp. smoked paprika*
- *3 bay leaves*
- *1LB b. new potatoes, halved*
- *3 cups water*
- *2 pounds fish fillets, such as rockfish, striped bass, or cod, cut into ½- to 1-inch dice*
- *8 medium eggs*

Direction: Preparation Time: 20 minutes Cooking Time: 21 minutes Servings: 8

✓ *Select the Sauté setting on an electric pressure cooker, and combine the broth, onions, garlic, tomato paste, red pepper flakes, paprika, and bay leaves. Cook for 2 minutes, or until the onions and garlic are translucent.*

✓ *Add the potatoes and 1 cup water.*

✓ *Close and lock the lid, and set the pressure valve to sealing.*

✓ *Change to the Manual/Pressure Cook setting, and cook for 3 minutes.*

✓ *Once cooking is complete, quick-release the pressure. Carefully remove the lid.*

✓ *Add the fish and enough water just to cover the fish.*

✓ *Close and lock the lid, and set the pressure valve to sealing.*

✓ *Select the Manual/Pressure Cook setting, and cook for 3 more minutes.*

✓ *Once cooking is complete, quick-release the pressure. Carefully remove the lid.*

✓ *Carefully crack the eggs one by one into the stew,*

keeping the yolks intact.

✓ *Close and lock the lid, and set the pressure valve to sealing.*

✓ *Select the Manual/Pressure Cook setting, and cook for 1 minute.*

✓ *Once cooking is complete, quick-release the pressure. Carefully remove the lid, discard the bay leaves, and serve in bowls.*

Nutrition: Calories: 218 Fat: 6g Protein: 28g

563)   *White Bean and Bacon Soup*

Ingredients:

- *3 cups chicken bouillon*
- *2 cups beans*
- *slices medium-cut bacon*
- *2 carrots*
- *2 celeries, stalks*
- *¾ cup onion*
- *1 ½ garlic cloves, chopped*
- *¼ tsp. pepper*
- *½ tsp. salt*
- *1 bay leaf*

Direction: Preparation Time: 20 minutes Cooking Time: 35 minutes Servings: 8

✓ *Before cooking, soak the beans in water for 8 hours.*

✓ *Place washed beans into the instant pot.*

✓ *Fry chopped bacon in a skillet over medium heat until it becomes crisp.*

✓ *Take bacon from the skillet and mill it into small pieces.*

✓ *Add chopped carrot, onion, celery, and garlic in skillet; cook until vegetables are tender.*

✓ *Shift cooked mixture and bacon into the instant pot.*

✓ *Add bouillon, salt, pepper, and bay leaf. Cook until beans are tender.*

Nutrition: Calories: 80 Protein: 2g Fat: 4g

564)   *Quick Kidney Bean Soup with Cheese*

Ingredients:

- *1 (15-oz) can no-salt-added kidney beans*
- *¼ cup shredded cheese (reduced-fat)*
- *1/3 cup Picante sauce*
- *1/3 cup green onions*
- *1 tsp. paprika (smoke*
- *d) 2/3 cup water*
- *2 tsp. extra virgin olive oil*

Direction: Preparation Time: 10 minutes Cooking Time: 15 minutes Servings: 8

✓ Mix drained and rinsed beans, Picante sauce, smoked paprika, and water in a small saucepan; bring to a boil. Reduce heat, simmer for 5 minutes.

✓ Remove from heat, and stir in oil.

✓ Top soup evenly with 2 tbsp. Cheese and chopped green onions.

Nutrition: Calories: 56 Protein: 4g Fat: 1g

565)   *Beef and Vegetable Soup*

Ingredients:

- lb. ground beef (extra-lean)
- 2 cups green bell pepper
- cups green cabbage
- 2 cups frozen mixed vegetables 1 cup onion
- 1 (14.5-oz) can stewed tomatoes (no-salt-added)
- 2.5 cups beef broth (low-sodium)
- ¼ cup ketchup
- tbsp. Worcestershire sauce
- 2 tbsp. extra virgin olive oil
- 1 dried bay leaf
- ¼ tsp. pepper
- ¾ tsp. salt

Direction: Preparation Time: 9 minutes Cooking Time: 21 minutes Servings: 8

✓ Cook beef for 2 minutes in the oven.

✓ Add chopped bell pepper and chopped onion, cook for 3 minutes.

✓ Add chopped cabbage, mixed vegetables, tomatoes, bay leaf, Worcestershire sauce, broth, and pepper; bring to a boil, cook 15 minutes.

✓ Add ketchup, oil, and salt

Nutrition: Calories: 175 Protein: 25g Fat: 7g

566)   *Butternut Soup*

Ingredients:

- 1 stalk celery
- 2 carrots
- 1 lb. butternut squash
- 1 onion
- olive oil
- ½ lb. waxy potatoes
- Salt to taste

Direction: Preparation Time: 10 minutes Cooking Time: 85 minutes Servings: 8

✓ Smooth the bottom of the oven with extra virgin olive oil, add the vegetables and fry for 10 minutes.

✓ Take butternut and cut it into cubes. Cut potatoes into chunks of the same size. Add them into the vegetable ingredients in the casserole, add a couple of tsp. of sea salt and 2 ½ cups boiling water, cover, and simmer for 1 hour.
Very carefully mash the soup in a blender in small batches, making sure the top of the mixer is secure.

✓ Taste for seasoning and serve drizzled with a few drops of olive oil and good balsamic vinegar. A crisp dice of apples on top make this look lovely and adds a very pleasing note of sweetness and texture.

Nutrition: Calories: 130 Protein: 10g Fat: 3g

567)   *Turkey Broth*

Ingredients:

- 6 to 7 lb. turkey or turkey parts
- 2 carrots
- 2 celery stalks
- 1 or 2 onions
- parsley
- bay leaves
- whole peppercorns
- salt to taste

Direction: Preparation Time: 16 minutes Cooking Time: 2 hours Servings: 8

✓ Buy a small turkey and wash it thoroughly. Plunk it into a large stockpot and add enough water to cover it. Turn up the heat and bring it almost to a boil.

✓ Skim off the foam that rises to the top, and keep skimming for about 7 minutes, until the foam stops coming. Add the onion, the carrots— washed and cut in half—the celery, some parsley, a bay leaf, and a handful of peppercorns. Add 2 tsp. of salt.

✓ Cook broth for about 2 hours. Strain the broth, discard the solids, let the broth cool to room temperature, and then chill overnight.

Nutrition: Calories: 180 Protein: 20 g Fat 8g

568)   *Chicken and Zoodle Soup*

Ingredients:

- 2 tbsp. extra-virgin olive oil
- 12 oz. (340g) chicken breast, cut into bite-sized pieces
- 2 carrots, chopped
- 2 celery stalks, chopped
- 1 onion, chopped
- 2 garlic cloves
- 1 tsp. dried thyme
- 6 cups low-sodium chicken broth
- 1 tsp. sea salt

- *2 medium zucchinis, spiralized*

Direction: Preparation Time: 10 minutes Cooking Time: 15 minutes Servings: 4

✓ *Heat the olive oil in a pot over medium-high heat until shimmering.*

✓ *Add the chicken and sear for 5 minutes or until well browned. Remove the cooked chicken from the pot and set it aside on a plate.*

✓ *Add the carrots, celery, and onion to the pot and sauté for 5 minutes or until tender.*

✓ *Add the garlic and sauté for 1 minute or until fragrant.*
Add the thyme, chicken broth, and salt. Bring to a boil, then reduce the heat to medium.

✓ *Put the chicken back to the pot and add the spiralized zucchini. Simmer for 2 minutes or until the zucchini is tender. Keep stirring during the simmering.*

✓ *Pour the soup into a large bowl and serve immediately.*

Nutrition: Calories: 292 Fat: 16.9g Protein: 25.8g

569) Ritzy Calabaza Squash Soup

Ingredients:

- *2 pounds (907g) calabaza squash, peeled and chopped*
- *1 large tomato, chopped*
- *1 medium onion, chopped*
- *1 medium green bell pepper, chopped*
- *1 scotch bonnet chili, deseeded and minced*
- *8 scallions, chopped*
- *3 sprigs fresh thyme*
1 tbsp. minced ginger root
- *8 cups low-sodium vegetable broth*
- *1 lime, juiced*
- *¼ cup chopped cilantro Salt, to taste*
- *¼ cup toasted pepitas*

Direction: Preparation Time: 15 minutes Cooking Time: 45 minutes Servings: 8

✓ *Put the calabaza squash, tomato, onion, bell pepper, scotch bonnet, scallions, thyme, and ginger roots in a saucepan, then pour in the vegetable broth.*

✓ *Bring to a boil over medium-high heat. Reduce the heat to low, then simmer for 45 minutes or until the vegetables are soft. Stir constantly.*

✓ *Add the lime juice, cilantro, and salt. Pour the soup in a large bowl, then discard the thyme sprigs and garnish with pepitas before serving.*

Nutrition: Calories: 50 Fat: 0.1g Protein: 20g

570) Creamy Squash Soup

Ingredients:

- *2 tbsp. extra-virgin olive oil*
- *1 medium onion, chopped*
- *1 ½ pounds (680g) buttercup squash, peeled, deseeded, and cut into 1- inch chunks*
- *4 cups vegetable broth*
- *½ tsp. Kosher salt*
- *¼ tsp. ground white pepper Ground nutmeg, to taste*

Direction: Preparation Time: 15 minutes Cooking Time: 33 minutes Servings: 6

✓ *Heat the olive oil in a pot over medium-high heat until shimmering.*

✓ *Add the onion and sauté for 3 minutes or until translucent.*

✓ *Add the buttercup squash, vegetable broth, salt, and pepper. Stir to mix well. Bring to a boil.*

✓ *Reduce the heat to low and simmer for 30 minutes or until the buttercup squash is soft.*

✓ *Pour the soup in a food processor, then pulse to purée until creamy and smooth.*

✓ *Pour the soup in a large serving bowl, then sprinkle with ground nutmeg and serve.*

Nutrition: Calories: 110 Fat: 5.0g Protein: 1.0g

571) Turkey, Barley and Vegetable Stock

Ingredients:

- *2 tbsp. avocado oil*
- *1 lb. (454g) ground turkey*
- *28 oz. (1.3kg) tomatoes, diced*
- *2 tbsp. sugar-free tomato paste*
- *4 cups low-sodium chicken broth*
- *1 (15 oz./425g) package frozen peppers and onions (about 2½ cups)*
- *1 (15 oz./425g) package frozen chopped carrots (about 2½ cups)*
- *1/3 cup dry barley*
- *2 bay leaves*
- *1 tsp. Kosher salt*
- *¼ tsp. freshly ground black pepper*

Direction: Preparation Time: 25 minutes Cooking Time: 3 hours and 7 minutes Servings: 8

✓ *Heat the avocado oil in a pot over medium-high heat.*

✓ *Add the turkey and sauté for 7 minutes or until lightly browned.*

✓ *Add the tomatoes, tomato paste, and chicken broth. Stir to mix well.*

✓ *Add the peppers and onions, carrots, barley, bay*

leaves, salt, and pepper. Stir to mix well.

✓ Bring to a boil. Reduce the heat to low, then cover the pot and simmer for 3 hours.

✓ Once the simmering is finished, allow to cool for 20 minutes, then discard the bay leaves and pour the soup in a large bowl to serve.

Nutrition: Calories: 253 Fat: 12.0g Protein: 19.0g

572) *Roasted Tomato and Bell Pepper Soup*

Ingredients:

* 2 tbsp. extra-virgin olive oil, plus more for coating the baking dish
* 16 plum tomatoes, cored and halved
* 4 celery stalks, coarsely chopped
* 4 red bell peppers, seeded, halved
* 4 garlic cloves, lightly crushed
* 1 sweet onion, cut into eighths
* Sea salt and freshly ground black pepper, to taste
* 6 cups low-sodium chicken broth
* tbsp. chopped fresh basil
* 2 oz. (57 g) goat cheese, grated

Direction: Preparation Time: 20 minutes Cooking Time: 35 minutes Servings: 6

✓ Preheat the oven to 400°F (205°C). Coat a large baking dish lightly with olive oil.

✓ Put the tomatoes in the oiled dish, cut-side down. Scatter the celery, bell peppers, garlic, and onion on top of the tomatoes. Drizzle with 2 tbsp—olive oil and season with salt and pepper.

✓ Roast in the preheated oven for about 30 minutes, or until the vegetables are fork-tender and slightly charred.

✓ Remove the vegetables from the oven. Let them rest for a few minutes until cooled slightly.

✓ Transfer to a food processor, along with the chicken broth, and purée until fully mixed and smooth.

✓ Pour the puréed soup into a medium saucepan and bring it to a simmer over medium-high heat.

✓ Sprinkle the basil and grated cheese on top before serving.

Nutrition: Calories: 187 Fat: 9.7g Protein: 7.8g

573) *Black Bean and Tomato Soup with Lime Yogurt*

Ingredients:

* 2 tbsp. avocado oil

* 1 medium onion, chopped
* 1 (10 oz./284g) can diced tomatoes and green chilies
* 1 pound (454 g) dried black beans, soaked in water for at least 8 hours, rinsed
* 1 tsp. ground cumin
* 3 garlic cloves, minced
* 6 cups chicken bone broth, vegetable broth, or Kosher water salt, to taste
* tbsp. freshly squeezed lime juice
* ¼ cup plain Greek yogurt

Direction: Preparation Time: 8 hours and 20 minutes Cooking Time: 93 minutes Servings: 8

✓ Heat the avocado oil in a nonstick skillet over medium heat until shimmering.

✓ Add the onion and sauté for 3 minutes or until translucent.

✓ Transfer the onion to a pot, then add the tomatoes and green chilies and their juices, black beans, cumin, garlic, broth, and salt. Stir to combine well.

✓ Bring to a boil over medium-high heat, then reduce the heat to low. Simmer for 1 hour and 30 minutes or until the beans are soft.

✓ Meanwhile, combine the lime juice with Greek yogurt in a small bowl. Stir to mix well.

✓ Pour the soup in a large serving bowl, then drizzle with lime yogurt before serving.

Nutrition: Calories: 285 Fat: 6.0g Protein: 19.0g

574) *Black Bean, Corn, and Chicken Soup*

Ingredients:

* 2 tbsp. olive oil
* ½ onion, diced
* 1 pound (454 g) boneless and skinless chicken breast, cut into ½-inch cubes
* ½ tsp. Adobo seasoning, divided
* ¼ tsp. black pepper
* 1 (15 oz./425g) can no-salt-added black beans, rinsed and drained
* 1 (14.5 oz./411g) can fire-roasted tomatoes
* ½ cup frozen corn
* ½ tsp. cumin
* 1 tbsp. chili powder
* 5 cups low-sodium chicken broth

Direction: Preparation Time: 10 minutes Cooking Time: 25 minutes Servings: 7

✓ Grease a stockpot with olive oil and heat over medium-high heat until shimmering.

✓ Add the onion and sauté for 3 minutes or until translucent.

✓ Add the chicken breast and sprinkle with Adobo

seasoning and pepper. Put the lid on and cook for 6 minutes or until lightly browned. Shake the pot halfway through the cooking time.

✓ Add the remaining ingredients. Reduce the heat to low and simmer for 15 minutes or until the black beans are soft.

✓ Serve immediately.

Nutrition: Calories: 170 Fat: 3.5g Protein: 20.0g

575) Slow Cooked Beef and Vegetables Roast

Ingredients:

- 1 tbsp. olive oil
- medium celery stalks, halved lengthwise and cut into 3-inch pieces
- 4 medium carrots, scrubbed, halved lengthwise, and cut into 3-inch pieces
- 1 medium onion, cut in eighths
- 1¼ pounds (567g) lean chuck roast, boneless, trimmed of fat
- 2 tsp. Worcestershire sauce
- 1 tbsp. balsamic vinegar
- 2 tbsp. water
- 1 tbsp. onion soup mix
- ½ tsp. ground black pepper

Direction: Preparation Time: 15 minutes Cooking Time: 4 hours Servings: 4

✓ Grease a slow cooker with olive oil.

✓ Put the celery, carrots, and onion in the slow cooker, then add the beef.

✓ Top them with Worcestershire sauce, balsamic vinegar, and water, then sprinkle with onion soup mix and black pepper.

✓ Cover and cook on high for 4 hours.

✓ Allow to cool for 20 minutes, then serve them on a large plate.

Nutrition: Calories: 250 Fat: 6g Protein: 33g

576) Comforting, Traditional, Split Pea Soup

Ingredients:

- 1 (8 oz.) pack of dried split peas
- 1 large chopped carrot
- 1 large chopped onion
- ½ a cup chopped celery
- ½ a cup low-sodium diced and cooked ham
- 2 cups low sodium chicken broth or stock
- 1 ½ cups fresh water

- Sea salt and black pepper to taste
- 1 bay leaf

Direction: Preparation Time: 10 minutes Cooking Time: 8 hours Servings: 2

✓ Place all the ingredients in your slow cooker

✓ Cook covered on the low setting for 8 hours or until the peas are tender and the soup has thickened

✓ Serve

Nutrition: Calories: 457 Fat 3.3g Protein: 36.4g

577) Hearty Vegetarian Minestrone

Ingredients:

- 1 cup vegetable stock or broth
- ¼ cup soaked white dried beans
- ¼ cup soaked red dried beans
- 3 medium, ripe, quartered Tomatoes
- 1 chunky diced onion
- 1 large chopped stick of celery leaves included
- 1 diced carrot
- ½ a cup chopped green beans
  ½ a cup chopped baby spinach
- 1 diced zucchini
- 3 finely diced cloves of garlic
- 1 tbsp. chopped parsley
- 1 tsp. oregano
- 1 sprigs thyme
- Sea salt and freshly cracked black pepper to taste
- Freshly shaved parmesan cheese for topping when serving

Direction: Preparation Time: 20 minutes Cooking Time: 7 hours Servings: 2

✓ Combine everything except the spinach leaves in your crockpot, put on the lid, and cook the soup for 4 to 5 hours on high or 7 to 8 hours on low Stir the baby spinach into the minestrone and cook for about another 15 minutes

✓ Sprinkle the herbs and Parmesan over and serve

Nutrition: Calories: 219 Fat: 8.9g Protein: 5.1g

578) Divine Lebanese Red Lentil Soup

Ingredients:

- 1 cup dry red lentils
- cups vegetable stock or broth
- 1 small chopped Yellow onion
- 1 small chopped red onion
- 1 chopped carrot
- 1 chopped stalk of celery leaves included
- 4 garlic cloves, minced

- 1 tsp. red wine vinegar 1 tbsp. olive oil
- 1 tsp. ground black cumin 1 tsp. paprika
- Cayenne pepper to taste 1 bay leaf
- Freshly chopped cilantro leaves for garnish A Lemon or lime sliced into wedges

Direction: Preparation Time: 16 minutes Cooking Time: 5 hours Servings: 2

✓ Sauté the yellow onion with the carrots and celery in the oil for a few minutes

✓ Add the garlic, paprika, cumin, and cayenne, then continue cooking until fragrant for about 2 minutes

✓ Pour the mixture into your crockpot and add the red lentils, stock, bay leaves, and a little salt. Stir and cover

✓ Cook covered on low for 4 to 5 hours Check the flavor and add more stock and salt if needed

✓ Once the lentils and vegetables have become tender, remove the bay leaf and blend in your blender until smooth. Taste and adjust the seasoning if needed

✓ Serve in bowls with the red onion, cilantro, and lemon wedges

Nutrition: Calories: 227 Fat: 7.9g Protein: 6g

579)   *Romantic Greek Lemon Chicken Soup*

Ingredients:

- ½ lb. skinless chicken breasts
- 1 small chopped Yellow onion
- 1 small chopped stick of celery leaves included
- 1 clove of minced garlic
- 1 cup low sodium, chicken stock, or broth
- 1 cups water
- 2 tbsp. fresh Lemon Juice
- 1 egg
- Sea salt and cracked black pepper to taste

Direction: Preparation Time: 16 minutes Cooking Time: 3 hours Servings: 2

✓ Place the chicken, celery, onion, garlic, stock, and water in your crockpot and season it with 1 tsp. of salt and ¼ of a tsp. of pepper.

✓ Cook, the chicken for about 3 hours on high or 4 to 5 hours on low.

✓ When the chicken is cooked through and tender, take it from the cooker and allow it to cool slightly.

✓ Slice the chicken into chunks and return it to the crockpot.

✓ Whisk the eggs lightly in a bowl with the lemon juice before tempering them by adding several drops of hot soup at a time while constantly beating the eggs. Keep beating the eggs while

adding a little hot soup until you have added about a cupful, then mix the eggs into the soup in your crockpot.

✓ Taste and if necessary, adjust the seasoning, then serve.

Nutrition: Calories: 167 Fat: 4g Protein: 20g

580)   *Home-Style Chicken and Mushroom Soup*

Ingredients:

- 1 cups chicken stock
- ½ a cup water
- 1 small chopped onion
- 1 clove minced garlic
- 1 tsp. unsalted butter or clarified butter
- 2 oz. sliced baby Portabella Mushrooms
- 1 cup shredded cooked chicken
- 1 tsp. Dijon mustard
- 1 tbsp. chopped fresh parsley
- Sea salt and black pepper to taste

Direction: Preparation Time: 10 minutes Cooking Time: 8 hours Servings: 2

✓ Sauté the onion in the butter until tender.

✓ Add the garlic and cook it for 60 seconds.

✓ Place everything in your crockpot and stir to combine.

✓ Cook on low for 6 to 8 hours or high for 3 to 4 hours.

✓ Add salt and pepper to taste and serve.

Nutrition: Calories: 305 Fat: 8.9g Protein: 47.9g

581)   *Fantastic Chicken Orzo Soup*

Ingredients:

- ¼ lb. chicken breasts, trimmed
- 2 cups low-sodium chicken stock or broth
- h 1 ripe chopped tomatoes
- 1 onion, halved and sliced
- 1 lemon, juiced and zested
- 1 tsp. Herbes de Provence or mixed Italian Herbs
- ½ a tsp. sea salt
- ½ a tsp. freshly cracked black pepper
- ¾ cup whole-wheat orzo
- 1/3 cup black or green olives stoned and quartered
- 1 tbsp. chopped fresh parsley for garnish

Direction: Preparation Time: 15 minutes Cooking Time: 4 hours Servings: 2

✓ Slice the chicken into 1-inch cubes.

✓ Place the chicken, tomatoes, onion, stock, lemon juice, and zest, herbs de Provence, sea salt, and black pepper in your crockpot.

✓ Cook covered on high for 2 hours or low for 4 hours.
Then stir in the olives and orzo and allow it to cook for a further 30 minutes.

✓ Allow the soup to cool slightly and serve it garnished with parsley.

Nutrition: Calories: 278 Fat: 5g Protein: 29g

582) Homely Italian Butternut Soup with Chicken and Salami

Ingredients:

- 1 cup peeled and cubed butternut squash
- ½ a cup chicken, chopped into 1-inch piece
- s 1 stick diced Celery
- 1 small diced carrot
- 1 small diced onion
- 1 garlic clove finely chopped
- 2 tsp. olive oil
- 1 cup chicken stock
- 1 cup diced tomatoes
- A pinch grated Nutmeg
- ¼ tsp. Italian Seasoning
- A pinch Red Pepper Flakes
- ¼ cup diced Salami
- ¼ cup milk
- green onion, sliced for garnishing

Direction: Preparation Time: 30 minutes Cooking Time: 8 hours Servings: 2

✓ Sauté the chicken using the oil in a pan or use the sauté option on your crockpot, until browned.

✓ Take out the chicken and let it cool if sautéed in the crockpot then add the squash, carrots, onions, and celery and sauté these for 3–4 minutes.

✓ Add the garlic and sauté until fragrant.

✓ Chop the chicken into cubes or strips and place everything except the salami and milk in your crockpot.

✓ Cook on high for 4 hours or low for 7 hours.

✓ Then add the milk and salami, then cook it for a further hour.

✓ Serve in individual soup bowls with sliced green onions as a garnish.

Nutrition: Calories: 121 Fat: 6.2g Protein: 5.5g

583) Delectable Chicken, Chorizo and Kale Soup

Ingredients:

- oz. pork chorizo without the casing (a fermented, cured, smoked sausage)
- 1 cloves sliced garlic
- 1 sliced onion
- 2 cups chicken stock
- 1 bay leaf
-
- 1 tsp. sweet paprika
- 1 medium diced potatoes
- 2 oz. thinly sliced baby kale
- Sea salt and freshly cracked black pepper to taste
-

Direction: Preparation Time: 20 minutes Cooking Time: 8 hours Servings: 2

✓ Preheat your crockpot on the sauté setting, then add the oil and sauté the onions until golden.

✓ Add the chorizo and the garlic, stir for about a minute and add the stock, bay leaf, and potatoes.

✓ Cook covered for 4 to 5 hours on high or 7 to 8 hours on low.

✓ About 30 minutes before serving, adjust the seasoning if necessary, add the kale, give a stir and cook again for about 10 minutes.

✓ Then remove half of the chorizo and the bay leaf.

✓ Using your immersion (stick blender) or benchtop blender, puree the soup, leaving just a few chunks.

✓ Place the remaining chorizo to the soup and serve.

Nutrition: Calories: 223 Fat: 9.1g Protein: 9.9g

584) Delightful Thick Beef and Vegetable Soup

Ingredients:

- ½ lb. Beef, diced
- ½ a cup fire-roasted tomatoes, diced
- 1 cup beef stock or broth
- 1 sliced carrot
- sliced celery stalks 1 small diced onion
- cloves minced garlic
- 2 tsp. crushed dried Rosemary
- 1 small bunch of baby spinach
- Sea salt and freshly cracked black pepper to taste
- 1 tsp. balsamic vinegar

Direction: Preparation Time: 16 minutes Cooking Time: 8 hours Servings: 2

✓ Turn your Sauté option on your crockpot

✓ *Add the oil and when hot, add the beef*

✓ *Sauté the beef, browning on all sides*

✓ *Add all the other ingredients except the baby spinach and vinegar and stir to mix*
Cook the soup covered until the beef is tender, on low for 7 to 8 hours

✓ *Just before serving, stir in the vinegar and baby spinach*

✓ *Allow the soup to stand for 10 minutes, so the spinach warms through and serve*

Nutrition: Calories: 547 Fat: 34.6g Protein: 43.7g

585)   *Dreamy Mediterranean Fish Soup*

Ingredients:

- ¼ lb. cod fillets, cubed
- ¼ lb. shrimp
- 1 small diced onion
- 1 small green diced capsicum
- 2 garlic cloves, minced
- ½ cup tomatoes, diced
- 1 cup chicken stock or broth
- ¼ cup tomato sauce
- ¼ cup canned mushrooms
- 1 tbsp. cup sliced black olives
- ¼ cup fresh orange juice
- ¼ cup dry white wine (nice drinking wine)
- 1 bay leaf
- 1 tsp. basil, dried
- ⅛ tsp. fennel seed, crushed
- ⅛ tsp. freshly cracked black pepper

Direction: Preparation Time: 30 minutes Cooking Time: 4 hours Servings: 2

✓ *Place everything except the fish and shrimp in your crockpot and cook for about 4 to 4½ hours*

✓ *Add the fresh fish 45 minutes before serving and the fresh shrimp 15 minutes before serving*

✓ *Remove the bay leaf and serve*

Nutrition: Calories: 207 Fat: 3.1g Protein: 28.9g

586)   *Mediterranean Calamari Stew*

Ingredients:

- ½ lb. calamari tubes
- 1 small diced onions
- 1 garlic clove, minced
- 1 chili pepper
- 1 tbsp. capers
- 6 large black olives
- 2 tbsp. tomato paste

- ½ cup tomatoes, diced
- 3 sprigs of fresh thyme
- 1 bay leaf
- Sea salt to taste
- Freshly cracked black pepper to taste
- 1 tbsp. olive oil

Direction: Preparation Time: 20 minutes Cooking Time: 4 hours Servings: 2

✓ *Cut the calamari tubes to about ⅛ inch thick*

✓ *Place the onions, thyme sprigs, bay leaves, chili, tomato paste, tomatoes, and garlic in your crockpot*

✓ *Cook covered on high for 2 ½ hours or low for 4 hours*

✓ *Dice the capers, finely and slice the olives into rings and add them with the calamari to your crockpot, then add these to your slow cooker with the calamari rings*

✓ *Cook covered on high another hour, then remove the bay leaves and thyme*

✓ *Taste and then serve*

Nutrition: Calories: 430 Fat: 21.4g Protein: 38.8g

587)   *Heavenly Vegan White Bean Stew*

Ingredients:

- ½ lb. white beans
- 1 small carrot, diced
- 1 small celery stalk
- 1 small onion, diced
- 1 garlic clove, minced
- 1 bay leaf
- ½ a tsp. dried Rosemary
- ½ a tsp. dried thyme
- ½ a tsp. dried oregano
- 3 to 6 cups fresh drinking water
- tbsp. Sea Salt, more or less to taste
- Freshly ground White Pepper, to taste
- ½ a cup tomatoes, diced
- or 3 cups (or more) of green leafy green vegetables (kale, chard, spinach)
- Couscous, polenta for serving

Direction: Preparation Time: 20 minutes Cooking Time: 10 hours Servings: 2

✓ *Place the soaked beans in your crockpot, covered with the water.*

✓ *Cook, covered, for 8 to 10 hours on low. Then add the carrots, onion, celery, garlic, bay leaf, and dried herbs. Cook, covered, on low for 4 to 7 When the beans are tender, add the tomatoes, salt, and pepper to taste. Add the greens 15 mins before serving. They can be served hot, warm, or cold over couscous, polenta, or bread.*

Nutrition: Calories: 336 Fat: 0.09g Protein: 233g

588) Kidney Bean Stew

Ingredients:

* *1lb cooked kidney beans*
* *1 cup tomato passata*
* *1 cup low sodium beef broth*
* *3tbsp Italian herbs*

Direction: Preparation time: 15 minutes

Cooking time: 15 minutes Servings: 2

✓ *Mix all the ingredients in your Instant Pot.*

✓ *Cook on Stew for 15 minutes.*
  Release the pressure naturally.

Nutrition: Calories: 270; Carbs: 16; Sugar: 3; Fat: 10; Protein: 23; GL: 8

589) Cabbage Soup

Ingredients:

* *1lb shredded cabbage*
* *1 cup low sodium vegetable broth*
* *1 shredded onion*
* *2tbsp mixed herbs*
* *1tbsp black pepper*

Direction: Preparation time: 15 minutes Cooking time: 35 minutes Servings: 2

✓ *Mix all the ingredients in your Instant Pot.*

✓ *Cook on Stew for 35 minutes.*
  Release the pressure naturally.

Nutrition: Calories: 60; Carbs: 2; Sugar: 0; Fat: 2; Protein: 4; GL: 1

590) Pumpkin Spice Soup

Ingredients:

* *1lb cubed pumpkin*
* *1 cup low sodium vegetable broth*
* *2tbsp mixed spice*

Direction: Preparation time: 10 minutes Cooking time: 35 minutes Servings: 2

✓ *Mix all the ingredients in your Instant Pot.*

✓ *Cook on Stew for 35 minutes.*
  Release the pressure naturally.

✓ *Blend the soup.*

Nutrition: Calories: 100; Carbs: 7; Sugar: 1; Fat: 2; Protein: 3; GL: 1

591) Cream of Tomato Soup

Ingredients:

* *1lb fresh tomatoes, chopped*
* *1.5 cups low sodium tomato puree*
* *1tbsp black pepper*

Direction: Preparation time: 15 minutes Cooking time: 15 minutes Servings: 2

✓ *Mix all the ingredients in your Instant Pot.*

✓ *Cook on Stew for 15 minutes.*
  Release the pressure naturally.

✓ *Blend.*

Nutrition: Calories: 20; Carbs: 2; Sugar: 1; Fat: 0; Protein: 3; GL: 1

592) Shiitake Soup

Ingredients:

* *1 cup shiitake mushrooms*
* *1 cup diced vegetables*
* *1 cup low sodium vegetable broth*
* *2tbsp 5 spice seasoning*

Direction: Preparation time: 15 minutes Cooking time: 35 minutes Servings: 2

✓ *Mix all the ingredients in your Instant Pot.*

✓ *Cook on Stew for 35 minutes.*
  Release the pressure naturally.

Nutrition: Calories: 70; Carbs: 5; Sugar: 1; Fat: 2; Protein: 2; GL: 1

593) Spicy Pepper Soup

Ingredients:

* *1lb chopped mixed sweet peppers*
* *1 cup low sodium vegetable broth*
* *3tbsp chopped chili peppers*
* *1tbsp black pepper*

Direction: Preparation time: 15 minutes

Cooking time: 15 minutes Servings: 2

✓ *Mix all the ingredients in your Instant Pot.*

✓ *Cook on Stew for 15 minutes.*
  Release the pressure naturally. Blend.

Nutrition: Calories: 100; Carbs: 11; Sugar: 4; Fat: 2; Protein: 3; GL: 6

594) Zoodle Won-Ton Soup

Ingredients:

* *1lb spiralized zucchini*
* *1 pack unfried won-tons*

- 1 cup low sodium beef broth
- 2tbsp soy sauce

Direction: Preparation time: 15 minutes Cooking time: 5 minutes Servings: 2

✓ Mix all the ingredients in your Instant Pot.
✓ Cook on Stew for 5 minutes.
  Release the pressure naturally.

Nutrition: Calories: 300; Carbs: 6; Sugar: 1; Fat: 9; Protein: 43; GL: 2

595)   Broccoli Stilton Soup

Ingredients:

- 1lb chopped broccoli
- 0.5lb chopped vegetables
- 1 cup low sodium vegetable broth
- 1 cup Stilton

Direction: Preparation time: 15 minutes

Cooking time: 35 minutes Servings: 2

✓ Mix all the ingredients in your Instant Pot.
✓ Cook on Stew for 35 minutes.
  Release the pressure naturally.
✓ Blend the soup.

Nutrition: Calories: 280; Carbs: 9; Sugar: 2; Fat: 22; Protein: 13; GL: 4

596)   Lamb Stew Recipe 2

Ingredients:

- 1lb diced lamb shoulder
- 1lb chopped winter vegetables
- 1 cup low sodium vegetable broth
- 1tbsp yeast extract
- 1tbsp star anise spice mix

Direction: Preparation time: 15 minutes Cooking time: 35 minutes Servings: 2

✓ Mix all the ingredients in your Instant Pot.
✓ Cook on Stew for 35 minutes.
  Release the pressure naturally.

Nutrition: Calories: 320; Carbs: 10; Sugar: 2; Fat: 8; Protein: 42; GL: 3

597)   Irish Stew

Ingredients:

- 1.5lb diced lamb shoulder
- 1lb chopped vegetables
- 1 cup low sodium beef broth
- 3 minced onions
- 1tbsp ghee

Direction: Preparation time: 15 minutes Cooking time: 35 minutes Servings: 2

✓ Mix all the ingredients in your Instant Pot.
✓ Cook on Stew for 35 minutes.
✓ Release the pressure naturally.

Nutrition: Calories: 330; Carbs: 9; Sugar: 2; Fat: 12; Protein: 49; GL: 3

598)   Sweet And Sour Soup

Ingredients:

- 1lb cubed chicken breast
- 1lb chopped vegetables
- 1 cup low carb sweet and sour sauce
- 0.5 cup diabetic marmalade

Direction: Preparation time: 15 minutes Cooking time: 35 minutes Servings: 2

✓ Mix all the ingredients in your Instant Pot.
✓ Cook on Stew for 35 minutes.
  Release the pressure naturally.

Calories: 78 Carbs: 5; Fat: 6; Protein: 12; GL: 1

599)   Meatball Stew

Ingredients:

- 1lb sausage meat
- 2 cups chopped tomato
- 1 cup chopped vegetables
- 2tbsp Italian seasonings
- 1tbsp vegetable oil

Direction: Preparation time: 15 minutes Cooking time: 25 minutes Servings: 2

✓ Roll the sausage into meatballs.
✓ Put the Instant Pot on Sauté and fry the meatballs in the oil until brown.
✓ Mix all the ingredients in your Instant Pot.
  Cook on Stew for 25 minutes.
✓ Release the pressure naturally.

Nutrition: Calories: 300; Carbs: 4; Sugar: 1; Fat: 12; Protein: 40; GL: 2

600)   Kebab Stew

Ingredients:

- 1lb cubed, seasoned kebab meat
- 1lb cooked chickpeas
- 1 cup low sodium vegetable broth
- 1tbsp black pepper

Direction: Preparation time: 15 minutes Cooking time: 35 minutes Servings: 2

✓ *Mix all the ingredients in your Instant Pot.*

✓ *Cook on Stew for 35 minutes.
Release the pressure naturally.*

Nutrition: Calories: 290; Carbs: 22; Sugar: 4; Fat: 10; Protein: 34; GL: 6

601)   *French Onion Soup*

Ingredients:

- *6 onions, chopped finely*
- *2 cups vegetable broth*
- *2tbsp oil*
- *2tbsp Gruyere*

Direction: Preparation time: 35 minutes Cooking time: 35 minutes Servings: 2

✓ *Place the oil in your Instant Pot and cook the onions on Sauté until soft and brown.*

✓ *Mix all the ingredients in your Instant Pot. Cook on Stew for 35 minutes.*

✓ *Release the pressure naturally.*

Nutrition: Calories: 110; Carbs: 8; Sugar: 3; Fat: 10; Protein: 3; GL: 4

602)   *Meatless Ball Soup*

Ingredients:

- *1lb minced tofu*
- *0.5lb chopped vegetables*
- *2 cups low sodium vegetable broth*
- *1tbsp almond flour*
- *salt and pepper*

Direction: Preparation time: 15 minutes Cooking time: 15 minutes Servings: 2

✓ *Mix the tofu, flour, salt and pepper.*
✓ *Form the meatballs.*
✓ *Place all the ingredients in your Instant Pot. Cook on Stew for 15 minutes.*
✓ *Release the pressure naturally.*

Nutrition: Calories: 240; Carbs: 9; Sugar: 3; Fat: 10; Protein: 35; GL: 5

603)   *Fake-On Stew*

Ingredients:

- *0.5lb soy bacon*
- *1lb chopped vegetables*
- *1 cup low sodium vegetable broth*
- *1tbsp nutritional yeast*

Direction: Preparation time: 15 minutes Cooking time: 25 minutes Servings: 2

✓ *Mix all the ingredients in your Instant Pot.*

✓ *Cook on Stew for 25 minutes.
Release the pressure naturally.*

Nutrition: Calories: 200; Carbs: 12; Sugar: 3; Fat: 7; Protein: 41; GL: 5

604)   *Chickpea Soup*

Ingredients:

- *1lb cooked chickpeas*
- *1lb chopped vegetables*
- *1 cup low sodium vegetable broth*
- *2tbsp mixed herbs*

Direction: Preparation time: 15 minutes Cooking time: 35 minutes Servings: 2

✓ *Mix all the ingredients in your Instant Pot.*

✓ *Cook on Stew for 35 minutes.
Release the pressure naturally.*

Nutrition: Calories: 310; Carbs: 20; Sugar: 3; Fat: 5; Protein: 27; GL: 5

605)   *Chicken Zoodle Soup*

Ingredients:

- *1lb chopped cooked chicken*
- *1lb spiralized zucchini*
- *1 cup low sodium chicken soup*
- *1 cup diced vegetables*

Direction: Preparation time: 15 minutes Cooking time: 35 minutes Servings: 2

✓ *Mix all the ingredients except the zucchini in your Instant Pot.*

✓ *Cook on Stew for 35 minutes.
Release the pressure naturally.*

✓ *Stir in the zucchini and allow to heat thoroughly.*

Nutrition: Calories: 250; Carbs: 5; Sugar: 0; Fat: 10; Protein: 40; GL: 1

SMOOTHIES & JUICES

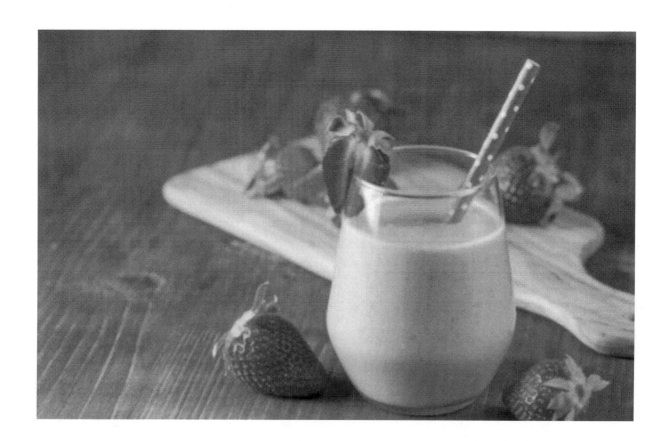

606) Choco-Nut Milkshake

Ingredients:

- cups unsweetened coconut, almond
- 1 banana, sliced and frozen
- ¼ cup unsweetened coconut flakes
- 1 cup ice cubes
- ¼ cup macadamia nuts, chopped
- 3 tbsp. sugar-free sweetener
- 2 tbsp. raw unsweetened cocoa powder
- Whipped coconut cream

Direction: Preparation Time: 10 minutes Cooking Time: 0 minute Servings: 2

- ✓ Place all ingredients into a blender and blend on high until smooth and creamy.
- ✓ Divide evenly between 4 "mocktail" glasses and top with whipped coconut cream, if desired.
- ✓ Add a cocktail umbrella and toasted coconut for added flair.
- ✓ Enjoy your delicious choco-nut smoothie!

Nutrition: Carbohydrates: 12g Protein: 3g Calories: 199

607) Pineapple & Strawberry Smoothie

Ingredients:

- 1 cup strawberries
- 1 cup pineapple, chopped
- ¾ cup almond milk
- 1 tbsp. almond butter

Direction: Preparation Time: 7 minutes Cooking Time: 0 minute Servings: 2

- ✓ Add all ingredients to a blender.
- ✓ Blend until smooth.
- ✓ Add more almond milk until it reaches your desired consistency.
- ✓ Chill before serving.

Nutrition: Calories: 255 Carbohydrate: 39g Protein: 5.6g

608) Cantaloupe Smoothie

Ingredients:

- ¾ cup carrot juice
- 4 cups cantaloupe, sliced into cubes
- Pinch of salt
- Frozen melon balls
- Fresh basil

Direction: Preparation Time: 11 minutes Cooking Time: 0 minute Servings: 2

- ✓ Add the carrot juice and cantaloupe cubes to a blender. Sprinkle with salt.
- ✓ Process until smooth.
- ✓ Transfer to a bowl.
- ✓ Chill in the refrigerator for at least 30 minutes.
- ✓ Top with the frozen melon balls and basil before serving.

Nutrition: Calories: 135 Carbohydrates: 31g Protein: 3.4g

609) Berry Smoothie with Mint

Ingredients:

- ¼ cup orange juice
- ½ cup blueberries
- ½ cup blackberries
- cup reduced-fat plain kefir
- 1 tbsp. honey
- 1tbsp. fresh mint leaves

Direction: Preparation Time: 7 minutes Cooking Time: 0 minute Servings: 2

- ✓ Add all the ingredients to a blender.
- ✓ Blend until smooth.
- ✓ Serve

Nutrition: Calories: 137 Carbohydrates: 27g Protein: 6g

610) Green Smoothie

Ingredients:

- 1 cup vanilla almond milk (unsweetened)
- ¼ ripe avocado, chopped
- 1 cup kale, chopped
- banana
- 2 tsp. honey
- 1tbsp. chia seeds
- 1 cup ice cubes

Direction: Preparation Time: 12 minutes Cooking Time: 0 minute Servings: 2

- ✓ Combine all the ingredients in a blender. Process until creamy.

Nutrition: Calories: 343 Carbohydrates: 14.7g Protein: 5.9g

611) Banana, Cauliflower & Berry Smoothie

Ingredients:

- cups almond milk (unsweetened)
- 1 cup banana, sliced

- ½ cup blueberries
- ½ cup blackberries
- cup cauliflower rice
- 2 tsp. maple syrup

Direction: Preparation Time: 9 minutes Cooking Time: 0 minute Servings: 2

✓ Pour almond milk into a blender.

✓ Stir in the rest of the ingredients.

✓ Process until smooth.

✓ Chill before serving.

Nutrition: Calories: 149 Carbohydrates: 29g Protein: 3g

612) Berry & Spinach Smoothie

Ingredients:

- 2 cups strawberries
- 1 cup raspberries
- 1 cup blueberries
- 1 cup fresh baby spinach leaves
- 1 cup pomegranate juice
- 3 tbsp. milk powder (unsweetened)

Direction: Preparation Time: 11 minutes Cooking Time: 0 minute Servings: 2

✓ Mix all the ingredients in a blender.

✓ Blend until smooth.

✓ Chill before serving.

Nutrition: Calories: 118 Carbohydrates; 25.7g Protein: 4.6g

613) Peanut Butter Smoothie with Blueberries

Ingredients:

- 2 tbsp. creamy peanut butter
- 1 cup vanilla almond milk (unsweetened)
- 6 oz. soft silken tofu
- ½ cup grape juice
- 1 cup blueberries
- Crushed ice

Direction: Preparation Time: 12 minutes Cooking Time: 0 minute Servings: 2

✓ Mix all the ingredients in a blender.

✓ Process until smooth.

Nutrition: Calories: 247 Carbohydrate 30g Protein: 10.7g

614) Peach & Apricot Smoothie

Ingredients:

- 1 cup almond milk (unsweetened)
- 1 tsp. honey
- ½ cup apricots, sliced
- ½ cup peaches, sliced
- ½ cup carrot, chopped
- 1 tsp. vanilla extract

Direction: Preparation Time: 11 minutes Cooking Time: 0 minute Servings: 2

✓ Mix milk and honey.

✓ Pour into a blender.

✓ Add the apricots, peaches, and carrots.

✓ Stir in the vanilla.

✓ Blend until smooth.

Nutrition: Calories: 153 Carbohydrate: 30g Protein: 32.6g

615) Tropical Smoothie

Ingredients:

- 1 banana, sliced
- 1 cup mango, sliced
- 1 cup pineapple, sliced
- 1 cup peaches, sliced
- 6 oz. nonfat coconut yogurt
- Pineapple wedges

Direction: Preparation Time: 8 minutes Cooking Time: 0 minute Servings: 2

✓ Freeze the fruit slices for 1 hour.

✓ Transfer to a blender.

✓ Stir in the rest of the ingredients except pineapple wedges.

✓ Process until smooth.

✓ Garnish with pineapple wedges.

Nutrition: Calories: 102 Carbohydrate: 22.6g Protein: 2.5g

616) Banana & Strawberry Smoothie

Ingredients:

- 1 banana, sliced
- 4 cups fresh strawberries, sliced
- 1 cup ice cubes
- 6 oz. yogurt
- kiwi fruit, sliced

Direction: Preparation Time: 7 minutes Cooking Time: 0 minute Servings: 2

✓ Add banana, strawberries, ice cubes, and yogurt in

a blender.
- ✓ Blend until smooth.
- ✓ Garnish with kiwi fruit slices and serve.

Nutrition: Calories: 54 Carbohydrate: 11.8g Protein: 1.7g

617) *Cantaloupe & Papaya Smoothie*

Ingredients:

- ¾ cup low-fat milk
- ½ cup papaya, chopped
- ½ cup cantaloupe, chopped
- ½ cup mango, cubed
- 4 ice cubes
- Lime zest

Direction: Preparation Time: 9 minutes Cooking Time: 0 minute Servings: 2

- ✓ Pour milk into a blender.
- ✓ Add the chopped fruits and ice cubes.
- ✓ Blend until smooth.
- ✓ Garnish with lime zest and serve.

Nutrition: Calories: 207 Carbohydrate: 18.4g Protein: 7.7g

618) *Watermelon & Cantaloupe Smoothie*

Ingredients:

- 2 cups watermelon, sliced
- 1 cup cantaloupe, sliced
- ½ cup nonfat yogurt
- ¼ cup orange juice

Direction: Preparation Time: 10 minutes Cooking Time: 0 minute Servings: 2

- ✓ Add all the ingredients to a blender.
- ✓ Blend until creamy and smooth.
- ✓ Chill before serving.

Nutrition: Calories: 114 Carbohydrate: 13g Protein: 4.8g

619) *Raspberry and Peanut Butter Smoothie*

Ingredients:

- 2 tbsp. peanut butter, smooth and natural
- 2 tbsp. skim milk
- 1 or 1 ½ cups raspberries, fresh
- 1 cup ice cubes
- 2 tsp. stevia

Direction: Preparation Time: 10 minutes Cooking

Time: 0 minute Servings: 2

- ✓ Situate all the ingredients in your blender. Set the
- ✓ mixer to puree. Serve

Nutrition: Calories: 170 Fat: 8.6g Carbohydrate: 20g

620) *Strawberry, Kale, and Ginger Smoothie*

Ingredients:

- 6 pcs. curly kale leaves, fresh and large with stems removed
- 2 tsp. grated ginger, raw and peeled
- ½ cup water, cold
- 3 tbsp. lime juice
- 2 tsp. honey
- 1 or 1 ½ cups strawberries, fresh and trimmed
- 1 cup ice cubes

Direction: Preparation Time: 13 minutes Cooking Time: 0 minute Servings: 2

- ✓ Position all the ingredients in your blender. Set to puree.
- ✓ Serve

Nutrition: Calories: 205 Fat: 2.9g Carbohydrates: 42.4g

621) *Green Detox Smoothie*

Ingredients:

- 2 cups baby spinach
- 2 cups baby kale
- 2 ribs celery, chopped
- 1 medium green apple, chopped
- 1 cup frozen sliced banana
- 1 cup almond milk
- 1 tbsp. grated fresh ginger
- 1 tbsp. chia seeds
- 1 tbsp. honey

Direction: Preparation Time: 10 minutes Cooking Time: 0 minutes Servings: 4

- ✓ Combine everything in a blender and blend until smooth.
- ✓ Serve.

Nutrition: Calories: 136 Fat: 1g Protein: 1g

622) *Cucumber Ginger Detox*

Ingredients:

- 1 ½ oz. spinach
- 1 orange, peeled
- ½ inch ginger, peeled

- *1 cup water*
- *1 cucumber, chopped*
- *½ avocado, chopped*
- *1 cup ice*
- *1 tsp. rosehips*

Direction: Preparation Time: 5 minutes Cooking Time: 0 minutes Servings: 2

✓ *Combine everything in the blender and blend until smooth.*
✓ *Serve.*

Nutrition: Calories: 144 Fat: 8g Protein: 3g

623)   *Green Protein: Smoothie*

Ingredients:

- *1 oz. kale*
- *4 oz. pineapple*
- *1 tbsp. pea protein*
- *1 cup water*
- *1 tangerine, peeled*
- *½avocado*
- *3 tbsp. almonds*
- *1 cup ice*

Direction: Preparation Time: 5 minutes Cooking Time: 0 minute Servings: 2

✓ *Except for the almonds, blend everything in the blender.*
✓ *Top with almonds and serve.*

Nutrition: Calories: 227 Fat: 15g Protein: 7g

624)   *Ginger Detox Twist*

Ingredients:

- *1 ½ oz. collard greens*
- *1 apple, chopped*
- *½ inch ginger*
- *1 cup water*
- *Persian cucumbers, chopped*
- *1 Meyer lemon, peeled*
- *½ tsp. chlorella*
- *1 cup ice*

Direction: Preparation Time: 5 minutes Cooking Time: 0 minute Servings: 2

✓ *Blend everything in a blender and serve.*

Nutrition: Calories: 114 Fat: 1g Protein: 5g

625)   *Classic Apple Detox Smoothie*

Ingredients:

- *1 ½ oz. baby spinach*
- *2 oz. celery, chopped*
- *1 lemon, juiced*
- *1 cup water*
- *1 apple, chopped*
- *1 mini cucumber, chopped*
- *½ inch ginger, peeled and chopped*
- *1 cup ice*

Direction: Preparation Time: 5 minutes Cooking Time: 0 minute Servings: 2

✓ *Blend everything in a blender and enjoy.*

Nutrition: Calories: 66 Fat: 0.1g Protein: 1g

626)   *Energy-Booting Green Smoothie*

Ingredients:

- *2 handfuls of greens*
- *½ seeded cucumber 1 apple*
- *1 burro banana*
- *½ tsp. Bromide Plus Powder*
- *1 tbsp. walnuts*
- *½ lb. soft-jelly coconut milk*

Direction: Preparation Time: 15 minutes Cooking Time: 0 minutes Servings: 4

✓ *To prepare your green smoothie, first, mix all the ingredients in a food processor.*
✓ *Pour into a glass and enjoy.*

Nutrition: Fat: 16.5g Protein: 2.9g Calories: 222

627)   *Zucchini Relaxing Smoothie*

Ingredients:

- *1 zucchini, chopped*
- *0.2 lb. herbal tea*
- *½ lb. soft jelly coconut water*

Direction: Preparation Time: 15 minutes Cooking Time: 10 minutes Servings: 4

✓ *To make your smoothie relaxed, first, brew the tea according to the instructions and let it cool.*
✓ *Combine all ingredients in a blender. Blend well.*
✓ *Pour into serving glasses and enjoy!*

Nutrition: Fat: 0.4g Protein: 1.1g Calories: 52

628)   *Magnesium-Boosting Smoothie*

Ingredients:

- *½ lb. fresh spring water*

- *0.7 lb. brazil nuts*
- *½ burro banana*
- *2 strawberries*
- *½ lb. figs*

Direction: Preparation Time: 10 minutes Cooking Time: 0 minutes Servings: 2

✓ *Mix all the ingredients using a high-speed mixer. Enjoy*

Nutrition: Calories: 182 Fat: 3g Protein: 2.8g

629)   *Detox Smoothie*

Ingredients:

- *½ avocado*
- *½ lb. homemade soft-jelly coconut milk*
- *1 handful "approved" greens, such as callaloo, watercress, or dandelion greens*
- *1 squeeze key lime*
- *1 tsp. Dr. Sebi'sBromide Plus Powder*

Direction: Preparation Time: 20 minutes Cooking Time: 0 minutes Servings: 4

✓ *Mix all the ingredients in a high-speed mixer.*
✓ *Fill in more water if the mixture is too concentrated. Enjoy.*

Nutrition: Calories: 202 Fat: 19.4g Protein: 2.4g

630)   *Immunity-Boosting Smoothie*

Ingredients:

- *1 mango*
- *1 Seville orange*
- *½ lb. brewed Dr. Sebi's Immune Support Herbal Tea*
- *1 tbsp. coconut oil*
- *1 tbsp. date sugar or agave syrup*
- *1 lime, juiced*

Direction: Preparation Time: 35 minutes Cooking Time: 20 minutes Servings: 2

✓ *Boil distilled water and pour 1 half tsp. Of Dr. Sebi's Immune Support Herbal Tea. Cook for about 15 minutes. Let cool, strain. Seville orange peel and mango cut into pieces.*
✓ *Mix all ingredients in a high-speed mixer. Add to serving glasses and enjoy!*

Nutrition: Calories: 97 Fat: 3.7g Protein: 9g

631)   *Blueberry and Strawberry Smoothie*

Ingredients:

- *6–7 strawberries, sliced*
- *½ lb. blueberries*

- *½ pint of almond milk*

Direction: Preparation Time: 5 minutes Cooking Time: 0 minutes Servings: 2

✓ *Add all ingredients to a blender jar. Blend until smooth. Add to serving glasses.*
✓ *Serve and enjoy.*

Nutrition: Calories: 107 Fat: 7g Protein: 4g

632)   *Blueberry and Apple Smoothie*

Ingredients:

- *Brae burn apple, or another kind of organic apple*
- *½-1 lb. brazil nuts*
- *½ lb. homemade walnut milk*
- *½ lb. blueberries*
- *½ lb. approved greens (dandelion greens, turnip greens, watercress, etc.)*
- *½ tbsp. date sugar or agave syrup*

Direction: Preparation Time: 25 minutes Cooking Time: 15 minutes Servings: 4

✓ *Incorporate all the ingredients in a high-speed mixer.*
✓ *Stir more water if the mixture is too concentrated.*

Nutrition: Calories: 181 Fat: 5.8g Protein: 3.8g

633)   *Blueberry Pie Smoothie*

Ingredients:

- *1 oz. fresh blueberries 1 burro banana*
- *1 glass coconut milk*
- *½ lb. cooked amaranth*
- *1 tsp. Bromide Plus Powder*
- *1 tbsp. homemade walnut butter*
- *1 tbsp. date sugar*

Direction: Preparation Time: 20 minutes Cooking Time: 0 minutes Servings: 2

✓ *Combine all the ingredients in a high-speed mixer.*
✓ *Fill in more water if too concentrated*

Nutrition: Calories: 413 Fat: 31.9g Protein: 5.8g

634)   *Cucumber and Carley Green Smoothie*

Ingredients:

- *1 lb. soft jelly coconut water 4 seeded cucumbers*
- *2–3 key limes*
- *1 bunch basil or sweet basil leaves*
- *½ tsp. Bromide Plus Powder*

Direction: Preparation Time: 10 minutes Cooking

Time: 0 minutes Servings: 4

✓ *Mix cucumbers, basil, and lime. If you don't have a juicer, treat them in a grinder with sweet coconut jelly.*

✓ *Transfer in a tall glass and stir in coconut water to make it smooth and add powdered bromide. Mix well and enjoy.*

Nutrition: Calories: 141 Fat: 7.4g Protein: 5g

635) *Fruity and Green Smoothie*

Ingredients:

- ½ cup lettuce
- 1 cup water
- 3 medium-size bananas
- 2 tsp. lime juice
- ½ cup raspberries
- ¼ tsp. ginger

Direction: Preparation Time: 10 minutes Cooking Time: 0 minute Servings: 2

✓ *Mash the banana and blend all ingredients for 30 seconds at a time.*

✓ *Serve in a cup and add some ice cubes or place them in a refrigerator.*

Nutrition: Calories: 98 Protein: 16g Fiber: 9.7g

636) *Strawberry-Pineapple Smoothie*

Ingredients:

- 1 cup solidified strawberries
- 1 cup hacked new pineapple
- ¾ cup chilled unsweetened almond milk, in addition to more if necessary
- 1 tbsp. almond spread

Direction: Preparation Time: 8 minutes Cooking Time: 0 minute Servings: 1

✓ *Consolidate strawberries, pineapple, almond milk, and almond margarine in a blender.*

✓ *Procedure until smooth, including more almond milk, if necessary, for wanted consistency. Serve right away.*

Nutrition: Calories: 255 Fat: 11.1g Protein: 5.6g

637) *Truly Green Smoothie*

Ingredients:

- 1 enormous ready banana
- 1 cup pressed child kale or coarsely cleaved develop kale
- 1 cup unsweetened vanilla almond milk

- ¼ ready avocado
- 1 tbsp. chia seeds
- 2 tsp. honey
- 1 cup ice 3D shapes

Direction: Preparation Time: 11 minutes Cooking Time: 0 minute Servings: 1

✓ *Consolidate banana, kale, almond milk, avocado, chia seeds, and honey in a blender. Mix on high until velvety and smooth.*

✓ *Include ice and mix until smooth.*

Nutrition: Calories: 343 Fat: 14.2g Protein: 5.9g

638) *Super Berry Smoothies*

Ingredients:

- 2 cups solidified unsweetened strawberries
- 1 cup solidified unsweetened raspberries
- 1 cup new blackberries or blueberries
- 1 cup new child spinach leaves
- 1 cup pomegranate juice
- 3 tbsp. sans sugar vanilla-season protein powder, soy protein powder, or nonfat dry milk powder

Direction: Preparation Time: 7 minutes Cooking Time: 0 minute Servings: 4

✓ *Consolidate strawberries, raspberries, blackberries, spinach, pomegranate juice, and protein powder in a blender. Spread and mix until smooth. Fill glasses to serve.*

Nutrition: Calories: 118 Fat: 0.7g Protein: 4.6g

639) *Pineapple-Grapefruit Detox Smoothie*

Ingredients:

- 1 cup plain coconut water
- 1 cup solidified diced pineapple
- 1 cup stuffed child spinach
- little grapefruit, stripped and portioned, in addition to any juice pressed from the films
- ½ tsp. ground new ginger
- 1 cup ice

Direction: Preparation Time: 12 minutes Cooking Time: 0 minute Servings: 2

✓ *Mix coconut water, pineapple, spinach, grapefruit, and any juices, ginger, and ice in a blender. Puree until smooth and foamy.*

Nutrition: Calories: 102 Fat: 0.2g Protein: 2g

640)   *Very Veggie Smoothies*

Ingredients:

- *2 cups ice shapes*
- *2 cups V8 V-Fusion Light peach mango juice*
- *1 ½ peach, divided and pitted*
- *½ banana*
- *2 chard leaves, ribs evacuated*
- *Mango wedges (optional)*

Direction: Preparation Time: 9 minutes Cooking Time: 0 minute Servings: 4

✓ *Mix ice 3D shapes, juice, peach, banana, and chard. Spread and mix until smooth. Serve right away. Whenever wanted, decorate with mango wedges.*

Nutrition: Calories: 68 Fat: 0.2g Protein: 0.8g

641)   *Super Hydrating Smoothie*

Ingredients:

- *½ lb. watermelon*
- *½ lb. raspberries*
- *¼ seeded cucumber*
- *1 key lime, juiced*
- *½ lb. soft jelly coconut water*

Direction: Preparation Time: 10 minutes Cooking Time: 0 minutes Servings: 4

✓ *To make the "Super Hydration" smoothie, peel the cucumber and cut it into small pieces. Mix all the ingredients in a fast blender. Let cool to drink. Enjoy.*

Nutrition: Calories: 41 Fat: 6g Carbohydrates: 9.3g Protein: 8g

642)   *Lettuce and Ginger Detox Smoothie*

Ingredients:

- *1 cup coconut water*
- *2 cups chopped Romaine lettuce*
- *1 small banana, peeled*
- *1 cup ginger tea, cooled*
- *6 tbsp. key lime juice*
- *½ cup whole blueberries, fresh*

Direction: Preparation Time: 5 minutes Cooking Time: 0 minute Servings: 2

✓ *With a high-powered blender, situate all the ingredients inside, in order. Close blender then pulses at high speed for 1 minute.*

Nutrition: Calories: 160 Fat: 0.8g Protein: 2g

643)   *Strawberry and Dates Smoothie*

Ingredients:

- *4 cups spring water*
- *2 small bananas, peeled*
- *5 whole strawberries*
- *3 Medjool dates, pitted*

Direction: Preparation Time: 5 minutes Cooking Time: 0 minute Servings: 2

✓ *Get a high-powered blender, and blend all the ingredients inside*

Nutrition: Calories: 219 Fat: 0.8g Protein: 1.6g

644)   *Kale and Ginger Smoothie*

Ingredients:

- *2 cups spring water*
- *1 cup kale leaves, fresh*
- *¼ cup key lime juice*
- *1 medium fresh apple, cored*
- *1-inch piece ginger, fresh*
- *1 cup sliced cucumber, fresh*
- *1 tbsp. sea moss gel*

Direction: Preparation Time: 5 minutes Cooking Time: 0 minute Servings: 2

✓ *Using a high-powered blender, turn it on, and situate all the ingredients.*
✓ *Close blender then pulses at high speed for 1 minute*

Nutrition: Calories: 65.5 Fat: 0.4g Protein: 0.7g

645)   *Arugula and Cucumber Smoothie*

Ingredients:

- *2 cups spring water*
- *1 large bunch callaloo, fresh*
- *¼ cup lime juice*
- *1 cup diced cucumber, fresh*
- *1 large bunch of arugulas, fresh*
- *¼ honey, fresh*
- *1-inch piece ginger, fresh*
- *1 pear, destemmed, diced*
- *6 Medjool dates, pitted*
- *1 tbsp. sea moss gel*

Direction: Preparation Time: 5 minutes Cooking Time: 0 minute Servings: 2

✓ *Take a high-powered blender, turn it on, and place all the ingredients inside.*
Close blender then pulses at high speed for 1 minute.

Nutrition: Calories: 369 Carbohydrates: 85g Protein: 5.5g

646)   Dandelion and Watercress Smoothie

Ingredients:

- 2 cups spring water
- 1 large bunch of dandelion greens, fresh
- ¼ cup key lime juice
- 1 cup watercress, fresh
- 3 baby bananas, peeled
- ½ cup fresh blueberries
- 1-inch piece of ginger, fresh
- 6 Medjool dates, pitted
- 1 tbsp. burdock root powder

Direction: Preparation Time: 5 minutes Cooking Time: 0 minute Servings: 2

✓ With a high-powered blender, switch it on, then place all the ingredients.

✓ Close blender then pulses at high speed for 1 minute.

Nutrition: Calories:418.5 Fats: 1.4g Protein: 5.2g

647)   Watermelon Smoothie

Ingredients:

- 4 cups watermelon, deseeded, cubed
- 4 key limes, juiced
- 4 cucumbers, deseeded, sliced

Direction: Preparation Time: 5 minutes Cooking Time: 0 minute Servings: 2

✓ I was using a high-powered blender, process all the ingredients inside.

✓ Cover then pulse at high speed for a minute

Nutrition: Calories: 123 Fats: 0.8g Protein: 2.5g

648)   Lettuce and Orange Smoothie

Ingredients:

- 1 cup coconut water
- 1 cup lettuce leaves, fresh
- 1 key lime, juiced
- 1 Seville orange, peeled
- 1 tbsp. bromide plus powder
- ½ a medium avocado, pitted

Direction: Preparation Time: 5 minutes Cooking Time: 0 minute Servings: 2

✓ With a high-powered blender, mix all the ingredients.

✓ Close and process at high speed for a minute

Nutrition: Calories: 140.5 Fats: 5.5g Protein: 3.2g

649)   Detox Apple Smoothie

Ingredients:

- 2 cups spring water
- 2 cups amaranth greens
- 2 medium fresh apples, cored
- 1 key lime, juiced
- ¼ avocado

Direction: Preparation Time: 5 minutes Cooking Time: 0 minute Servings: 2

✓ With a high-powered blender, combine all the ingredients

✓ Cover then process at high speed for 1 minute

Nutrition: Calories: 141 Fats: 2.8g Protein: 1.4g

650)   Berries and Hemp Seeds Smoothie

Ingredients:

- 1 cup spring water
- 2 cups fresh lettuce
- 1 medium banana, peeled
- 1 cup mixed berries, fresh
- 1 Seville orange, peeled
- 1 tbsp. hemp seeds
- ¼ avocado, pitted

Direction: Preparation Time: 5 minutes Cooking Time: 0 minute Servings: 2

✓ Get a high-powered blender, then mix all the ingredients inside

Nutrition: Calories: 216 Fats: 5.5g Protein: 5.4g

651)   Pear, Berries, and Quinoa Smoothie

Ingredients:

- 2 cups spring water
- ½ avocado, pitted
- 2 fresh pears, chopped
- ½ cup cooked quinoa
- ¼ cup fresh whole blueberries

Direction: Preparation Time: 5 minutes Cooking Time: 0 minute Servings: 2

✓ Get a high-powered blender, then blend all the ingredients

Nutrition: Calories: 325.5 Fats: 7.3g Protein: 7.3g

652)   Mango and Banana Smoothie

Ingredients:

- 1 cup spring water

- *2 cups greens*
- *½ banana, peeled*
- *1 fresh mango, peeled, destoned, sliced*

Direction: Preparation Time: 5 minutes Cooking Time: 0 minute Servings: 2

✓ *Get a high-powered blender and combine all the ingredients for 1 minute*

Nutrition: Calories: 134.5 Fats: 1g Protein: 1.7g

653) *Berries and Sea Moss Smoothie*

Ingredients:

- *1 cup coconut water*
- *2 cups lettuce leaves*
- *1 banana, peeled*
- *1 cup mixed berries*
- *1 tbsp. sea moss*
- *2 key limes, juiced*

Direction: Preparation Time: 5 minutes Cooking Time: 0 minute Servings: 2

✓ *Get a high-powered blender then pulse all the ingredients for a minut*

Nutrition: Calories: 163 Fats: 0.9g Protein: 3.7g

654) *Raspberry and Chard Smoothie*

Ingredients:

- *2 cups coconut water*
- *2 cups Swiss chards*
- *2 key limes, juiced*
- *2 cups fresh whole raspberries*

Direction: Preparation Time: 5 minutes Cooking Time: 0 minute Servings: 2

✓ *Using a high-powered blender, switch it on, then incorporate all the ingredients inside*

Nutrition: Calories: 137.5 Fats: 1.4g Protein: 3.4g

655) *Apple, Berries, and Kale Smoothie*

Ingredients:

- *1 cup spring water*
- *1 cup mixed berries*
- *2 cups kale leaves, fresh*
- *1 large apple, cored*

Direction: Preparation Time: 5 minutes Cooking Time: 0 minute Servings: 2

✓ *Using a high-powered blender, turn it on, then process all the ingredients inside*

Nutrition: Calories: 112 Fats: 0.7g Protein: 2g

656) *Strawberry Smoothie*

Ingredients:

- *5 Strawberries, medium*
- *6 Ice Cubes*
- *1 cup Soy Milk, unsweetened*
- *1/2 cup Greek Yoghurt, low-fat*

Direction: Preparation Time: 5 Minutes Cooking Time: 5 Minutes Servings: 1

✓ *Place strawberries, yogurt, milk, and ice cubes in a high-speed blender.*

✓ *Blend them for 2 to 3 minutes or until you get a smooth and luscious smoothie.*
Transfer to a serving glass and enjoy it.

Nutrition: Calories 167Kcal; Carbohydrates 11g; Proteins 16g; Fat 6g; Sodium 161mg

657) *Berry Mint Smoothie*

Ingredients:

- *1 tbsp. Low-carb Sweetener of your choice*
- *1 cup Kefir or Low Fat-Yoghurt*
- *2 tbsp. Mint*
- *¼ cup Orange*
- *1 cup Mixed Berries*

Direction: Preparation Time: 5 Minutes Cooking Time: 5 Minutes Servings: 2

✓ *Place all of the ingredients in a high-speed blender, and then blend it until smooth.*

✓ *Transfer the smoothie to a serving glass and enjoy it.*

Nutrition: Calories: 137Kcal; Carbohydrates: 11g; Proteins: 6g; Fat: 1g; Sodium: 64mg

658) *Greenie Smoothie*

Ingredients:

- *1 1/2 cup Water*
- *1 tsp. Stevia*
- *1 Green Apple, ripe*
- *1 tsp. Stevia*
- *1 Green Pear, chopped into chunks*
- *1 Lime*
- *2 cups Kale, fresh*
- *¾ tsp. Cinnamon*
- *12 Ice Cubes*
- *20 Green Grapes*
- *1/2 cup Mint, fresh*

Direction: Preparation Time: 5 Minutes Cooking Time: 5 Minutes Servings: 2

✓ *Pour water, kale, and pear in a high-speed blender and blend them for 2 to 3 minutes until mixed. Stir in all the remaining ingredients and blend until it becomes smooth.*

✓ *Transfer the smoothie to the serving glass.*

Nutrition: Calories: 123Kcal; Carbohydrates: 27g; Proteins: 2g; Fat: 2g; Sodium: 30mg

659) *Coconut Spinach Smoothie*

Ingredients:

- *1 ¼ cup Coconut Milk*
- *2 Ice Cubes*
- *2 tbsp. Chia Seeds*
- *1 scoop of Protein Powder, preferably vanilla*
- *1 cup Spin*

Direction: Preparation Time: 5 Minutes

Cooking Time: 5 Minutes Servings: 2

✓ *Pour coconut milk along with spinach, chia seeds, protein powder, and ice cubes in a high-speed blender.*

✓ *Blend for 2 minutes to get a smooth and luscious smoothie.*

✓ *Serve in a glass and enjoy it.*

Nutrition: Calories 251Kcal; Carbs 10.9g; Proteins 20.3g; Fat 15.1g; Sodium: 102mg

660) *Oats Coffee Smoothie*

Ingredients:

- *1 cup Oats, uncooked & grounded*
- *2 tbsp. Instant Coffee*
- *3 cup Milk, skimmed*
- *2 Banana, frozen & sliced into chunks*
- *2 tbsp. Flax Seeds, grounded*

Direction: Preparation Time: 5 Minutes

Cooking Time: 5 Minutes Servings: 2

✓ *Place all of the ingredients in a high-speed blender and blend for 2 minutes or until smooth and luscious.*

✓ *Serve and enjoy.*

Nutrition: Calories: 251Kcal; Carbs 10.9g; Proteins: 20.3g; Fat: 15.1g; Sodium: 102mg

661) *Veggie Smoothie*

Ingredients:

- *¼ of 1 Red Bell Pepper, sliced*
- *1/2 tbsp. Coconut Oil*
- *1 cup Almond Milk, unsweetened*

- *¼ tsp. Turmeric 4 Strawberries, chopped*
- *Pinch of Cinnamon*
- *1/2 of 1 Banana, preferably frozen*

Direction: Preparation Time: 5 Minutes

Cooking Time: 5 Minutes Servings: 1

✓ *Combine all the ingredients required to make the smoothie in a high-speed blender. Blend for 3 minutes to get a smooth and silky mixture.*

✓ *Serve and enjoy.*

Nutrition: Calories: 169cal; Carbs: 17g; Proteins: 2.3g; Fat: 9.8g; Sodium: 162mg

662) *Avocado Smoothie*

Ingredients:

- *1 Avocado, ripe & pit removed*
- *2 cups Baby Spinach*
- *2 cups Water*
- *1 cup Baby Kale*
- *1 tbsp. Lemon Juice*
- *2 sprigs of Mint*
- *1/2 cup Ice Cubes*

Direction: Preparation Time: 10 Minutes

Cooking Time: 0 Minutes Servings: 2

✓ *Place all the ingredients needed to make the smoothie in a high-speed blender then blend until smooth.*

✓ *Transfer to a serving glass and enjoy it.*

Nutrition: Calories: 214cal; Carbohydrates: 15g; Proteins: 2g; Fat: 17g; Sodium: 25mg

663) *Orange Carrot Smoothie*

Ingredients:

- *1 1/2 cups Almond Milk*
- *¼ cup Cauliflower, blanched & frozen*
- *1 Orange*
- *1 tbsp. Flax Seed*
- *1/3 cup Carrot, grated*
- *1 tsp. Vanilla Extract*

Direction: Preparation Time: 5 Minutes

Cooking Time: 0 Minutes Servings: 1

✓ *Mix all the ingredients in a high-speed blender and blend for 2 minutes or until you get the desired consistency.*

✓ *Transfer to a serving glass and enjoy it.*

Nutrition: Calories: 216cal; Carbohydrates: 10g; Proteins: 15g; Fat: 7g; Sodium: 25mg

664)   Blackberry Smoothie

Ingredients:

- *1 1/2 cups Almond Milk*
- *¼ cup Cauliflower, blanched & frozen*
- *1 Orange*
- *1 tbsp. Flax Seed*
- *1/3 cup Carrot, grated*
- *1 tsp. Vanilla Extract*

Direction: Preparation Time: 5 Minutes Cooking Time: 0 Minutes Servings: 1

✓ *Place all the ingredients needed to make the blackberry smoothie in a high-speed blender and blend for 2 minutes until you get a smooth mixture. Transfer to a serving glass and enjoy it.*

Nutrition: Calories: 275cal; Carbohydrates: 9g; Proteins: 11g; Fat: 17g; Sodium: 73mg

665)   Key Lime Pie Smoothie

Ingredients:

- *1/2 cup Cottage Cheese*
- *1 tbsp. Sweetener of your choice*
- *1/2 cup Water*
- *1/2 cup Spinach*
- *1 tbsp. Lime Juice*
- *1 cup Ice Cubes*

Direction: Preparation Time: 5 Minutes Cooking Time: 0 Minutes Servings: 1

✓ *Spoon in the ingredients to a high-speed blender and blend until silky smooth.*

✓ *Transfer to a serving glass and enjoy it.*

Nutrition: Calories: 180cal; Carbohydrates: 7g; Proteins: 36g; Fat: 1 g; Sodium: 35mg

666)   Cinnamon Roll Smoothie

Ingredients:

- *1 tsp. Flax Meal or oats, if preferred*
- *1 cup Almond Milk*
- *1/2 tsp. Cinnamon*
- *2 tbsp. Protein Powder*
- *1 cup Ice*
- *¼ tsp. Vanilla Extract*
- *4 tsp. Sweetener of your choice*

Direction: Preparation Time: 5 Minutes Cooking Time: 0 Minutes Servings: 1

✓ *Pour the milk into the blender, followed by the protein powder, sweetener, flax meal, cinnamon,*

vanilla extract, and ice.
Blend for 40 seconds or until smooth.

✓ *Serve and enjoy.*

Nutrition: : Calories: 145cal; Carbs: 1.6g; Proteins: 26.5g; Fat: 3.25g; Sodium: 30mg

667)   Strawberry Cheesecake Smoothie

Ingredients:

- *¼ cup Soy Milk, unsweetened*
- *1/2 cup Cottage Cheese, low-fat*
- *1/2 tsp. Vanilla Extract*
- *2 oz. Cream Cheese*
- *1 cup Ice Cubes*
- *1/2 cup Strawberries*
- *4 tbsp. Low-carb Sweetener of your choice*

Direction: Preparation Time: 5 Minutes Cooking Time: 0 Minutes Servings: 1

✓ *Add all the ingredients for making the strawberry cheesecake smoothie to a high-speed blender until you get the desired smooth consistency.*

✓ *Serve and enjoy.*

Nutrition: Calories: 347cal; Carbs: 10.05g; Proteins: 17.5g; Fat: 24g; Sodium: 45mg

668)   Peanut Butter Banana Smoothie

Ingredients:

- *¼ cup Greek Yoghurt, plain*
- *1/2 tbsp. Chia Seeds*
- *1/2 cup Ice Cubes*
- *1/2 of 1 Banana*
- *1/2 cup Water*
- *1 tbsp. Peanut Butter*

Direction: Preparation Time: 5 Minutes

Cooking Time: 2 Minutes Servings: 1

✓ *Place all the ingredients needed to make the smoothie in a high-speed blender and blend to get a smooth and luscious mixture.*

✓ *Transfer the smoothie to a serving glass and enjoy it.*

Nutrition: Calories: 202cal; Carbohydrates: 14g; Proteins: 10g; Fat: 9g; Sodium: 30mg

669)   Avocado Turmeric Smoothie

Ingredients:

- *1/2 of 1 Avocado*
- *1 cup Ice, crushed*

- ¾ cup Coconut Milk, full-fat
- 1 tsp. Lemon Juice
- ¼ cup Almond Milk
- 1/2 tsp. Turmeric
- 1 tsp. Ginger, freshly grated

Direction: Preparation Time: 5 Minutes

Cooking Time: 2 Minutes Servings: 1

✓ Place all the ingredients, excluding the crushed ice in a high-speed blender and blend for 2 to 3 minutes or until smooth.

✓ Transfer to a serving glass and enjoy it.

Nutrition: Calories: 232cal; Carbs: 4.1g; Proteins: 1.7g; Fat: 22.4g; Sodium: 25mg

670)   *Blueberry Smoothie*

Ingredients:

- 1 tbsp. Lemon Juice
- 1 ¾ cup Coconut Milk, full-fat
- 1/2 tsp. Vanilla Extract
- 3 oz. Blueberries, frozen

Direction: Preparation Time: 5 Minutes

Cooking Time: 2 Minutes Servings: 2

✓ Combine coconut milk, blueberries, lemon juice, and vanilla extract in a high-speed blender.

✓ Blend for 2 minutes for a smooth and luscious smoothie.
Serve and enjoy.

671)   *Matcha Green Smoothie*

Ingredients:

- ¼ cup Heavy Whipping Cream
- 1/2 tsp. Vanilla Extract
- 1 tsp. Matcha Green Tea Powder
- 2 tbsp. Protein Powder
- 1 tbsp. Hot Water
- 1 ¼ cup Almond Milk, unsweetened
- 1/2 of 1 Avocado, medium

Direction: Preparation Time: 5 Minutes

Cooking Time: 2 Minutes Servings: 2

✓ Place all the ingredients in the high-blender for one to two minutes.

✓ Serve and enjoy.

Nutrition: Calories: 229cal; Carbs: 1.5g; Proteins: 14.1g; Fat: 43g; Sodium: 35mg

DESSERT

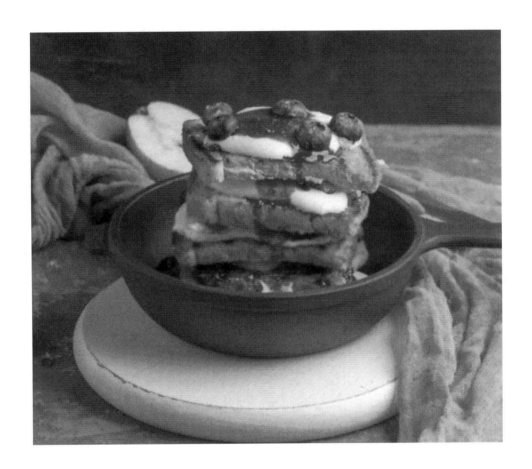

672)   *Slow Cooker Peaches*

Ingredients:

- 4 cups peaches, sliced
- 2/3 cup rolled oats
- 1/3 cup Bisques
- 1/4 teaspoon cinnamon
- 1/2 cup brown sugar
- 1/2 cup granulated sugar

Direction: Preparation Time: 10 minutesCooking time: 4 hours 20 minutes Servings: 4-6

✓ Spray the slow cooker pot with a cooking spray.

✓ Mix oats, Bisques, cinnamon and all the sugars in the pot.

✓ Add peaches and stir well to combine. Cook on low for 4-6 hours.

Nutrition: 617 calories; 3.6 g fat; 13 g total carbs; 9 g protein

673)   *Pumpkin Custard*

Ingredients:

- 1/2 cup almond flour
- 4 eggs
- 1 cup pumpkin puree
- 1/2 cup stevia/erythritol blend, granulated
- 1/8 teaspoon sea salt
- 1 teaspoon vanilla extract or maple flavoring
- 4 tablespoons butter, ghee, or coconut oil melted
- 1 teaspoon pumpkin pie spice

Direction: Preparation Time: 10 minutesCooking time: 2 hours 30 minutes Servings: 6

✓ Grease or spray a slow cooker with butter or coconut oil spray.

✓ In a medium mixing bowl, beat the eggs until smooth. Then add in the sweetener.

✓ To the egg mixture, add in the pumpkin puree along with vanilla or maple extract.

✓ Then add almond flour to the mixture along with the pumpkin pie spice and salt. Add melted butter, coconut oil or ghee.
Transfer the mixture into a slow cooker. Close the lid. Cook for 2-2 ¾ hours on low.

✓ When through, serve with whipped cream, and then sprinkle with little nutmeg if need be. Enjoy!

✓ Set slow-cooker to the low setting. Cook for 2-2.45 hours, and begin checking at the two-hour mark. Serve warm with stevia sweetened whipped cream and a sprinkle of nutmeg.

Nutrition: 147 calories; 12 g fat; 4 g total carbs; 5 g protein

674)   *Blueberry Lemon Custard Cake*

Ingredients:

- 6 eggs, separated
- 2 cups light cream
- 1/2 cup coconut flour
- 1/2 teaspoon salt
- 2 teaspoon lemon zest
- 1/2 cup granulated sugar substitute
- 1/3 cup lemon juice
- 1/2 cup blueberries fresh
- 1 teaspoon lemon liquid stevia

Direction: Preparation Time: 10 minutesCooking time: 3 hours Servings: 12

✓ Into a stand mixer, add the egg whites and whip them well until stiff peaks have formed; set aside.

✓ Whisk the yolks together with the remaining ingredients except blueberries, to form batter.

✓ When done, fold egg whites into the formed batter a little at a time until slightly combined.
Grease the crockpot and then pour in the mixture. Then sprinkle batter with the blueberries.

✓ Close the lid then cook for 3 hours on low. When the cooking time is over, open the lid and let cool for an hour, and then let chill in the refrigerator for at least 2 hours or overnight.

✓ Serve cold with little sugar free whipped cream and enjoy!

Nutrition: 165 calories; 10 g fat; 14 g total carbs; 4 g protein

675)   *Sugar Free Carrot Cake*

Ingredients:

- 2 eggs
- 1 1/2 almond flour
- 1/2 cup butter, melted
- ¼ cup heavy cream
- 1 teaspoon baking powder
- 1 teaspoon vanilla extract or almond extract, optional
- 1 cup sugar substitute
- 1 cup carrots, finely shredded
- 1 teaspoon cinnamon
- ¼ teaspoon nutmeg
- 1/8 teaspoon allspice
- 1 teaspoon ginger
- 1/2 teaspoon baking soda
- For cream cheese frosting:
- 1 cup confectioner's sugar substitute
- ¼ cup butter, softened

- *1 teaspoon almond extract*
- *4 oz. cream cheese, softened*

Direction: Cooking time: 4 hours Servings: 8 Ingredients

✓ *Grease a loaf pan well and then set it aside.*

✓ *Using a mixer, combine butter together with eggs, vanilla, sugar substitute and heavy cream in a mixing bowl, until well blended.*

✓ *Combine almond flour together with baking powder, spices and the baking soda in another bowl until well blended.*

✓ *When done, combine the wet ingredients together with the dry ingredients until well blended, and then stir in carrots.*
Pour the mixer into the prepared loaf pan, and then place the pan into a slow cooker on a trivet. Add 1 cup water inside.

✓ *Cook for about 4-5 hours on low. Be aware that the cake will be very moist.*

✓ *When the cooking time is over, let the cake cool completely.*

✓ *To prepare the cream cheese frosting: blend the cream cheese together with extract, butter and powdered sugar substitute until frosting is formed.*

✓ *Top the cake with the frosting.*

Nutrition: 299 calories; 25.4 g fat; 15 g total carbs; 4 g protein

676) *Sugar Free Chocolate Molten Lava Cake*

Ingredients:

- *3 egg yolks*
- *1 1/2 cups Swerve sweetener, divided*
- *1 teaspoon baking powder*
- *1/2 cup flour, gluten free*
- *3 whole eggs*
- *5 tablespoons cocoa powder, unsweetened, divided*
- *4 oz. chocolate chips, sugar free*
- *1/2 teaspoon salt*
- *1/2 teaspoon vanilla liquid stevia*
- *1/2 cup butter, melted, cooled*
- *2 cups hot water*
- *1 teaspoon vanilla extract*

Direction: Preparation Time: 10 minutes Cooking time: 3 hours Servings: 12

✓ *Grease the crockpot well with cooking spray.*

✓ *Whisk 1 ¼ cups of swerve together with flour, salt, baking powder and 3 tablespoons cocoa powder in a bowl.*

✓ *Stir the cooled melted butter together with eggs,*

yolks, liquid stevia and the vanilla extract in a separate bowl.

✓ *When done, add the wet ingredients to the dry ingredient until nicely combined, and then pour the mixture into the prepared crockpot.*
Then top the mixture in the crockpot with chocolate chips.

✓ *Whisk the rest of the swerve sweetener and the remaining cocoa powder with the hot water, and then pour this mixture over the chocolate chips top.*

✓ *Close the lid and cook for 3 hours on low. When the cooking time is over, let cool a bit and then serve. Enjoy!*

Nutrition: 157 calories; 13 g fat; 10.5 g total carbs; 3.9 g protein

677) *Chocolate Quinoa Brownies*

Ingredients:

- *2 eggs*
- *3 cups quinoa, cooked*
- *1 teaspoon vanilla liquid stevia*
- *1 ¼ chocolate chips, sugar free*
- *1 teaspoon vanilla extract*
- *1/3 cup flaxseed ground*
- *¼ teaspoon salt*
- *1/3 cup cocoa powder, unsweetened*
- *1/2 teaspoon baking powder*
- *1 teaspoon pure stevia extract*
- *1/2 cup applesauce, unsweetened*
- *Sugar- frees frosting:*
- *¼ cup heavy cream*
- *1 teaspoon chocolate liquid stevia*
- *¼ cup cocoa powder, unsweetened*
- *1/2 teaspoon vanilla extract*

Direction: Preparation Time: 10 minutes Cooking time: 2 hours Servings: 16

✓ *Add all the ingredients to a food processor. Then process until well incorporated.*

✓ *Line a crockpot with parchment paper, and then spread the batter into the lined pot.*

✓ *Close the lid and cook for 4 hours on LOW or 2 hours on HIGH. Let cool.*
Prepare the frosting. Whisk all the ingredients together and then microwave for 20 seconds. Taste and adjust on sweetener if desired.

✓ *When the frosting is ready, stir it well again and then pour it over the sliced brownies.*

✓ *Serve and enjoy!*

Nutrition: 133 calories; 7.9 g fat; 18.4 g total carbs; 4.3 g protein

678)   *Keto Chocolate Bombs*

Ingredients:

- 2 cups smooth peanut butter
- ¾ cup coconut of flour
- ½ cup sticky sweetener
- 2 cups sugar-free chocolate chips

Direction: Preparation Time: 30 minutes Cooking Time: 0 minutes Servings: 12

✓ Start by lining a large tray with parchment paper and set it aside.

✓ In a large mixing bowl, combine all your ingredients together except for the chocolate chips, and combine your ingredients very well until it is completely combined

✓ If your batter is too thick or is crumbly, you may add a small quantity of milk or water

✓ With both your hands, try forming small balls from the batter and arrange it over an already prepared lined tray and freeze for about 10 minutes

✓ While your peanut butter balls are in the freezer, melt the sugar-free chocolate chips in the microwave for about 30 seconds to about 1 minute

✓ Remove the peanut butter from the freezer; then carefully and gently dip each of the balls into the melted chocolate

✓ Repeat the same process until all the chocolate balls are covered in chocolate and arrange over a platter

✓ Once you finish covering all the balls, place the balls in the refrigerator for about 20 minutes or just until the chocolate firms up

✓ Serve and enjoy your delicious chocolate balls

Nutrition: Calories: 95 Fat: 9.7g Protein: 3g

679)   *Blueberry Crisp*

Ingredients:

- 1/4 cup butter, melted
- 24 oz. blueberries, frozen
- 3/4 teaspoon salt
- 1 1/2 cups rolled oats, coarsely ground
- 3/4 cup almond flour, blanched
- 1/4 cup coconut oil, melted
- 6 tablespoons sweetener
- 1 cup pecans or walnuts, coarsely chopped

Direction: Preparation Time: 10 minutes

Cooking time: 3-4 hours Servings: 10

✓ Using a non-stick cooking spray, spray the slow cooker pot well.

✓ Into a bowl, add ground oats and chopped nuts along with salt, blanched almond flour, brown sugar, stevia granulated sweetener, and then stir in

the coconut/butter mixture. Stir well to combine. When done, spread crisp topping over blueberries. Cook for 3-4 hours, until the mixture has become bubbling hot and you can smell the blueberries.

✓ Serve while still hot with the whipped cream or ice cream if desired. Enjoy!

Nutrition: 261 calories; 16.6 g fat; 32 g total carbs; 4 g protein

680)   *Maple Custard*

Ingredients:

- 1 teaspoon maple extract
- 2 egg yolks
- 1 cup heavy cream
- 1/2 teaspoon cinnamon
- 2 eggs
- 1/2 cup whole milk
- 1/4 teaspoon salt
- 1/4 cup Sukrin Gold or any sugar-free brown sugar substitute

Direction: Preparation Time: 10 minutesCooking time: 2 hours Servings: 6

✓ Combine all ingredients together in a blender, process well.

✓ Grease 6 ramekins and then pour the batter evenly into each ramekin.

✓ To the bottom of the slow cooker, add 4 ramekins and then arrange the remaining 2 against the side of a slow cooker and not at the top of the bottom ramekins.
Close the lid and cook on high for 2 hours, until the center is cooked through but the middle is still jiggly.

✓ Let cool at room temperature for an hour after removing from the slow cooker, and then chill in the fridge for at least 2 hours.

✓ Serve and enjoy with a sprinkle of cinnamon and little sugar-free whipped cream.

Nutrition: 190 calories; 18 g fat; 2 g total carbs; 4 g protein

681)   *Raspberry Cream Cheese Coffee Cake*

Ingredients:

- 1 1/4 almond flour
- 2/3 cup water
- 1/2 cup Swerve
- 3 eggs
- 1/4 cup coconut flour

- *1/4 cup protein powder*
- *1/4 teaspoon salt*
- *1/2 teaspoon vanilla extract*

For the Filling:

- *1 1/2 cup fresh raspberries*
- *8 oz. cream cheese*
- *1 large egg*
- *1/3 cup powdered Swerve*
- *2 tablespoon whipping cream*
- *1 1/2 teaspoon baking powder*
- *6 tablespoons butter, melted*

Direction: Preparation Time: 10 minutes Cooking time: 4 hours Servings: 12

✓ *Grease the slow cooker pot. Prepare the cake batter. In a bowl, combine almond flour together with coconut flour, sweetener, baking powder, protein powder and salt, and then stir in the melted butter along with eggs and water until well combined. Set aside.*

✓ *Prepare the filling.*

✓ *Beat cream cheese thoroughly with the sweetener until have smoothened, and then beat in whipping cream along with the egg and vanilla extract until well combined.*
Assemble the cake. Spread around 2/3 of batter in the slow cooker as you smoothen the top using a spatula or knife.

✓ *Pour cream cheese mixture over the batter in the pan, evenly spread it, and then sprinkle with raspberries. Add the rest of the batter overfilling.*

✓ *Cook for 3-4 hours on low. Let cool completely.*

✓ *Serve and enjoy!*

Nutrition: 239 calories; 19.18 g fat; 6.9 g total carbs; 7.5 g protein

682) *Pumpkin Pie Bars*

Ingredients:

- *For the Crust:*
- *3/4 cup coconut, shredded*
- *4 tablespoons butter, unsalted, softened*
- *1/4 cup cocoa powder, unsweetened*
- *1/4 teaspoon salt*
- *1/2 cup raw sunflower seeds or sunflower seed flour*
- *1/4 cup confectioners Swerve*

Filling:

- *2 teaspoons cinnamon liquid stevia*
- *1 cup heavy cream*
- *1 can pumpkin puree*
- *6 eggs*

- *1 tablespoon pumpkin pie spice*
- *1/2 teaspoon salt*
- *1 tablespoon vanilla extract*
- *1/2 cup sugar-free chocolate chips, optional*

Direction: Preparation Time: 10 minutes

Cooking time: 3 hours Servings: 16

✓ *Add all the crust ingredients to a food processor. Then process until fine crumbs are formed.*

✓ *Grease the slow cooker pan well. When done, press crust mixture onto the greased bottom.*

✓ *In a stand mixer, combine all the ingredients for the filling, and then blend well until combined. Top the filling with chocolate chips if using, and then pour the mixture onto the prepared crust.*

✓ *Close the lid and cook for 3 hours on low. Open the lid and let cool for at least 30 minutes, and then place the slow cooker into the refrigerator for at least 3 hours.*

✓ *Slice the pumpkin pie bar and serve it with sugar-free whipped cream. Enjoy!*

Nutrition: 169 calories; 15 g fat; 6 g total carbs; 4 g protein

683) *Dark Chocolate Cake*

Ingredients:

- *1 cup almond flour*
- *3 eggs*
- *2 tablespoons almond flour*
- *1/4 teaspoon salt*
- *1/2 cup Swerve Granular*
- *3/4 teaspoon vanilla extract*
- *2/3 cup almond milk, unsweetened*
- *1/2 cup cocoa powder*
- *6 tablespoons butter, melted*
- *1 1/2 teaspoon baking powder*
- *3 tablespoon unflavored whey protein powder or egg white protein powder*
- *1/3 cup sugar-free chocolate chips, optional*

Direction: Preparation Time: 10 minutes Cooking time: 3 hours Servings: 10

✓ *Grease the slow cooker well.*

✓ *Whisk the almond flour together with cocoa powder, sweetener, whey protein powder, salt and baking powder in a bowl. Then stir in butter along with almond milk, eggs and the vanilla extract until well combined, and then stir in the chocolate chips if desired.*

✓ *When done, pour into the slow cooker. Allow cooking for 2-2 1/2 hours on low.*

✓ *When through, turn off the slow cooker and let the cake cool for about 20-30 minutes.*

✓ When cooled, cut the cake into pieces and serve warm with lightly sweetened whipped cream. Enjoy!

Nutrition: 205 calories; 17 g fat; 8.4 g total carbs; 12 g protein

684)   Lemon Custard

Ingredients:

* 2 cups whipping cream or coconut cream
* 5 egg yolks
* 1 tablespoon lemon zest
* 1 teaspoon vanilla extract
* 1/4 cup fresh lemon juice, squeezed
* 1/2 teaspoon liquid stevia
* Lightly sweetened whipped cream

Direction: Preparation Time: 10 minutes Cooking time: 3 hours Servings: 4

✓ Whisk egg yolks together with lemon zest, liquid stevia, lemon zest and vanilla in a bowl, and then whisk in heavy cream.

✓ Divide the mixture among 4 small jars or ramekins.

✓ To the bottom of a slow cooker add a rack, and then add ramekins on top of the rack and add enough water to cover half of the ramekins.
Close the lid and cook for 3 hours on low. Remove ramekins.

✓ Let cool to room temperature, and then place into the refrigerator to cool completely for about 3 hours.

✓ When through, top with the whipped cream and serve. Enjoy!

Nutrition: 319 calories; 30 g fat; 3 g total carbs; 7 g protein

685)   Coffee & Chocolate Ice Cream

Ingredients:

* 3 cups brewed coffee
* ½ cup low-calorie chocolate flavored syrup
* ¾ cup low fat half and half

Direction: Preparation Time: 4 minutes Cooking Time: 0 minutes Servings: 15

✓ Mix the ingredients in a bowl.

✓ Pour into popsicle molds. Freeze for 4 hours.

Nutrition: Calories 21 Total Fat 0 g Saturated Fat 0 g Cholesterol 1 mg Sodium 28 mg Total Carbohydrate 4 g Dietary Fiber 0 g Total Sugars 3 g Protein 0 g Potassium 450 mg

686)   Choco Banana Bites

Ingredients:

* 2 bananas, sliced into rounds
* ¼ cup dark chocolate cubes

Direction: Preparation Time: 2 hours and 5 minutes Cooking Time: 5 minutes Servings: 4

✓ Melt chocolate in the microwave or in a saucepan over medium heat.

✓ Coat each banana slice with melted chocolate.

✓ Place on a metal pan. Freeze for 2 hours.

Nutrition: Calories 102 Total Fat 3 g Saturated Fat 2 g Cholesterol 0 mg Sodium 4 mg Total Carbohydrate 20 g Dietary Fiber 2 g Total Sugars 13 g Protein 1 g Potassium 211 mg

687)   Blueberries with Yogurt

Ingredients:

* 1 cup nonfat Greek yogurt
* ¼ cup blueberries
* ¼ cup almonds

Direction: Preparation Time: 5 minutes Cooking Time: 0 minute Serving: 1

✓ Add yogurt and blueberries to a food processor. Pulse until smooth. Top with almonds before serving.

Nutrition: **Calories 154 Total Fat 1 g Saturated Fat 0 g Cholesterol 11 mg Sodium 81 mg Total Carbohydrate 13 g Dietary Fiber 1 g Total Sugars 11 g Protein 23 g Potassium 346 mg**

688)   Roasted Mangoes

Ingredients:

* 2 mangoes, peeled and sliced into cubes
* 2 tablespoons coconut flakes
* 2 teaspoons crystallized ginger, chopped
* 2 teaspoons orange zest

Direction: Preparation Time: 5 minutes Cooking Time: 10 minutes Servings: 4

✓ Preheat your oven to 350 degrees F. Put the mango cubes in custard cups.
Top with the ginger and orange zest—Bake in the oven for 10 minutes.

Nutrition: Calories 89 Total Fat 2 g Saturated Fat 1 g Cholesterol 0 mg Sodium 14 mg Total Carbohydrate 20 g Dietary Fiber 2 g Total Sugars 17 g Protein 1 g Potassium 177 mg

689) *Figs with Yogurt*

Ingredients:

- 8 oz. low fat yogurt
- ½ teaspoon vanilla
- 2 figs, sliced
- 1 tablespoon walnuts, toasted and chopped
- Lemon zest

Direction: Preparation Time: 8 hours and 5 minutes Cooking Time: 0 minutes Servings: 2

✓ Refrigerate yogurt in a bowl for 8 hours.

✓ After 8 hours, take it out of the refrigerator and stir in yogurt and vanilla.
Stir in the figs. Sprinkle walnuts and lemon zest on top before serving.

Nutrition: Calories 157 Total Fat 4 g Saturated Fat 1 g Cholesterol 7 mg Sodium 80 mg Total Carbohydrate 24 g Dietary Fiber 2 g Total Sugars 1 g Protein 7 g Potassium 557mg

690) *Grilled Peaches*

Ingredients:

- 1 cup balsamic vinegar
- ⅛ teaspoon ground cinnamon
- 1 tablespoon honey
- 3 peaches, pitted and sliced in half
- 2 teaspoons olive oil
- 6 gingersnaps, crushed

Direction: Preparation Time: 5 minutes Cooking Time: 3 minutes Servings: 6

✓ Pour the vinegar into a saucepan. Bring it to a boil—lower heat and simmer for 10 minutes.

✓ Remove from the stove. Stir in cinnamon and honey.
Coat the peaches with oil—grill peaches for 2 to 3 minutes.

✓ Drizzle each one with syrup. Top with the gingersnaps.

Nutrition: Calories 135 Total Fat 3 g Saturated Fat 1 g Cholesterol 0 mg Sodium 42 mg Total Carbohydrate 25 g Dietary Fiber 2 g Total Sugars 18 g Protein 1 g Potassium 251 mg

691) *Fruit Salad*

Ingredients:

- 8 oz. light cream cheese
- 6 oz. Greek yogurt
- 1 tablespoon honey
- 1 teaspoon orange zest
- 1 teaspoon lemon zest
- 1 orange, sliced into sections
- 3 kiwi fruit, peeled and sliced 1 mango, cubed
- 1 cup blueberries

Direction: Preparation Time: 5 minutes Cooking Time: 0 minute Servings: 6

✓ Beat cream cheese using an electric mixer.

✓ Add yogurt and honey. Beat until smooth.

✓ Stir in the orange and lemon zest.
Toss the fruits to mix.

✓ Divide in glass jars. Top with the cream cheese mixture.

Nutrition: Calories 131 Total Fat 3 g Saturated Fat 2 g Cholesterol 9 mg Sodium 102 mg Total Carbohydrate 23 g Dietary Fiber 3 g Total Sugars 18 g Protein 5 g Potassium 234 mg

692) *Strawberry & Watermelon Pops*

Ingredients:

- ¾ cup strawberries, sliced
- 2 cups watermelon, cubed
- ¼ cup lime juice
- 2 tablespoons brown sugar
- ⅛ teaspoon salt

Direction: Preparation Time: 6 hours and 10 minutes Cooking Time: 0 minutes Servings: 6

✓ Put the strawberries inside popsicle molds. In a blender, pulse the rest of the ingredients until well mixed.

✓ Pour the puree into a sieve before pouring it into the molds. Freeze for 6 hours.

Nutrition: Calories 57 Total Fat 0 g Saturated Fat 0 g Cholesterol 0 mg Sodium 180 mg Total Carbohydrate 14 g Dietary Fiber 2 g Total Sugars 11 g Protein 1 g Potassium 180 mg

693) *Frozen Vanilla Yogurt*

Ingredients:

- 3 cups fat-free plain Greek yogurt
- 4-6 drops liquid stevia
- 1 teaspoon organic vanilla extract
- ¼ cup fresh strawberries, hulled and sliced

Direction: Preparation Time: 10 mins Servings: 6

✓ In a bowl, add all the ingredients except strawberries and mix until well combined.

✓ Transfer the mixture into an ice cream maker and process it according to the manufacturer's directions.

✓ Transfer the mixture into a bowl and freeze, covered for about 30-40 minutes or until desired consistency.

Garnish with strawberry slices and serve. **Meal Prep Tip:** *Line a cookie sheet with parchment paper. With a cookie scooper, place the yogurt portion onto the prepared cookie sheet.*

✓ *Freeze overnight. Remove from the freezer and transfer the frozen yogurt balls into an airtight container. Store in freezer up to 1 week. Remove from the freezer and set aside for 15-20 minutes before serving.*

Nutrition: Calories 74 Total Fat 0.3 g Saturated Fat 0 g Cholesterol 4mg Total Carbs 5.6 g Sugar 4.9 g Fiber 0.1 g Sodium 58 mg Potassium 10 mg Protein 12 g

694)   *Spinach Sorbet*

Ingredients:

- 3 cups fresh spinach, chopped
- 1 tablespoon fresh basil leaves
- ½ of avocado, peeled, pitted and chopped
- ¾ cup unsweetened almond milk
- 20 drops liquid stevia
- 1 teaspoon almonds, chopped very finely
- 1 teaspoon organic vanilla extract 1 cup ice cubes

Direction: Preparation Time: 15 minutes Servings: 4

✓ *In a blender, add all ingredients and pulse until creamy and smooth.*

✓ *Transfer into an ice cream maker and process according to manufacturer's directions. Transfer into an airtight container and freeze for at least 4-5 hours before serving.* **Meal Prep Tip:** *Transfer the sorbet into a shallow, flat container.*

✓ *With plastic wrap, cover the ice cream and store it in the back of the freezer.*

Nutrition: Calories 70 Total Fat 5.9 g Saturated Fat 1.1 g Cholesterol 0 mg Total Carbs 3.6 g Sugar 0.4 g Fiber 2.4 g Sodium 53 mg Potassium 290 mg Protein 1.4 g

695)   *Avocado Mousse*

Ingredients:

- 2 ripe Haas avocados, peeled, pitted and chopped roughly
- 1 teaspoon liquid stevia
- 1 teaspoon organic vanilla extract Pinch of salt

Direction: Preparation Time: 15 minutes Servings: 3

✓ *In a high-speed blender, add all the ingredients and pulse until smooth.*

✓ *Transfer the pudding into a serving bowl. Cover the bowl and refrigerate to chill for at least 2 hours before serving.*

Meal Prep Tip:

✓ *Transfer the mousse into an airtight container.*

✓ *Cover the containers and refrigerate for about 1 day.*

Nutrition: Calories 277 Total Fat 26.1 g Saturated Fat 5.5 g Cholesterol 0 mg Total Carbs 11.7 g Sugar 0.9 g Fiber 8 g Sodium 59 mg Potassium 652 mg Protein 2.6g

696)   *Strawberry Mousse*

Ingredients:

- 1½ cups fresh strawberries, hulled
- 1 2/3 cups chilled unsweetened almond milk
- 2-3 drops liquid stevia
- 1 teaspoon organic vanilla extract

Direction: Preparation Time: 15 minutes Servings: 6

✓ *In a food processor, add all the ingredients and pulse until smooth.*

✓ *Transfer into serving bowls and serve.*

Meal Prep Tip:

✓ *Transfer the mousse into an airtight container.*

✓ *Cover the containers and refrigerate for up to 3 days.*

Nutrition: Calories 25 Total Fat 1.1g Saturated Fat 0.1 g Cholesterol 0 mg Total Carbs 3.4 g Sugar 1.9 g Fiber 1 g Sodium 50 mg Potassium 109 mg Protein 0.5 g

697)   *Blueberries Pudding*

Ingredients:

- 1 small avocado, peeled, pitted and chopped
- 1 cup frozen blueberries
- ¼ teaspoon fresh ginger, grated freshly
- 1 teaspoon lime zest, grated finely
- 2 tablespoons fresh lime juice
- 10 drops liquid stevia
- 5 tablespoons filtered water

Direction: Preparation Time: 10 mins Servings: 3

✓ *In a blender, add all the ingredients and pulse till creamy and smooth.*

✓ *Transfer into serving bowls and serve.*

Meal Prep Tip:

✓ *Transfer the pudding into an airtight container.*

✓ *Cover the containers and refrigerate for up to 2 days.*

Nutrition: Calories 166 Total Fat 13.3 g Saturated Fat 4.2.8 g Cholesterol 0 mg Total Carbs 13.1 g Sugar 5.2 g Fiber 5.8 g Sodium 4 mg Potassium 331 mg Protein 1.7 g

698) Raspberry Chia Pudding

Ingredients:

- 1½ cups unsweetened almond milk
- 1¼ cups fresh raspberries
- ½ cup chia seeds
- 1 tablespoon flax meal
- 3-4 drops liquid stevia
- 2 teaspoons organic vanilla extract

Direction: Preparation Time: 10 mins Servings: 4

✓ In a blender, add the almond milk and raspberries and pulse until smooth.

✓ Transfer the milk mixture into a large bowl.

✓ Add the remaining ingredients except for raspberries and stir until well combined. Refrigerate to chill for at least 1 hour before serving.

Meal Prep Tip:

✓ Transfer the pudding into an airtight container.

✓ Cover the containers and refrigerate for about 1 day.

Nutrition: Calories 107 Total Fat 7.2 g Saturated Fat 0.5 g Cholesterol 0 mg Total Carbs 12.1 g Sugar 2 g Fiber 8.4 g Sodium 68 mg Potassium 246 mg Protein 4.2 g

699) Brown Rice Pudding

Ingredients:

- 2 cups low-fat milk
- 1/3 cup Erythritol
- 1½ teaspoons organic vanilla extract
- ¼ teaspoon ground cinnamon
- 1 egg
- 2 cups cooked brown rice

Direction: Preparation Time: 15 minutes Cooking Time: 30 minutes Servings: 4

✓ In a medium pan, add the milk, Erythritol, vanilla extract and cinnamon over medium-high heat and bring to a boil, stirring continuously. Remove from the heat.

✓ In a large bowl, add the egg and beat it well. Slowly, add the hot milk mixture a little bit at a time and beat until well combined. In the same pan, add the milk mixture and rice and

✓ Place the 2 cups of cooked rice into the pan used to cook the milk mixture and stir to combine.

✓ Place the pan over medium-high heat and bring to a boil, stirring continuously. Reduce heat to low and simmer for about 15-20 minutes, stirring after every 5 minutes. Remove from the heat and transfer into a bowl. With wax paper, cover the top of the pudding and refrigerate to chill before serving.

Meal Prep Tip:

✓ Transfer the pudding into an airtight container. Cover the containers and refrigerate for up to 2 days.

Nutrition: Calories 416 Total Fat 4.8 g Saturated Fat 1.6 g Cholesterol 47 mg Total Carbs 78 g Sugar 6 g Fiber 3.3 g Sodium 73 mg Potassium 455 mg Protein 12.5 g

700) Lemon Cookies

Ingredients: Preparation Time: 10 minutes Cooking Time: 12 minutes Servings: 6

- ¼ cup unsweetened applesauce
- 1 cup cashew butter
- 1 teaspoon fresh lemon zest, grated finely
- 2 tablespoons fresh lemon juice
- Pinch of sea salt

Direction: Preparation Time: 18 mins Servings: 4

✓ Preheat the oven to 350 degrees F. Line a large cookie sheet with parchment paper. In a food processor, add all ingredients and pulse until smooth. With a tablespoon, place the mixture onto a prepared cookie sheet in a single layer—Bake for about 12 minutes or until golden brown.

✓ Remove from oven and place the cookie sheet onto a wire rack to cool for about 5 minutes.

✓ Carefully invert the cookies onto a wire rack to cool completely before serving.

Meal Prep Tip:

Store these cookies in an airtight container by placing parchment papers between the cookies to avoid sticking. These cookies can be stored in the refrigerator for up to 2 weeks.

Nutrition: Calories 257 Total Fat 21.9 g Saturated Fat 4.2 g Cholesterol 0 mg Total Carbs 13.1 g Sugar 1.2 g Fiber 1 g Sodium 47 mg Potassium 248 mg Protein 7.6 g

701) Yogurt Cheesecake

Ingredients:

- 2½ cups fat-free plain Greek yogurt
- 6-8 drops liquid stevia
- 3 egg whites
- 1/3 cup cacao powder
- ¼ cup arrowroot starch
- 1 teaspoon organic vanilla extract
- Pinch of sea salt

Direction: Preparation Time: 15 minutes Cooking Time: 35 minutes Servings: 8

- ✓ Preheat the oven to 35 degrees F. Grease a 9-inch cake pan.
- ✓ In a large bowl, add all ingredients and mix until well combined.
- ✓ Place the mixture into the prepared pan evenly. Bake for about 30-35 minutes. Remove from oven and let it cool completely. Refrigerate to chill for about 3-4 hours or until set completely.
- ✓ Cut into 8 equal sized slices and serve.

Meal Prep Tip:

- ✓ With foil pieces, wrap the cheesecake slices and refrigerate for about 1-3 days. Reheat in the microwave before serving.

Nutrition: Calories 74 Total Fat 0.9g Saturated Fat 0.4 g Cholesterol 2 mg Total Carbs 8.5 g Sugar 3 g Fiber 1.1 g Sodium 89 mg Potassium 21 mg Protein 9.5 g

702)   *Flourless Chocolate Cake*

Ingredients:

- 1/2 Cup of stevia
- 12 ounces of unsweetened baking chocolate
- 2/3 Cup of ghee
- 1/3 Cup of warm water
- ¼ Teaspoon of salt
- 4 large pastured eggs
- 2 cups of boiling water

Direction: Preparation time: 10 minutes Cooking time: 45 minutes Yield: 6 Servings

- ✓ Line the bottom of a 9-inch pan of a springform with parchment paper.
- ✓ Heat the water in a small pot; then add the salt and the stevia over the water until wait until the mixture becomes completely dissolved.
- ✓ Melt the baking chocolate into a double boiler or simply microwave it for about 30 seconds.
- ✓ Mix the melted chocolate and the butter in a large bowl with an electric mixer.
- ✓ Beat in your hot mixture; then crack in the egg and whisk after adding each of the eggs.
- ✓ Pour the obtained mixture into your prepared spring form tray. Wrap the springform tray with foil paper.
- ✓ Place the spring form tray in a large cake tray and add boiling water right to the outside; make sure the depth doesn't exceed 1 inch.
- ✓ Bake the cake into the water bath for about 45 minutes at a temperature of about 350 F.
- ✓ Remove the tray from the boiling water and transfer it to a wire to cool.
- ✓ Let the cake chill overnight in the refrigerator.

- ✓ Serve and enjoy your delicious cake!

Nutrition: Calories: 295| Fat: 26g | Carbohydrates: 6g | Fiber: 4g |Protein: 8g

703)   *Raspberry Cake With White Chocolate Sauce*

Ingredients:

- 5 Ounces of melted cacao butter
- 2 Ounces of grass-fed ghee
- 1/2 Cup of coconut cream
- 1 Cup of green banana flour
- 3 Teaspoons of pure vanilla
- 4 large eggs
- 1/2 Cup of as Lakanto Monk Fruit
- 1 teaspoon of baking powder
- 2 Teaspoons of apple cider vinegar
- 2 Cup of raspberries
- For the white chocolate sauce:
- 3 and 1/2 ounces of cacao butter
- 1/2 Cup of coconut cream
- 2 Teaspoons of pure vanilla extract
- 1 Pinch of salt

Direction: Preparation time: 15 minutes Cooking time: 60 minutes Yield: 5-6 Servings

- ✓ Preheat your oven to a temperature of about 280 degrees Fahrenheit.
- ✓ Combine the green banana flour with the pure vanilla extract, the baking powder, the coconut cream, the eggs, the cider vinegar and the monk fruit and mix very well.
- ✓ Leave the raspberries aside and line a cake loaf tin with baking paper.
- ✓ Pour the batter into the baking tray and scatter the raspberries over the top of the cake.
- ✓ Place the tray in your oven and bake it for about 60 minutes; in the meantime, prepare the sauce by Directions for sauce:
- ✓ Combine the cacao cream, the vanilla extract, the cacao butter and the salt in a saucepan over low heat.
- ✓ Mix all your ingredients with a fork to make sure the cacao butter mixes very well with the cream.
- ✓ Remove from the heat and set aside to cool a little bit, but don't let it harden.
- ✓ Drizzle with the chocolate sauce.
- ✓ Scatter the cake with more raspberries.
- ✓ Slice your cake; then serve and enjoy it!

Nutrition: Calories: 323| Fat: 31.5g | Carbohydrates: 9.9g | Fiber: 4g |Protein: 5g

704) Ketogenic Lava Cake

Ingredients:

- 2 Oz of dark chocolate; you should at least use chocolate of 85% cocoa solids
- 1 Tablespoon of super-fine almond flour
- 2 Oz of unsalted almond butter
- 2 large eggs

Direction: Preparation time: 10 minutes Cooking time: 10 minutes Yield: 2 Servings

- ✓ Heat your oven to a temperature of about 350 Fahrenheit.
- ✓ Grease 2 heatproof ramekins with almond butter.
- ✓ Now, melt the chocolate and the almond butter and stir very well.
- ✓ Beat the eggs very well with a mixer.
- ✓ Add the eggs to the chocolate and the butter mixture and mix very well with almond flour and the swerve; then stir.
- ✓ Pour the dough into 2 ramekins.
- ✓ Bake for about 9 to 10 minutes.
- ✓ Turn the cakes over plates and serve with pomegranate seeds!

Nutrition: Calories: 459| Fat: 39g | Carbohydrates: 3.5g | Fiber: 0.8g |Protein: 11.7g

705) Ketogenic Cheese Cake

Ingredients:

- For the Almond Flour Cheesecake Crust:
- 2 Cups of Blanched almond flour
- 1/3 Cup of Almond Butter
- 3 Tablespoons of Erythritol (powdered or granular)
- 1 teaspoon of Vanilla extract

For the Keto Cheesecake Filling:

- 32 Oz of softened Cream cheese
- 1 and ¼ cups of powdered erythritol
- 3 Large Eggs
- 1 Tablespoon of Lemon juice
- 1 teaspoon of Vanilla extract

Direction: Preparation time: 15 minutes Cooking time: 50 minutes Yield: 6 Servings

- ✓ Preheat your oven to a temperature of about 350 degrees F.
- ✓ Grease a springform pan of 9¨ with cooking spray or just line its bottom with parchment paper.
- ✓ In order to make the cheesecake crust, stir in the melted butter, almond flour, vanilla extract and erythritol in a large bowl.
- ✓ The dough will get will be a bit crumbly, so press it

into the bottom of your prepared tray.

- ✓ Bake for about 12 minutes; then let cool for about 10 minutes.
  In the meantime, beat the softened cream cheese and the powdered sweetener at a low speed until it becomes smooth.
- ✓ Crack in the eggs and beat them in at a low to medium speed until it becomes fluffy. Make sure to add one a time.
- ✓ Add in the lemon juice and the vanilla extract and mix at a low to medium speed with a mixer.
- ✓ Pour your filling into your pan right on top of the crust. You can use a spatula to smooth the top of the cake.
- ✓ Bake for about 45 to 50 minutes.
- ✓ Remove the baked cheesecake from your oven and run a knife around its edge.
- ✓ Let the cake cool for about 4 hours in the refrigerator.

Nutrition: Calories: 325| Fat: 29g | Carbohydrates: 6g | Fiber: 1g |Protein: 7g

706) Cake with Whipped Cream Icing

Ingredients:

- ¾ Cup Coconut flour
- ¾ Cup of Swerve Sweetener
- 1/2 Cup of Cocoa powder
- 2 Teaspoons of Baking powder
- 6 Large Eggs
- 2/3 Cup of Heavy Whipping Cream
- 1/2 Cup of Melted almond Butter

For the whipped cream Icing:

- 1 Cup of Heavy Whipping Cream
- ¼ Cup of Swerve Sweetener
- 1 teaspoon of Vanilla extract
- 1/3 Cup of Sifted Cocoa Powder

Direction: Preparation time: 20 minutes Cooking time: 25 minutes Yield: 7 Servings

- ✓ Pre-heat your oven to a temperature of about 350 F.
- ✓ Grease an 8x8 cake tray with cooking spray.
- ✓ Add the coconut flour, the Swerve sweetener; the cocoa powder, the baking powder, the eggs, the melted butter; and combine very well with an electric or a hand mixer.
- ✓ Pour your batter into the cake tray and bake for about 25 minutes.
- ✓ Remove the cake tray from the oven and let cool for about 5 minutes.
  For the Icing:
- ✓ Whip the cream until it becomes fluffy; then add in the Swerve, the vanilla and the cocoa powder.
- ✓ Add the Swerve, the vanilla and the cocoa powder;

then continue mixing until your ingredients are very well combined.

✓ Frost your baked cake with the icing; then slice it; serve and enjoy your delicious cake!

Nutrition: Calories: 357| Fat: 33g | Carbohydrates: 11g | Fiber: 2g |Protein: 8g

707)   *Walnut-Fruit Cake*

Ingredients:

- 1/2 Cup of almond butter (softened)
- ¼ Cup of so Nourished granulated erythritol
- 1 Tablespoon of ground cinnamon
- 1/2 Teaspoon of ground nutmeg
- ¼ Teaspoon of ground cloves
- 4 large pastured eggs
- 1 teaspoon of vanilla extract
- 1/2 Teaspoon of almond extract
- 2 cups of almond flour
- 1/2 Cup of chopped walnuts
- ¼ Cup of dried of unsweetened cranberries
- ¼ Cup of seedless raisins

Direction: Preparation time: 18 minutes Cooking time: 20 minutes Yield: 9 Servings

✓ Preheat your oven to a temperature of about 350 F and grease an 8-inch baking tin of round shape with coconut oil.

✓ Beat the granulated erythritol at a high speed until it becomes fluffy.

✓ Add the cinnamon, the nutmeg, and the cloves; then blend your ingredients until they become smooth.

✓ Crack in the eggs and beat very well by adding one at a time, plus the almond extract and the vanilla. Whisk in the almond flour until it forms a smooth batter then fold in the nuts and the fruit.

✓ Spread your mixture into your prepared baking pan and bake it for about 20 minutes.

✓ Remove the cake from the oven and let cool for about 5 minutes.

✓ Dust the cake with powdered erythritol.

✓ Serve and enjoy your cake!

Nutrition: Calories: 250| Fat: 11g | Carbohydrates: 12g | Fiber: 2g |Protein: 7g

708)   *Ginger Cake*

Ingredients:

- 1/2 Tablespoon of unsalted almond butter to grease the pan
- 4 large eggs
- ¼ Cup coconut milk
- 2 Tablespoons of unsalted almond butter

- 1 and 1/2 teaspoons of stevia
- 1 Tablespoon of ground cinnamon
- 1 Tablespoon of natural unweeded cocoa powder
- 1 Tablespoon of fresh ground ginger
- 1/2 Teaspoon of kosher salt
- 1 and 1/2 cups of blanched almond flour
- 1/2 Teaspoon of baking soda

Direction: Preparation time: 15 minutes Cooking time: 20 minutes Yield: 9 Servings

✓ Preheat your oven to a temperature of 325 F.

✓ Grease a glass baking tray of about 8X8 inches generously with almond butter.

✓ In a large bowl, whisk all together with the coconut milk, the eggs, the melted almond butter, the stevia, the cinnamon, the cocoa powder, the ginger and the kosher salt.
Whisk in the almond flour, then the baking soda and mix very well.

✓ Pour the batter into the prepared pan and bake for about 20 to 25 minutes.

✓ Let the cake cool for about 5 minutes; then slice; serve and enjoy your delicious cake.

Nutrition: Calories: 175| Fat: 15g | Carbohydrates: 5g | Fiber: 1.9g |Protein: 5g

709)   *Ketogenic Orange Cake*

Ingredients:

- 2 and 1/2 cups of almond flour
- 2 Unwaxed washed oranges
- 5 Large separated eggs
- 1 teaspoon of baking powder
- 2 Teaspoons of orange extract
- 1 Teaspoon of vanilla bean powder
- 6 Seeds of cardamom pods crushed
- 16 drops of liquid stevia; about 3 teaspoons
- 1 Handful of flaked almonds to decorate

Direction: Preparation time: 10 minutes

Cooking time: 50 minutes Yield: 8 Servings

✓ Preheat your oven to a temperature of about 350 Fahrenheit.

✓ Line a rectangular bread baking tray with parchment paper.

✓ Place the oranges into a pan filled with cold water and cover it with a lid.

✓ Bring the saucepan to a boil, then let simmer for about 1 hour and make sure the oranges are totally submerged.

✓ Make sure the oranges are always submerged to remove any taste of bitterness.

✓ Cut the oranges into halves, then remove any seeds, and drain the water and set the oranges aside to cool down.

Cut the oranges in half and remove any seeds, then puree it with a blender or a food processor.

✓ Separate the eggs; then whisk the egg whites until you see stiff peaks forming.

✓ Add all your ingredients except for the egg whites to the orange mixture and add in the egg whites; then mix.

✓ Pour the batter into the cake tin and sprinkle with the flaked almonds right on top.

✓ Bake your cake for about 50 minutes.

✓ Remove the cake from the oven and set it aside to cool for 5 minutes.

✓ Slice your cake; then serve and enjoy its incredible taste!

Nutrition: Calories: 164| Fat: 12g | Carbohydrates: 7.1 | Fiber: 2.7g |Protein: 10.9g

710) *Lemon Cake*

Ingredients:

- 2 medium lemons
- 4 Large eggs
- 2 Tablespoons of almond butter
- 2 Tablespoons of avocado oil
- 1/3 cup of coconut flour
- 4-5 tablespoons of honey (or another sweetener of your choice)
- 1/2 tablespoon of baking soda

Direction: Preparation time: 20 minutes Cooking time: 20 minutes Yield: 9 Servings

✓ Preheat your oven to a temperature of about 350 F.

✓ Crack the eggs in a large bowl and set two egg whites aside.

✓ Whisk the 2 whites of eggs with the egg yolks, the honey, the oil, the almond butter, the lemon zest and the juice and whisk very well together.

✓ Combine the baking soda with the coconut flour and gradually add this dry mixture to the wet ingredients and keep whisking for a couple of minutes.

Beat the two eggs with a hand mixer and beat the egg into foam. Add the white egg foam gradually to the mixture with a silicone spatula.

✓ Transfer your obtained batter to tray covered with a baking paper.

✓ Bake your cake for about 20 to 22 minutes.

✓ Let the cake cool for 5 minutes; then slice your cake.

✓ Serve and enjoy your delicious cake!

Nutrition: Calories: 164| Fat: 12g | Carbohydrates: 7.1 | Fiber: 2.7g |Protein: 10.9g

711) *Mocha Pops*

Ingredients:

- 3 cups brewed coffee
- ½ cup low calorie chocolate flavored syrup
- ¾ cup low-fat half and half

Direction: Preparation Time: 4 minutes Cooking Time: 0 minutes Servings: 15

✓ Mix the ingredients in a bowl.

✓ Pour into popsicle molds. Freeze for 4 hours.

Nutrition: Calories 21 Total Fat 0 g Saturated Fat 0 g Cholesterol 1 mg Sodium 28 mg Total Carbohydrate 4 g Dietary Fiber 0 g Total Sugars 3 g Protein 0 g Potassium 450 mg

712) *Cinnamon Cake*

Ingredients:

- For the Cinnamon Filling:
- 3 Tablespoons of Swerve Sweetener
- 2 Teaspoons of ground cinnamon

 For the Cake:

- 3 cups of almond flour
- ¾ Cup of Swerve Sweetener
- ¼ Cup of unflavoured whey protein powder
- 2 teaspoon of baking powder
- 1/2 Teaspoon of salt
- 3 large pastured eggs
- 1/2 Cup of melted coconut oil
- 1/2 Teaspoon of vanilla extract
- 1/2 Cup of almond milk
- 1 Tablespoon of melted coconut oil
- For the cream cheese Frosting:
- 3 Tablespoons of softened cream cheese
- 2 Tablespoons of powdered Swerve Sweetener
- 1 Tablespoon of coconut heavy whipping cream
- 1/2 Teaspoon of vanilla extract

Direction: Preparation time: 15 minutes Cooking time: 35 minutes Yield: 8 Servings

✓ Preheat your oven to a temperature of about 325 F and grease a baking tray of 8x8 inches.

✓ For the filling, mix the Swerve and the cinnamon in a mixing bowl and mix very well; then set it aside.

✓ For the preparation of the cake, whisk all together with the almond flour, the sweetener, the protein powder, the baking powder, and the salt in a mixing bowl.

✓ Add in the eggs, the melted coconut oil and the vanilla extract and mix very well.

✓ Add in the almond milk and keep stirring until your ingredients are very well combined.

Spread about half of the batter in the prepared pan; then sprinkle with about two thirds of the filling mixture.

✓ *Spread the remaining mixture of the batter over the filling and smooth it with a spatula.*

✓ *Bake for about 35 minutes in the oven.*

✓ *Brush with the melted coconut oil and sprinkle with the remaining cinnamon filling.*

✓ *Prepare the frosting by beating the cream cheese, the powdered erythritol, the cream and the vanilla extract in a mixing bowl until it becomes smooth.*

✓ *Drizzle frost over the cooled cake.*

✓ *Slice the cake; then serve and enjoy your cake!*

Nutrition: Calories: 222| Fat: 19.2g | Carbohydrates: 5.4g | Fiber: 1.5g |Protein: 7.3g

713)   *Fruit Kebab*

Ingredients:

* 3 apples
* ¼ cup orange juice
* 1 ½ lb. watermelon
* ¾ cup blueberries

Direction: Preparation Time: 30 minutes Cooking Time: 0 minutes Servings: 12

✓ *Use a star-shaped cookie cutter to cut out stars from the apple and watermelon.*

✓ *Soak the apple stars in orange juice. Thread the apple stars, watermelon stars and blueberries into skewers.*

✓ *Refrigerate for 30 minutes before serving.*

Nutrition: Calories 52 Total Fat 0 g Saturated Fat 0 g Cholesterol 0 mg Sodium 1 mg Total Carbohydrate 14 g Dietary Fiber 2 g Total Sugars 10 g Protein 1 g Potassium 134 mg

714)   *Chocolate & Raspberry Ice Cream*

Ingredients:

* ¼ cup almond milk
* 2 egg yolks
* 2 tablespoons cornstarch
* ¼ cup honey
* ¼ teaspoon almond extract
* ⅛ teaspoon salt
* 1 cup fresh raspberries
* 2 oz. dark chocolate, chopped
* ¼ cup almonds, slivered and toasted

Direction: Preparation Time: 12 hours and 20 minutes Cooking Time: 0 minutes Servings: 8

✓ *Mix almond milk, egg yolks, cornstarch and honey*

in a bowl.

✓ *Pour into a saucepan over medium heat.*

✓ *Cook for 8 minutes.*

✓ *Strain through a sieve. Stir in salt and almond extract.*

✓ *Chill for 8 hours.*

✓ *Put into an ice cream maker.*

✓ *Follow manufacturer's directions.*

✓ *Stir in the rest of the ingredients.*

✓ *Freeze for 4 hours.*

Nutrition: Calories 142 Total Fat 7 g Saturated Fat 2 g Cholesterol 70 mg Sodium 87 mg Total Carbohydrate 18 g Dietary Fiber 2 g Total Sugars 13 g Protein 3 g Potassium 150 mg

715)   *Salad Preparation*

Ingredients:

* 8 oz. light cream cheese 6 oz. Greek yogurt
* 1 tablespoon honey
* 1 teaspoon orange zest
* 1 teaspoon lemon zest
* 1 orange, sliced into sections
* 3 kiwi fruit, peeled and sliced
* 1 mango, cubed 1 cup blueberries

Direction: Time: 5 minutes Cooking Time: 0 minute

Servings: 6

✓ *Beat cream cheese using an electric mixer. Add yogurt and honey.*

✓ *Beat until smooth. Stir in the orange and lemon zest. Toss the fruits to mix. Divide in glass jars. Top with the cream cheese mixture.*

Nutrition: Calories 131 Total Fat 3 g Saturated Fat 2 g Cholesterol 9 mg Sodium 102 mg Total Carbohydrate 23 g Dietary Fiber 3 g Total Sugars 18 g Protein 5 g Potassium 234 mg

MORE RECIPES

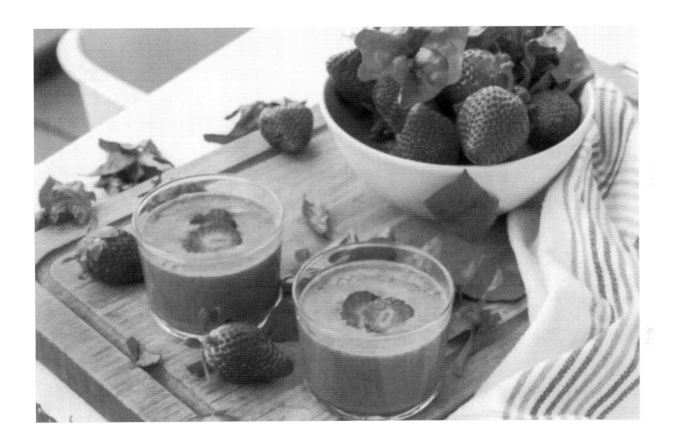

716)   Lemon Rooibos Iced Tea

Ingredients:

- 4 bags natural, unflavored rooibos tea
- 4 cups boiling water
- 3 tbsp. freshly squeezed lemon juice
- 30–40 drops liquid stevia

Direction: Preparation Time: 10 minutes Cooking Time: 0 minute Servings: 4

✓ Situate tea bags into a teapot and pour the boiling water over the bags.

✓ Set aside to room temperature, then refrigerate the tea until it is ice-cold.

✓ Remove the tea bags. Squeeze them gently.

✓ Add the lemon juice and liquid stevia to taste, and stir until well mixed.

✓ Serve immediately, preferably with ice cubes and some nice garnishes, like lemon wedges.

Nutrition: Calories: 70 Carbs: 16g Protein: 1g

717)   Lemon Lavender Iced Tea

Ingredients:

- 2 bags natural, unflavored rooibos tea
- 2 oz lemon chunks without peel and pith, seeds removed
- 1 tsp. dried lavender blossoms placed in a tea ball
- 4 cups water, at room temperature
- 20–40 drops liquid stevia

Direction: Preparation Time: 15minutes Cooking Time: 0 minute Servings: 4

✓ Place the tea bags, lemon chunks, and the tightly-closed tea ball with the lavender blossoms in a 1.5 qt (1.5 l) pitcher.

✓ Pour in the water.

✓ Refrigerate overnight.

✓ Remove the tea bags, lemon chunks, and the tea ball with the lavender on the next day. Squeeze the tea bags gently to save as much liquid as possible.

✓ Add liquid stevia to taste and stir until well mixed.

✓ Serve immediately with ice cubes and lemon wedges.

Nutrition: Calories: 81 Carbs: 12g Protein: 3g

718)   Cherry Vanilla Iced Tea

Ingredients:

- 4 bags natural, unflavored rooibos tea
- 4 cups boiling water
- 2 tbsp. freshly squeezed lime juice
- 1–2 tbsp. cherry flavoring
- 30–40 drops (or to taste) liquid vanilla stevia

Direction: Preparation Time: 12 minutes Cooking Time: 0 minute Servings: 4

✓ Place tea bags into a tea pot and pour the boiling water over the bags.

✓ Put aside the tea cool down first, then refrigerate the tea until it is ice- cold.

✓ Remove the tea bags. Squeeze them lightly. Add the lime juice, cherry flavoring, and vanilla stevia and stir until well mixed.

✓ Serve immediately, preferably with ice cubes and some nice garnishes like lime wedges and fresh cherries.

Nutrition: Calories: 89 Carbs: 14g Protein: 2g

719)   Elegant Blueberry Rose Water Iced Tea

Ingredients:

- 2 bags herbal blueberry tea
- 4 cups boiling water
- 20 drops liquid stevia
- 1 tbsp. rose water

Direction: Preparation Time: 12 minutes Cooking Time: 0 minute Servings: 4

✓ Position tea bags into a teapot and pour the boiling water over the bags.

✓ Allow the tea to cool down first, then refrigerate the tea until it is ice-cold.

✓ Remove the tea bags. Press them gently.

✓ Add the liquid stevia and the rose water and stir until well mixed.

✓ Serve immediately, preferably with ice cubes and some nice garnishes, like fresh blueberries or natural rose petals

Nutrition: Calories: 75 Carbs: 10g Protein: 2g

720)   Melba Iced Tea

Ingredients:

- 1 bag herbal raspberry tea
- 1 bag herbal peach tea
- 4 cups boiling water
- 10 drops liquid peach stevia
- 20–40 drops (or to taste) liquid vanilla stevia

Direction: Preparation Time: 10 minutes Cooking Time: 0 minute Servings: 4

✓ Pour the boiling water over the tea bags.

✓ Leave tea cool down at room temperature, then refrigerate the tea until it is ice-cold.

✓ *Remove the tea bags. Press lightly.*

✓ *Add the peach stevia and stir until well mixed.*

✓ *Add vanilla stevia to taste and stir until well mixed.*

✓ *Serve immediately, preferably with ice cubes and some nice garnishes, like vanilla bean, fresh raspberries, or peach slices.*

Nutrition: Calories: 81 Carbs: 14g Protein: 4g

721) *Merry Raspberry Cherry Iced Tea*

Ingredients:

* *2 bags herbal raspberry tea*
* *4 cups boiling water*
* *1 tsp. stevia-sweetened cherry-flavored drink mix*
* *1 tsp. freshly squeezed lime juice*
* *10–20 drops (or to taste) liquid stevia*

Direction: Preparation Time: 11 minutes Cooking Time: 0 minute Servings: 4

✓ *Put the tea bags into a tea pot and fill in boiling water over the bags.*

✓ *Let the tea cool down first to room temperature, then chill until it is ice-cold.*

✓ *Discard tea bags. Squeeze them.*

✓ *Add the cherry-flavored drink mix and the lime juice and stir until the drink mix is dissolved.*

✓ *Add liquid stevia to taste and stir until well mixed.*

✓ *Serve immediately, preferably with ice cubes or crushed ice, and some nice garnishes, like fresh raspberries and cherries.*

Nutrition: Calories: 82 Carbs: 11g Protein: 4g

722) *Vanilla Kissed Peach Iced Tea*

Ingredients:

* *2 bags herbal peach te*
* *4 cups boiling water*
* *1 tsp. vanilla extract*
* *1 tsp. freshly squeezed lemon juice*
* *30–40 drops (or to taste) liquid stevia*

Direction: Preparation Time: 13 minutes Cooking Time: 0 minute Servings: 4

✓ *Soak tea bags over boiling water.*

✓ *Allow to cool down at room temperature, then refrigerate the tea until it is ice-cold.*

✓ *Remove and press tea bags.*

✓ *Add the vanilla extract and the lemon juice and stir until well mixed.*

✓ *Add liquid stevia to taste and stir until well mixed.*

✓ *Serve immediately, preferably with ice cubes and some nice garnishes, like peach slices.*

Nutrition: Calories: 88 Carbs: 14g Protein: 3g

723) *Xtreme Berried Iced Tea*

Ingredients:

* *bags herbal Wild Berry Tea*
* *4 cups = 950 ml boiling water*
* *2 tsp. freshly squeezed lime juice*
* *40 drops berry-flavored liquid stevia*
* *10 drops (or to taste) liquid stevia*

Direction: Preparation Time: 10 minutes Cooking Time: 0 minute Servings: 4

✓ *Submerge tea bags into boiling water.*

✓ *Set aside to cool down, then refrigerate the tea until it is ice-cold.*

✓ *Pull out tea bags. Squeeze.*

✓ *Add the lime juice and the berry stevia and stir until well mixed.*

✓ *Add liquid stevia to taste and stir until well mixed.*

✓ *Serve immediately.*

Nutrition: Calories: 76 Carbohydrates: 14g Protein: 4g

724) *Refreshingly Peppermint Iced Tea*

Ingredients:

* *4 bags peppermint tea*
* *4 cups = 950 ml boiling water*
* *2 tsp. stevia-sweetened lime-flavored drink mix*
* *1 cup = 240 ml ice-cold sparkling water*

Direction: Preparation Time: 15 minutes Cooking Time: 0 minute Servings: 5

✓ *Immerse tea bags in boiling water.*

✓ *Set aside before cooling until it is ice-cold.*

✓ *Take out tea bags then press.*

✓ *Add the lime-flavored drink mix and stir until it is properly dissolved.*

✓ *Add the sparkling water and stir very gently.*

✓ *Serve immediately, preferably with ice cubes, mint leaves, and lime wedges.*

Nutrition: Calories: 78 Carbohydrates: 17g Protein: 4g

725) *Lemongrass Mint Iced Tea*

Ingredients:

* *1 stalk lemongrass, chopped in 1-inch*
* *½ cup chopped, loosely packed mint sprigs*
* *4 cups boiling water*

Direction: Preparation Time: 12 minutes Cooking Time: 0 minute Servings: 4

✓ Put the lemongrass and the mint into a teapot and pour the boiling water over them.

✓ Let cool down first to room temperature, then refrigerate until the tea is ice-cold.

✓ Filter out the lemongrass and the mint.

✓ Add liquid vanilla stevia to taste if you prefer some sweetness and stir until well mixed.

✓ Serve immediately, preferably with ice cubes and some nice garnishes, like mint sprigs, and lemongrass stalks.

Nutrition: Calories: 89 Carbs: 17g Protein: 5g

726) *Spiced Tea*

Ingredients:

- 2 bags Bengal Spice tea
- 2 tsp. freshly squeezed lemon juice
- 1 packet zero-carb vanilla stevia
- packet zero-carb stevia
- 4 cups boiling water

Direction: Preparation Time: 8 minutes Cooking Time: 0 minute Servings: 4

✓ Put the tea bags, lemon juice, and both stevia into a tea pot.

✓ Pour in the boiling water.

✓ Put aside to cool over room temperature, then refrigerate.

✓ Pull away tea bags then squeeze them.

✓ Stir gently.

✓ Serve immediately, preferably with ice cubes or crushed ice and some lemon wedges or slices.

Nutrition: Calories: 91 Carbs: 16g Protein: 1g

727) *Infused Pumpkin Spice Latte*

Ingredients:

- 2 cups almond milk
- ¼ cup coconut cream
- 2 tsp. cannabis coconut oil
- ¼ cup pure pumpkin, canned
- ½ tsp. vanilla extract
- 1 ½ tsp. pumpkin spice
- ½ cup coconut whipped cream
- 1 pinch salt

Direction: Preparation Time: 11 minutes Cooking Time: 0 minute Servings: 2

✓ Place all ingredients except the coconut whipped cream, in a pan over a medium-low heat stove.

✓ Whisk well and allow to simmer but don't boil! Simmer for about 5 minutes.

✓ Pour into mugs and serve.

Nutrition: Calories: 94 Carbs: 17g Protein: 3g

728) *Infused Turmeric-Ginger Tea*

Ingredients:

- 1 cup water
- ½ cup coconut milk 1 tsp. Cannabis oil
- ½ tsp. ground turmeric
- ¼ cup fresh ginger root, sliced
- 1 pinch Stevia or maple syrup, to taste

Direction: Preparation Time: 9 minutes Cooking Time: 0 minute Servings: 1

✓ Combine all ingredients in a small saucepan over medium heat.

✓ Heat until simmer and turn heat low.

✓ Take the pan off the heat after 2 minutes

✓ Let it cool, strain mixture into cup or mug.

Nutrition: Calories: 98 Carbohydrates: 14g Protein: 2g

729) *Infused London Fog*

Ingredients:

- 1 cup hot water
- 1 Earl Grey teabag
- 1 tsp. cannabis coconut oil
- ¼ cup almond milk
- ¼ tsp. vanilla extract
- 1 pinch Stevia or sugar, to taste

Direction: Preparation Time: 17 minutes Cooking Time: 0 minute Servings: 2

✓ Fill up half a mug with boiling water.

✓ Add tea bag; if you prefer your tea strong, add 2.

✓ Add cannabis oil and stir well.

✓ Add almond milk to fill your mug and stir through with the vanilla extract

✓ Use Stevia or sugar to sweeten your Earl Grey to taste.

Nutrition: Calories: 79 Carbs: 14g Protein: 2g

730) *Infused Cranberry-Apple Snug*

Ingredients:

- ½ cup fresh cranberry juice
- ½ cup fresh apple juice, cloudy
- ½ stick cinnamon
- 2 whole cloves
- ¼ lemon, sliced

- *pinch Stevia or sugar, to taste*
- *cranberries for garnish (optional)*

Direction: Preparation Time: 10 minutes Cooking Time: 0 minute Servings: 1

✓ *Combine all ingredients in a small saucepan over medium heat.*
✓ *Heat until simmer and turn heat low.*
✓ *Let it cool, strain the mixture into a mug.*
✓ *Serve with cinnamon sticks and cranberries in a mug.*

Nutrition: Calories: 88 Carbs: 15g Protein: 3g

731) Creole Seasoning

Ingredients:

- *2 tbsp. garlic powder*
- *2 tbsp. dried basil*
- *1 tbsp. sweet paprika*
- *1 tbsp. smoked paprika*
- *1 tbsp. freshly ground black pepper*
- *1 tbsp. onion powder*
- *1 tbsp. cayenne pepper*
- *1 tbsp. dried thyme*
- *1 tbsp. dried oregano*
- *1 tsp. ground red sweet pepper*

Direction: Preparation Time: 9 minutes Cooking Time: 41 minutes Servings: 6

✓ *In an airtight container, combine the garlic powder, basil, sweet paprika, smoked paprika, black pepper, onion powder, cayenne, thyme, oregano, and sweet pepper.*

Nutrition: Calories: 15 Carbs: 0.1g Protein: 1.1g

732) BBQ Sauce

Ingredients:

- *1¼ cup tomato purée*
- *1½ cup white vinegar*
- *1 tbsp. yellow mustard*
- *1 tsp. mustard seeds*
- *1 tsp. ground turmeric*
- *1 tsp. Sweet paprika*
- *tsp. garlic powder*
- *1 tsp. celery seeds*
- *½ tsp. cayenne pepper*
- *½ tsp. onion powder*
- *½ tsp. freshly ground black pepper*

Direction: Preparation Time: 6 minutes Cooking Time: 15 minutes

✓ *In a medium pot, combine the tomato purée, vinegar, mustard, mustard seeds, turmeric, paprika, garlic powder, celery seeds, cayenne, onion powder, and black pepper. Simmer over low heat for 15 minutes, or until the flavors come together.*
✓ *Remove the sauce from the heat, and let cool for 5 minutes. Transfer to a blender, and purée until smooth.*

Nutrition: Calories: 10 Carbs: 0.2g Protein: 0.3g

733) Chicken Gravy

Ingredients:

- *2 cups low-sodium chicken broth, divided*
- *4 tbsp. whole-wheat flour, divided*
- *1 medium yellow onion, chopped*
- *½ bunch fresh thyme, roughly chopped*
- *2 garlic cloves, minced*
- *1 bay leaf*
- *½ tsp. celery seeds*
- *Freshly ground black pepper, to taste*
- *1 tsp. Worcestershire sauce*

Direction: Preparation Time: 6 minutes Cooking Time: 15 minutes Servings: 2

✓ *In a shallow stockpot, combine ½ cup broth, and 1 tbsp. whole-wheat flour and cook over medium-low heat, whisking until the flour is dissolved. Continue to add about ½ cup broth and the remaining 3 tbsp. flour in increments for about 2 minutes, or until a thick sauce is formed.*
✓ *Add the onion, thyme, garlic, bay leaf, and ½ cup broth, stirring well.*
✓ *Add the celery seeds, pepper, Worcestershire sauce, and remaining ½ cup broth. Stir and cook for 2 to 3 minutes, or until the gravy is thickened. Discard the bay leaf.*
✓ *Serve spooned over Baked Chicken Stuffed with Collard Greens or your protein of choice.*

Nutrition: Calories: 17 Carbohydrates: 0.1g Protein: 1,1g

734) Ranch Dressing

Ingredients:

- *8 oz. (227g) fat-free plain Greek yogurt*
- *¼ cup low-fat buttermilk*
- *1 tbsp. garlic powder*
- *1 tbsp. dried dill*
-
- *1 tbsp. dried chives*
- *1 tbsp. onion powder*

- 1 tbsp. dried parsley
- Pinch freshly ground black pepper

Direction: Preparation Time: 6 minutes Cooking Time: 0 minutes Servings: 9

✓ In a shallow, medium bowl, combine the Greek yogurt and buttermilk.

✓ Stir in the garlic powder, dill, chives, onion powder, parsley, and pepper and mix well.

✓ Serve with animal protein or vegetable of your choice, or place in an airtight container.

Nutrition: Calories: 30 Fat: 0.1g Protein: 3.0g

735)   Greek or Italian Vinaigrette

Ingredients:

Greek:
- ¼ cup extra virgin olive oil
- 3 garlic cloves, minced
- 1 tbsp. freshly squeezed lemon juice
- 1 tbsp. red wine vinegar
- 1 tsp. dried marjoram
- 1 tsp. dried oregano
- ½ tsp. lemon zest
- ¼ tsp. sea salt

Italian:
- ¼ cup extra-virgin olive oil
- 2 tbsp. red wine vinegar
- 1tsp. Dijon mustard
- 2 tsp. Italian seasoning
- 1 garlic clove, finely minced
- 1 tbsp. minced shallot
- ¼ tsp. sea salt
- ⅛ tsp. freshly ground black pepper

Direction: Preparation Time: 6 minutes Cooking Time: 0 minutes Servings: 4

✓ Stir together all ingredients in a medium bowl until completely mixed and emulsified.

Nutrition: Calories: 129 Fat: 14.3g Protein: 0.2g

736)   Quick Peanut Sauce

Ingredients:

- ¼ cup peanut butter
- 1 lime, juiced
- 1 tbsp. honey
- 1 minced garlic clove
- 1 tbsp. reduced-sodium soy sauce
- 1 tbsp. peeled fresh ginger, grated
- Pinch red pepper flakes

Direction: Preparation Time: 6 minutes Cooking Time: 0 minutes Servings: 4

✓ Put all ingredients in a medium bowl and whisk until well blended.

Nutrition: Calories: 120 Fat: 8.3g Protein: 4.2g

737)   Creamy Lemon Sauce

Ingredients:

- 1 cup half-and-half
- 1 tbsp. unsalted butter
- 2 tbsp. Parmesan cheese, shredded
- 1 tsp. freshly squeezed lemon juice
- ¼ tsp. garlic powder

Direction: Preparation Time: 6 minutes Cooking Time: 5 minutes Servings: 2

✓ Add all ingredients to a saucepan and cook over medium-low heat for about 3 to 5 minutes, stirring frequently, or until the sauce is heated through.

✓ Remove from the heat to a bowl. Let it cool for a few minutes before serving.

Nutrition: Calories: 55 Fat: 5.2g Protein: 3g

738)   Lemony Dill and Yogurt Dressing

Ingredients:

- 2 tbsp. mayonnaise
- 1 tsp. freshly squeezed lemon juice
- 1 tsp. fresh dill, chopped
- ½ cup plain Greek yogurt
- ¼ tsp. garlic powder
- ¼ tsp. salt

Direction: Preparation Time: 6 minutes Cooking Time: 0 minutes Servings: 6

✓ Combine all the ingredients in a bowl. Stir to mix well

Nutrition: Calories: 36 Fat: 1.0g Protein: 3.2g

739)   Fresh Cucumber Dip

Ingredients:

- 1 medium cucumber, peeled and grated
- ¼ tsp. salt
- 1 cup plain Greek yogurt
- 2 garlic cloves, minced
- 1 tbsp. freshly squeezed lemon juice
- 1 tbsp. extra-virgin olive oil
- ¼ tsp. freshly ground black pepper

Direction: Preparation Time: 9 minutes Cooking Time: 0 minutes Servings: 2

✓ Put the cucumber in a colander, then sprinkle with salt. Set aside.

✓ Combine the remaining ingredients in a bowl. Stir to mix well.

✓ Wrap the cucumber in a muslin cloth and squeeze the liquid out as much as possible.

✓ Put the cucumber in the bowl of mixture, then stir to mix well.

✓ Wrap the bowl in plastic and refrigerate to marinate for 2 hours.

Nutrition: Calories: 50 Fat: 3.0g Protein: 4.05g

740) Avocado Cilantro Dressing

Ingredients:

- 1 large avocado, peeled and pitted
- ½ cup plain Greek yogurt
- ¾ cup fresh cilantro
- 1 tbsp. water
- 2 tsp. freshly squeezed lime juice
- ⅛ tsp. garlic powder
- Pinch salt

Direction: Preparation Time: 6 minutes Cooking Time: 0 minutes Servings: 2

✓ Process the avocado, yogurt, cilantro, water, lime juice, garlic powder, and salt in a blender until creamy and emulsified.

✓ Chill for at least 30 minutes in the refrigerator to let the flavors blend.

Nutrition: Calories: 92 Fat: 6.8g Protein: 4.1g

741) Lemon Tahini Dressing with Honey

Ingredients:

- ½ cup water
- ¾ cup unsalted tahini
- 1/3 cup freshly squeezed lemon juice
- 3 tbsp. honey
- ½ tsp. salt

Direction: Preparation Time: 6 minutes Cooking Time: 0 minutes Servings: 2

✓ Mix together the water, tahini, lemon juice, honey, and salt in a medium bowl, and stir vigorously until well incorporated.

✓ Store the leftover dressing in an airtight container in the fridge for up to 2 weeks and shake before using.

Nutrition: Calories: 168 Fat: 13.1g Protein: 4.7g

742) Red Pepper and Chickpea Spread

Ingredients:

- 1 (16 oz./454g) jar roasted red bell peppers
- cup canned low-sodium chickpeas, drained and rinsed
- ½ small jalapeño pepper, deseeded and stemmed
- 2 tbsp. water
- 2 tbsp. extra-virgin olive oil
- 1 to 2 tsp. freshly squeezed lime juice
- ¼ tsp. garlic powder
- ½ tsp. salt
- ¼ tsp. ground cumin
- ⅛ tsp. freshly ground black pepper

Direction: Preparation Time: 6 minutes Cooking Time: 0 minutes Servings: 2

✓ In a food processor, add the bell peppers, chickpeas, jalapeño pepper, water, oil, lime juice, garlic powder, salt, cumin, and black pepper, and pulse until the mixture has a spreadable consistency.

✓ Transfer to an airtight container and store in the fridge for up to 1 week.

Nutrition: Calories: 52 Fat: 2.8g Protein: 1.1g

743) Spicy Asian Dipping Sauce

Ingredients:

- 1/3 cup low-fat mayonnaise
- 1 to 2 tsp. hot sauce, to your liking
- 2 tsp. rice vinegar
- 1 tsp. sesame oil

Direction: Preparation Time: 6 minutes Cooking Time: 0 minutes Servings: 2

✓ Stir together the mayo, hot sauce, rice vinegar, and oil in a small bowl until thoroughly smooth.

✓ Chill for at least 30 minutes to blend the flavors.

Nutrition: Calories: 54 Fat: 4.7g Protein: 0

744) Easy Thai Peanut Sauce

Ingredients:

- ½ cup natural peanut butter
- 2 tbsp. rice vinegar
- 4 tsp. sesame oil
- 2 to 4 tsp. freshly squeezed lime juice, to your liking
- 2 to 2½ tsp. hot sauce (optional)

- 1 tsp. low-sodium soy sauce
- 1 tsp. chopped peeled fresh ginger
- 1 tsp. honey

Direction: Preparation Time: 6 minutes Cooking Time: 0 minutes Servings: 6

✓ Mix together the peanut butter, rice vinegar, sesame oil, lime juice, hot sauce (if desired), soy sauce, ginger, and honey in a small bowl, and whisk to combine well.
You can store it in an airtight container in the fridge for up to 2 weeks.

Nutrition: Calories: 206 Fat: 16.7g Protein: 7.9g

745) *Chimichurri*

Ingredients:

- ½ cup Italian parsley
- ¼ cup extra-virgin olive oil
- ¼ cup fresh cilantro, stems removed
- 1 lemon, zested
- 2 tbsp. red wine vinegar
- ½ tsp. sea salt
- 1 garlic clove, minced
- ¼ tsp. red pepper flakes

Direction: Preparation Time: 6 minutes Cooking Time: 0 minutes Servings: 4

✓ Process all the ingredients in a food processor until smooth.
✓ Store in an airtight container in the fridge for up to 2 days or in the freezer for 6 months.

Nutrition: Calories: 124 Fat: 13.7g Protein: 0.1g

746) *Apricot-Orange Oat Bites*

Ingredients:

- 1 cup rolled oats
- 1½ cups pitted dates
- ½ cup dried apricots
- ½ cup almond butter
- 2/3 cup shredded coconut
- 1 orange, zested (about 1 tbsp.)
- 1 orange, juiced (about 3 tbsp.)
- 1 tsp. vanilla extract

Direction: Preparation Time: 9 minutes Cooking Time: 5 minutes Servings: 10

✓ Preheat the oven to 350°F. Line a baking sheet with parchment paper.
✓ Place the oats on the baking sheet and toast them until they are browned, about 5 minutes. Let them cool for 10 minutes.

✓ While the oats are toasting, put the dates in a food processor or blender, and pulse until smooth.
✓ Add the toasted oats, apricots, almond butter, coconut, orange zest and juice, and vanilla extract to the processor. Continue pulsing until the mixture is smooth and forms a ball. Transfer it to a medium bowl.
✓ Using clean hands, form 1 tbsp. batter into a 2-inch ball and place in a resealable container. Repeat for the remaining batter, making a total of 20 balls.
✓ Cover the container and refrigerate to allow the balls to set, at least 15 minutes.

Nutrition: Calories: 117 Fat: 5g Protein: 3g

747) *No-Bake Maple Cinnamon Bars*

Ingredients:

- 1 cup pitted dates
- 1 cup raw unsalted cashews
- ¼ cup 100% maple syrup
- 1 tsp. ground cinnamon
- 3 tbsp. dried cranberries
- Cooking spray

Direction: Preparation Time: 16 minutes Cooking Time: 0 minutes Servings: 8

✓ Line an 8-by-8-inch baking dish with parchment paper.
✓ In a food processor or blender, add the dates, cashews, maple syrup, and cinnamon. Blend until the mixture reaches a paste-like consistency. Transfer to a medium bowl.
✓ Add the cranberries to the mixture and gently fold until they are incorporated.
✓ Add the mixture to the baking dish and evenly spread it. Using clean hands, press down on the mixture. Cover and refrigerate until the bars set, about 1 hour. Slice into 2-inch bars.

Nutrition: Calories: 97 Fat: 4g Protein: 2g

748) *Honey Ricotta with Strawberries*

Ingredients:

- 1 cup part-skim ricotta cheese
- 2 tbsp. honey
- ¼ cup unsalted cashews, chopped
- 3 cups strawberries, halved

Direction: Preparation Time: 9 minutes Cooking Time: 0 minutes Servings: 4

✓ In a small bowl, combine the ricotta, honey, and cashews.
✓ Place ¼ cup the ricotta mixture and ¾ cup strawberries in each of 4 resealable containers.

Nutrition: Calories: 201 Fat: 9g Protein: 9g

749) *Homemade Trail Mix*

Ingredients:

- *½ cup raw almonds*
- *10 dried apricots*
- *3 tbsp. dried tart cherries*
- *3 tbsp. dark chocolate chips*
- *2 tbsp. unsalted sunflower seeds*

Direction: Preparation Time: 6 minutes Cooking Time: 0 minutes Servings: 4

✓ *In a medium bowl, add the almonds, apricots, cherries, chocolate chips, and sunflower seeds. Toss to combine*

Nutrition: Calories: 216 Fat: 15g Protein: 6g

750) *Crudité with Herbed Yogurt Dip*

Ingredients:

- *1 cup nonfat plain Greek yogurt*
- *¼ cup chopped fresh basil*
- *¼ cup chopped fresh parsley*
- *½ lemon, juiced (about 1 tbsp.)*
- *1 garlic clove, minced*
- *¼ tsp. salt*
- *⅛ tsp. freshly ground black pepper*
- *2 cups baby carrots*
- *celery stalks, sliced into 3-inch-long matchsticks*
- *1 cup cherry tomatoes*
- *1 red or yellow bell pepper, sliced into 2-inch-thick pieces (1 cup)*

Direction: Preparation Time: 16 minutes Cooking Time: 0 minutes Servings: 4

✓ *In a small bowl, add the Greek yogurt, basil, parsley, lemon juice, garlic, salt, and black pepper. Stir to combine.*

✓ *Spoon ¼ cup the dip into small resealable containers and serve with the vegetables on the side.*

Nutrition: Calories: 80 Fat: 1g Protein: 7g

751) *Chili-Roasted Chickpeas*

Ingredients:

- *Cooking spray*
- *2 (15 oz.) cans reduced-sodium chickpeas, drained and rinsed*
- *1 tbsp. coconut oil*
- *1 tbsp. chili powder*
- *2 tsp. cumin*
- *½ tsp. salt*

Direction: Preparation Time: 16 minutes Cooking

Time: 45 minutes Servings: 6

✓ *Preheat the oven to 400°F. Coat a baking sheet with the cooking spray.*

✓ *In a medium bowl, add the chickpeas, coconut oil, chili powder, cumin, and salt. Toss to combine.*

✓ *Spread the chickpeas in a single layer on the baking sheet. Roast until the chickpeas appear to split apart, 40 to 45 minutes. Let the chickpeas cool for 10 minutes.*

Nutrition: Calories: 113 Fat: 4g Protein: 5g

752) *Thyme-Roasted Almonds*

Ingredients:

- *1½ cups raw almonds*
- *2 tbsp. olive oil*
- *1 tbsp. dried thyme*
- *½ tsp. kosher salt*

Direction: Preparation Time: 6 minutes Cooking Time: 9 minutes Servings: 6

✓ *Preheat the oven to 400°F.*

✓ *In a small bowl, add the almonds, olive oil, thyme, and salt. Toss to evenly coat almonds.*

✓ *Spread the almonds in a single layer on the baking sheet. Bake until the almonds are slightly browned and fragrant, about 8 minutes. Let the almonds cool for 10 minutes.*

Nutrition: Calories: 238 Fat: 21g Protein: 8g

753) *Cinnamon Cocoa Popcorn*

Ingredients:

- *3 tbsp. coconut oil*
- *½ cup popcorn kernels Cooking spray*
- *1 tbsp. unsweetened cocoa powder*
- *1 tsp. ground cinnamon*
- *tbsp. granulated sugar*
- *1 tsp. sea salt*

Direction: Preparation Time: 6 minutes Cooking Time: 5 minutes Servings: 4

✓ *In a medium pot over medium-low heat, heat the coconut oil. Add 3 popcorn kernels, and when 1 of the kernels pops, add the rest of them. Cover and shake the pot occasionally to prevent burning. Once the popcorn is popped, transfer the popcorn to a large mixing bowl.*

✓ *Spray the popcorn with the cooking spray. Using clean hands, toss the popcorn to mix it thoroughly. Sprinkle it with the cocoa powder, cinnamon, sugar, and salt, and mix until the popcorn is thoroughly coated.*

Nutrition: Calories: 188 Fat: 12g Protein: 3g

754) *Fruit Salad with Mint*

Ingredients:

- ½ cantaloupe, cubed
- 2 cups strawberries, hulled and sliced lengthwise
- 1 cup blueberries, blackberries, or raspberries
- 1 cup seedless green or red grapes
- ¼ cup freshly squeezed orange juice
- 2 tbsp. chopped fresh mint
- 1 tsp. vanilla extract

Direction: Preparation Time: 16 minutes Cooking Time: 0 minutes Servings: 4

✓ In a large bowl, combine the cantaloupe, strawberries, blueberries, and grapes.

✓ In a small bowl, whisk together the orange juice, mint, and vanilla extract. Pour this over the fruit and toss to evenly coat.

755) *Herbed Vinaigrette*

Nutrition: Calories: 93 Fat: 1g Protein: 2g

Ingredients:

- ¼ cup extra-virgin olive oil
- 2 tbsp. freshly squeezed orange juice
- ½ tsp. 100% maple syrup
- 2 tsp. chopped fresh parsley
- 1 tsp. chopped fresh rosemary
- ¼ tsp. salt

Direction: Preparation Time: 9 minutes Cooking Time: 0 minutes Servings: 6

✓ In a small bowl, whisk together the olive oil, orange juice, maple syrup, parsley, rosemary, and salt until well combined

Nutrition: Calories: 123 Fat: 14g Protein: 0.1g

756) *Mason Jar Key Lime Parfaits*

Ingredients:

- 1¼ cups nonfat plain Greek yogurt, divided
- 1 lime, juiced (about 2 tbsp.)
- 1 lime, zested
- 1 tbsp. 100% maple syrup
- ½ cup Homemade Granola

Direction: Preparation Time: 9 minutes Cooking Time: 0 minutes Servings: 2

✓ In a small bowl, whisk together the Greek yogurt, lime juice and zest, and maple syrup.

✓ In each of 2 Mason jars, layer 5 tbsp. the Greek yogurt followed by 2 tbsp. the Homemade Granola. Repeat for a second layer. Cover and refrigerate.

Nutrition: Calories: 246 Fat: 4g Protein: 18g

757) *Sriracha Hummus*

Ingredients:

- 1 (15 oz.) can reduced-sodium chickpeas, drained and rinsed
- 1 garlic clove, minced
- 3 tbsp. tahini
- 1½ lemons, juiced (about 3 tbsp.)
- ½ to 1 tsp. sriracha
- ½ tsp. salt
- ¼ tsp. freshly ground black pepper
- ¼ cup extra-virgin olive oil
- 2 tbsp. water

Direction: Preparation Time: 9 minutes Cooking Time: 0 minutes Servings: 2

✓ In a food processor or blender, add the chickpeas, garlic, tahini, lemon juice, the desired amount of sriracha, salt, and black pepper, and process until well combined.

✓ With the machine running, slowly drizzle in the olive oil and water and continue processing until well incorporated, and the hummus is creamy.

Nutrition: Calories: 107 Fat: 5g Protein: 5g

758) *Rosemary Beet Chips*

Ingredients:

- Cooking spray
- 2 pounds beets, peeled
- 1 tbsp. olive oil
- 2 tsp. dried rosemary
- ½ tsp. salt
- ⅛ tsp. freshly ground black pepper

Direction: Preparation Time: 9 minutes Cooking Time: 21 minutes Servings: 4

✓ Preheat the oven to 375ºF. Coat a baking sheet with the cooking spray.

✓ Using a mandolin or a chef's knife, slice the beets as thin as possible and in a uniform size. The slices should almost curl up.

✓ Put the beet slices in a large bowl and drizzle them with olive oil, rosemary, salt, and black pepper. Toss gently to combine.

✓ Place the beets in a single layer on the baking sheet. Bake until the beets are crispy, about 15 to 20 minutes.

Nutrition: Calories: 130 Fat: 4g Protein: 4g

759) *Herbed Vinaigrette*

Ingredients:

- ¼ cup extra-virgin olive oil

- *2 tbsp. freshly squeezed orange juice*
- *½ tsp. 100% maple syrup*
- *2 tsp. chopped fresh parsley*
- *1 tsp. chopped fresh rosemary*
- *¼ tsp. salt*

Direction: Preparation Time: 9 minutes Cooking Time: 0 minutes Servings: 6

✓ *In a small bowl, whisk together the olive oil, orange juice, maple syrup, parsley, rosemary, and salt until well combined.*

Nutrition: Calories: 123 Fat: 14g Protein: 0.1g

760)   *Sriracha-Lime Kale Chips*

Ingredients:

- *Cooking spray*
- *¼ cup olive oil*
- *1 tsp. sriracha*
- *1 lime, zested*
- *lime, juiced (about 2 tbsp.)*
- *1 tsp. kosher salt*
- *½ tsp. freshly ground black pepper*
- *1 (10 oz.) bag torn kale*

Direction: Preparation Time: 16 minutes Cooking Time: 11 minutes Servings: 6

✓ *Preheat the oven to 400°F. Coat 2 baking sheets with the cooking spray.*

✓ *In a large bowl, whisk together the olive oil, sriracha, lime juice, and zest, salt, and black pepper.*

✓ *Add the kale to the bowl and toss until it is well coated with the dressing. Spread the kale in single, even layers on the baking sheets.*

✓ *Bake until the kale is crisp, about 10 minutes. Let cool for 10 minutes.*

Nutrition: Calories: 102 Fat: 9g Protein: 1g

761)   *Kale Pesto*

Ingredients:

- *2 cups baby kale*
- *4 cups basil leaves*
- *¼ cup extra-virgin olive oil*
- *1 garlic clove, chopped*
- *1 lemon, juiced (about 2 tbsp.)*
- *½ tsp. salt*

Direction: Preparation Time: 9 minutes Cooking Time: 0 minutes Servings: 6

✓ *In a food processor or blender, add the kale, basil, olive oil, garlic, lemon juice, and salt. Purée until it*

forms a paste.

Nutrition: Calories: 96 Fat: 9g Protein: 2g

762)   *White Balsamic Vinaigrette*

Ingredients:

- *1 garlic clove, minced*
- *2 tbsp. white balsamic vinegar*
- *½ tsp. Dijon mustard*
- *¼ tsp. salt*
- *¼ tsp. freshly ground black pepper*
- *¼ cup extra-virgin olive oil*

Direction: Preparation Time: 6 minutes Cooking Time: 0 minutes Servings: 6

✓ *In a small bowl, whisk together the garlic, vinegar, mustard, salt, and black pepper. Slowly drizzle in the olive oil while whisking vigorously to emulsify the dressing.*

Nutrition: Calories: 155 Fat: 17g Protein: 0.2g

763)   *Lighter Blue Cheese Dressing*

Ingredients:

- *½ cup nonfat plain Greek yogurt*
- *½ ounce crumbled blue cheese (about 1 heaping tbsp.)*
- *1 tsp. white balsamic vinegar*
- *1 tsp. freshly squeezed lemon juice*
- *1 garlic clove, smashed*
- *¼ tsp. salt*
- *⅛ tsp. freshly ground black pepper*

Direction: Preparation Time: 6 minutes Cooking Time: 15 minutes Servings: 6

✓ *In a blender or food processor, add Greek yogurt, blue cheese, vinegar, lemon juice, garlic, salt, and black pepper. Blend until smooth and creamy.*

Nutrition: Calories: 45 Fat: 2g Protein: 4g

764)   *Soy-Sesame Dressing*

Ingredients:

- *2 tbsp. reduced-sodium soy sauce*
- *2 tbsp. seasoned rice vinegar*
- *1 garlic clove, minced*
- *1 tsp. toasted sesame oil*
- *1 tsp. honey*
- *1/3 cup canola oil*

Direction: Preparation Time: 6 minutes Cooking Time: 0 minutes Servings: 6

✓ *In a small bowl, whisk together the soy sauce,*

vinegar, garlic, sesame oil, and honey. Slowly drizzle in the canola oil, while whisking vigorously to combine.

Nutrition: Calories: 122 Fat: 3g Protein: 0.1g

765)   *Asian Peanut Sauce*

Ingredients:

- ½ cup light coconut milk
- ¾ cup creamy peanut butter
- 3 tbsp. reduced-sodium soy sauce
- 1½ limes, juiced (about 3 tbsp.)
- 2 tbsp. chopped shallots
- 1 garlic clove, chopped
- 1 tbsp. brown sugar
- 2 tbsp. water, or more if needed

Direction: Preparation Time: 16 minutes Cooking Time: 0 minutes Servings: 6

✓ *In a blender or food processor add the coconut milk, peanut butter, soy sauce, lime juice, shallots, garlic, and brown sugar. Blend until smooth.*

✓ *Add the water to achieve your desired thickness.*

Nutrition: Calories: 130 Fat: 10g Protein: 5g

766)   *Thai Marinade*

Ingredients:

- 1¼ cups light coconut milk
- 2 tbsp. reduced-sodium soy sauce
- 2 tbsp. brown sugar
- 1 lime, juiced
- 1 lime, zested
- 1 tbsp. curry powder
- 1 tsp. ground coriander
- 1 garlic clove, minced
- 1 tsp. minced fresh ginger
- ¼ tsp. salt
- ⅛ tsp. freshly ground black pepper

Direction: Preparation Time: 16 minutes Cooking Time: 0 minutes Servings: 6

✓ *In a large bowl, whisk together the coconut milk, soy sauce, brown sugar, lime juice and zest, curry powder, coriander, garlic, ginger, salt, and black pepper until the sugar has dissolved.*

Nutrition: Calories: 78 Fat: 4g Protein: 2g

767)   *Coffee-Steamed Carrots*

Ingredients:

- 1 cup brewed coffee

- 1 tsp. light brown sugar
- ½ tsp. Kosher salt
- Freshly ground black pepper
- 1 lb. baby carrots
- Fresh parsley, chopped
- 1 tsp. grated lemon zest

Direction: Preparation Time: 10 minutes Cooking Time: 3 minutes Servings: 4

✓ *Pour the coffee into the electric pressure cooker. Stir in the brown sugar, salt, and pepper. Add the carrots.*

✓ *Close the pressure cooker. Set to sealing.*

✓ *Cook on high pressure for minutes.*

✓ *Once complete, click Cancel and quickly release the pressure.*

✓ *Once the pin drops, open and remove the lid.*

✓ *Using a slotted spoon, portion carrots to a serving bowl. Topped with the parsley and lemon zest, and serve.*

Nutrition: Calories: 51 Carbohydrates: 12g Fiber: 4g

768)   *Rosemary Potatoes*

Ingredients:

- 1 lb. red potatoes
- 1 cup vegetable stock
- 2 tbsp. olive oil
- 2 tbsp. Rosemary sprigs

Direction: Preparation Time: 5 minutes Cooking Time: 25 minutes Servings: 2

✓ *Situate potatoes in the steamer basket and add the stock into the Instant Pot.*

✓ *Steam the potatoes in your Instant Pot for 15 minutes.*

✓ *Depressurize and pour away the remaining stock. Set to sauté and add the oil, rosemary, and potatoes.*

✓ *Cook until brown.*

Nutrition: Calories: 195 Carbohydrates: 31g Fat: 1g

769)   *Corn on the Cob*

Ingredients:

- 6 ears corn

Direction: Preparation Time: 10 minutes Cooking Time: 5 minutes Servings: 12

✓ *Take off husks and silk from the corn. Cut or break each ear in half.*

✓ *Pour 1 cup of water into the bottom of the electric pressure cooker. Insert a wire rack or trivet.*

✓ *Place the corn upright on the rack, cut-side down. Seal lid of the pressure cooker.*

✓ *Cook on high pressure for 5 minutes.*

✓ *When it's complete, select Cancel and quickly release the pressure.*

✓ *When the pin drops, unlock and take off the lid.*

✓ *Pull out the corn from the pot—season as desired and serve immediately.*

Nutrition: Calories: 62 Carbohydrates: 14g Fiber: 1g

770) *Chili Lime Salmon*

Ingredients:

- *For Sauce:*
- *1 jalapeno pepper*
- *1 tbsp. chopped parsley*
- *1 tsp. minced garlic*
- *½ tsp. cumin*
- *½ tsp. paprika*
- *tbsp. lime juice*
- *1 tbsp. olive oil*

For Fish:

- *salmon fillets, each about 5 oz.*
- *1 cup water*
- *½ tsp. salt*
- *⅛ tsp. ground black pepper*
- *½ tsp. lime zest*
- *1 tbsp. honey*
- *1 tbsp. water*

Direction: Preparation Time: 6 minutes Cooking Time: 10 minutes Servings: 2

✓ *Prepare salmon and for this, season salmon with salt and black pepper until evenly coated.*

✓ *Plug in instant pot, insert the inner pot, pour in water, then place steamer basket and place seasoned salmon on it.*

✓ *Seal the instant pot with its lid, press the 'steam' button, then press the 'timer' to set the cooking time to 5 minutes and cook on high pressure, for 5 minutes.*

✓ *Transfer all the ingredients for the sauce to a bowl, whisk until combined, and set aside until required.*

✓ *When the timer beeps, press the 'cancel' button and do a quick pressure release until the pressure nob drops down.*

✓ *Open the instant pot, then transfer salmon to a serving plate and drizzle generously with prepared sauce.*

✓ *Serve straight away.*

Nutrition: Calories: 305 Carb: 29g Fiber: 6g

771) *Collard Greens*

Ingredients:

- *2 lb. chopped collard greens*
- *¾ cup chopped white onion*
- *1 tsp. onion powder*
- *tsp. garlic powder*
- *1 tsp. salt*
- *tsp. brown sugar*
- *½ tsp. ground black pepper*
- *½ tsp. red chili powder*
- *¼ tsp. crushed red pepper flakes*
- *3 tbsp. apple cider vinegar*
- *2 tbsp. olive oil*
- *14.5 oz. vegetable broth*
- *½ cup water*

Direction: Preparation Time: 5 minutes Cooking Time: 6 hours Servings: 12

✓ *Plug-in instant pot, insert the inner pot, add onion and collard, and then pour in vegetable broth and water.*

✓ *Close the instant pot with its lid, seal, press the 'slow cook' button, then press the 'timer' to set the cooking time to 6 hours at a high heat setting.*

✓ *When the timer beeps, press the 'cancel' button and do natural pressure release until the pressure nob drops down. Open the instant pot, add remaining ingredients and stir until mixed.*

✓ *Then press the 'sauté/simmer' button and cook for 3 to minutes or more until collards reach to desired texture. Serve straight away.*

Nutrition: Calories: 49 Carbs: 2.3g Fiber: 0.5g

772) *Mashed Pumpkin*

Ingredients:

- *2 cups chopped pumpkin*
- *½ cup water*
- *2 tbsp. powdered sugar-free sweetener of choice*
- *1 tbsp. cinnamon*

Direction: Preparation Time: 9 minutes Cooking Time: 15 minutes Servings: 2

✓ *Place the pumpkin and water in your Instant Pot.*

✓ *Seal and cook on Stew for 15 minutes. Remove and mash with the sweetener and cinnamon.*

Nutrition: Calories: 12 Carbohydrates: 3g Sugar: 1g

773) *Parmesan-Topped Acorn Squash*

Ingredients:

- *1 acorn squash (about 1 pound)*

- 1 tbsp. extra-virgin olive oil
- tsp. dried sage leaves, crumbled
- ¼ tsp. freshly grated nutmeg
- ⅛ tsp. Kosher salt
- ⅛ tsp. freshly ground black pepper
- 2 tbsp. freshly grated Parmesan cheese

Direction: Preparation Time: 8 minutes Cooking Time: 20 minutes Servings: 4

✓ Chop acorn squash in half lengthwise and remove the seeds. Cut each half in half for a total of 4 wedges. Snap off the stem if it's easy to do.

✓ In a small bowl, combine the olive oil, sage, nutmeg, salt, and pepper. Brush the cut sides of the squash with the olive oil mixture.

✓ Fill 1 cup water into the electric pressure cooker and insert a wire rack or trivet.

✓ Place the squash on the trivet in a single layer, skin-side down.
Set the lid of the pressure cooker on sealing.

✓ Cook on high pressure for 20 minutes.

✓ Once done, press cancel and quickly release the pressure.

✓ Once the pin drops, open it.

✓ Carefully remove the squash from the pot, sprinkle with the Parmesan, and serve.

Nutrition: Calories: 85 Carbohydrates: 12g Fiber: 2g

774)   *Quinoa Tabbouleh*

Ingredients:

- 1 cup quinoa, rinsed
- large English cucumber
- 2 scallions, sliced
- cups cherry tomatoes, halved
- 2/3 cup chopped parsley
- ½ cup chopped mint
- ½ tsp. minced garlic
- ½ tsp. salt
- ½ tsp. ground black pepper
- 2 tbsp. lemon juice
- ½ cup olive oil

Direction: Preparation Time: 8 minutes Cooking Time: 16 minutes Servings: 6

✓ Plugin instant pot, insert the inner pot, add quinoa, then pour in water and stir until mixed.

✓ Close the instant pot with its lid and turn the pressure knob to seal the pot.

✓ Select the 'manual' button, then set the 'timer' to 1 minute and cook in high pressure, it may take 7 minutes.

✓ Once the timer stops, select the 'cancel' button and do natural pressure release for 10 minutes, and

then do quick pressure release until pressure nob drops down.

✓ Open the instant pot, fluff quinoa with a fork, then spoon it on a rimmed baking sheet, spread quinoa evenly and let cool.

✓ Meanwhile, place lime juice in a small bowl, add garlic, and stir until just mixed.

✓ Then add salt, black pepper, and olive oil and whisk until combined.

✓ Transfer cooled quinoa to a large bowl, add remaining ingredients, then drizzle generously with the prepared lime juice mixture, and toss until evenly coated.

✓ Taste quinoa to adjust seasoning and then serve.

Nutrition: Calories: 283 Carbs: 30.6g Fiber: 3.4g

775)   *Wild Rice Salad with Cranberries and Almonds*

Ingredients:

For The Rice:

- 2 cups wild rice blend, rinsed
- 1 tsp. kosher salt
- 2½ cups Vegetable Broth
- For The Dressing:
- ¼ cup extra-virgin olive oil
- ¼ cup white wine vinegar
- 1½ tsp. grated orange zest
- 1 medium orange, juiced (about ¼ cup)
- 1 tsp. honey or pure maple syrup

For The Salad:

- ¾ cup unsweetened dried cranberries
- ½ cup sliced almonds, toasted
- Freshly ground black pepper

Direction: Preparation Time: 6 minutes Cooking Time: 25 minutes Servings: 18

✓ To make the rice.

✓ In the electric pressure cooker, combine the rice, salt, and broth.

✓ Close and lock the lid. Set the valve to sealing.

✓ Cook on high pressure for 25 minutes.

✓ When the cooking is complete, hit Cancel and allow the pressure to release naturally for 1 minute, then quickly release any remaining pressure.

✓ Once the pin drops, unlock and remove the lid.

✓ Let the rice cool briefly, then fluff it with a fork.

✓ To make the dressing.

✓ While the rice cooks, make the dressing: In a small jar with a screw-top lid, combine the olive oil, vinegar, zest, juice, and honey. (If you don't have a jar, whisk the ingredients together in a small bowl.)

Shake to combine.
✓ *To make the salad.*
✓ *Mix rice, cranberries, and almonds.*
✓ *Add the dressing and season with pepper.*
✓ *Serve warm or refrigerate.*

Nutrition: Calories: 126 Carbs: 18g Fiber: 2g

776) *Low Fat Roasties*

Ingredients:

- *1 lb. roasting potatoes*
- *1 garlic clove*
- *1 cup vegetable stock*
- *2 tbsp. olive oil*

Direction: Preparation Time: 8 minutes Cooking Time: 25 minutes Servings: 2

✓ *Position potatoes in the steamer basket and add the stock into the Instant Pot.*
✓ *Steam the potatoes in your Instant Pot for 15 minutes.*
✓ *Depressurize and pour away the remaining stock.*
✓ *Set to sauté and add the oil, garlic, and potatoes. Cook until brown.*

Nutrition: Calories: 201 Carbohydrates: 3g Fat: 6g

777) *Roasted Parsnips*

Ingredients:

- *1 lb. parsnips*
- *1 cup vegetable stock*
- *2 tbsp. herbs*
- *2 tbsp. olive oil*

Direction: Preparation Time: 9 minutes Cooking Time: 25 minutes Servings: 2

✓ *Put the parsnips in the steamer basket and add the stock into the Instant Pot.*
✓ *Steam the parsnips in your Instant Pot for 15 minutes.*
✓ *Depressurize and pour away the remaining stock.*
✓ *Set to sauté and add the oil, herbs, and parsnips.*
✓ *Cook until golden and crisp.*

Nutrition: Calories: 130 Carbs: 14g Protein: 4g

778) *Lower Carb Hummus*

Ingredients:

- *½ cup dry chickpeas*
- *1 cup vegetable stock*
- *1 cup pumpkin puree*
- *2 tbsp. smoked paprika*

- *Salt and pepper to taste*

Direction: Preparation Time: 9 minutes Cooking Time: 60 minutes Servings: 2

✓ *Soak the chickpeas overnight.*
✓ *Place the chickpeas and stock in the Instant Pot.*
✓ *Cook on Beans for 60 minutes.*
✓ *Depressurize naturally.*
✓ *Blend the chickpeas with the remaining ingredients.*

Nutrition: Calories: 135 Carbohydrates: 18g Fat: 3g

779) *Sweet and Sour Red Cabbage*

Ingredients:

- *2 cups Spiced Pear Applesauce*
- *1 small onion, chopped*
- *½ cup apple cider vinegar*
- *½ tsp. kosher salt*
- *1 head red cabbage*

Direction: Preparation Time: 7 minutes Cooking Time: 10 minutes Servings: 8

✓ *In the electric pressure cooker, combine the applesauce, onion, vinegar, salt, and cup water. Stir in the cabbage.*
✓ *Seal the lid of the pressure cooker.*
✓ *Cook on high pressure for 10 minutes. When the cooking is complete, hit Cancel and quickly release the pressure.*
✓ *Once the pin drops, unlock and remove the lid.*
✓ *Spoon into a bowl or platter and serve.*

Nutrition: Calories: 91 Carbohydrates: 18g Fiber: 4g

780) *Pinto Beans*

Ingredients:

- *2 cups pinto beans, dried*
- *1 medium white onion*
- *1 ½ tsp. minced garlic*
- *¾ tsp. salt*
- *¼ tsp. ground black pepper*
- *1 tsp. red chili powder*
- *¼ tsp. cumin*
- *1 tbsp. olive oil*
- *1 tsp. chopped cilantro*
- *5 ½ cup vegetable stock*

Direction: Preparation Time: 6 minutes Cooking Time: 55 minutes Servings: 10

✓ *Plug-in instant pot, insert the inner pot, press sauté/simmer button, add oil and when hot, add* onion and garlic and cook for 3 minutes or until onions begin to soften.

✓ Add remaining ingredients, stir well, then press the cancel button, shut the instant pot with its lid, and seal the pot.

✓ Click the 'manual' button, then press the 'timer' to set the cooking time to 45 minutes and cook at high pressure.

✓ Once done, click the 'cancel' button and do natural pressure release for 10 minutes until the pressure nob drops down. Open the instant pot, spoon beans into plates, and serve

Nutrition: Calories: 107 Carbs: 11.7g Fiber: 4g

781) *Parmesan Cauliflower Mash*

Ingredients:

* 1 head cauliflower
* ½ tsp. Kosher salt
* ½ tsp. garlic pepper
* 2 tbsp. plain Greek yogurt
* ¾ cup freshly grated Parmesan cheese
* 1 tbsp. unsalted butter or ghee (optional)
* Chopped fresh chives

Direction: Preparation Time: 19 minutes Cooking Time: 5 minutes Servings: 4

✓ Pour cup water into the electric pressure cooker and insert a steamer basket or wire rack.

✓ Place the cauliflower in the basket.

✓ Cover lid of the pressure cooker to seal.

✓ Cook on high pressure for 5 minutes.

✓ Once complete, hit Cancel and quickly release the pressure.

✓ When the pin drops, remove the lid.

✓ Remove the cauliflower from the pot and pour out the water. Return the cauliflower to the pot and add the salt, garlic pepper, yogurt, and cheese. Use an immersion blender to purée or mash the cauliflower in the pot.

✓ Spoon into a serving bowl, and garnish with butter (if using) and chives.

Nutrition: Calories: 141 Carbohydrates: 12g Fiber: 4g

782) *Steamed Asparagus*

Ingredients:

* 1 lb. fresh asparagus, rinsed and tough ends trimmed
* 1 cup water

Direction: Preparation Time: 3 minutes Cooking Time: 2 minutes Servings: 4

✓ Place the asparagus into a wire steamer rack, and set it inside your Instant Pot.

✓ Add water to the pot. Close and seal the lid, turning the steam release valve to the "Sealing" position.

✓ Select the "Steam" function to cook on high pressure for 2 minutes.

✓ Once done, do a quick pressure release of the steam.

✓ Lift the wire steamer basket out of the pot and place the asparagus onto a serving plate.

✓ Season as desired and serve.

Nutrition: Calories: 22 Carbs: 4g Protein: 2g

783) *Squash Medley*

Ingredients:

* 2 lbs. mixed squash
* ½ cup mixed veg
* 1 cup vegetable stock
* 2 tbsp. olive oil
* 2tbsp. mixed herbs

Direction: Preparation Time: 10 minutes Cooking Time: 20 minutes. Servings: 2

✓ Put the squash in the steamer basket and add the stock into the Instant Pot.

✓ Steam the squash in your Instant Pot for 10 minutes.

✓ Depressurize and pour away the remaining stock. Set to sauté and add the oil and remaining ingredients.

✓ Cook until a light crust forms.

Nutrition: Calories: 100 Carbohydrates: 10g Fat: 6g

784) *Eggplant Curry*

Ingredients:

* 3 cups chopped eggplant
* 1 thinly sliced onion
* 1 cup coconut milk
* 3 tbsp. curry paste
* 1 tbsp. oil or ghee

Direction: Preparation Time: 15 minutes Cooking Time: 20 minutes Servings: 2

✓ Select Instant Pot to sauté and put the onion, oil, and curry paste.

✓ Once the onion is soft, stir in the remaining ingredients and seal.

✓ Cook on Stew for 20 minutes. Release the pressure naturally

Nutrition: Calories: 33 Carbs: 4g Protein: 5g

785) *Lentil and Eggplant Stew*

Ingredients:

- *1 lb. eggplant*
- *1 lb. dry lentils*
- *1 cup chopped vegetables*
- *1 cup low sodium vegetable broth*

Direction: Preparation Time: 15 minutes Cooking Time: 35 minutes Servings: 2

✓ *Incorporate all the ingredients in your Instant Pot. Cook on Stew for 35 minutes.*
✓ *Release the pressure naturally and serve.*

Nutrition: Calories: 310 Carbohydrates: 22g Fat: 10g

786) *Tofu Curry*

Ingredients:

- *2 cups cubed extra firm tofu*
- *2 cups mixed stir fry vegetables*
- *½ cup soy yogurt*
- *3 tbsp. curry paste 1*
- *tbsp. oil or ghee*

Direction: Preparation Time: 15 minutes Cooking Time: 20 minutes Servings: 2

✓ *Set the Instant Pot to sauté and add the oil and curry paste.*
✓ *Once soft, place the remaining ingredients except for the yogurt and seal.*
  Cook on Stew for 20 minutes.
✓ *Release the pressure naturally and serve with a scoop of soy yogurt.*

Nutrition: Calories: 300 Carbohydrates: 9g Fat: 14g

787) *Lentil and Chickpea Curry*

Ingredients:

- *2 cups dry lentils and chickpeas*
- *1 thinly sliced onion*
- *1 cup chopped tomato*
- *3 tbsp. curry paste*
- *1 tbsp. oil or ghee*

Direction: Preparation Time: 15 minutes Cooking Time: 20 minutes Servings: 2

✓ *Press Instant Pot to sauté and mix onion, oil, and curry paste.*
✓ *Once the onion is cooked, stir the remaining ingredients and seal.*
✓ *Cook on Stew for 20 minutes.*
✓ *Release the pressure naturally and serve.*

Nutrition: Calories: 360 Carbohydrates: 26g Fat: 19g

788) *Split Pea Stew*

Ingredients:

- *1 cup dry split peas*
- *1 lb. chopped vegetables*
- *1 cup mushroom soup*
- *2 tbsp. old bay seasoning*

Direction: Preparation Time: 5 minutes Cooking Time: 35 minutes Servings: 2

✓ *Incorporate all the ingredients in Instant Pot, cook for 33 minutes*
✓ *Release the pressure naturally*

Nutrition: Calories: 300 Carbohydrates: 7g Fat: 2g

789) *Fried Tofu Hotpot*

Ingredients:

- *½ lb. fried tofu*
- *1 lb. chopped Chinese vegetable mix*
- *1 cup low sodium vegetable broth*
- *2 tbsp. 5 spice seasoning*
- *1 tbsp. smoked paprika*

Direction: Preparation Time: 15 minutes Cooking Time: 15 minutes Servings: 2

✓ *Combine all the ingredients in your Instant Pot, set on Stew for 15 minutes.*
✓ *Release the pressure naturally and serve.*

Nutrition: Calories: 320 Carbohydrates: 11g Fat: 23g

790) *Chili Sin Carne*

Ingredients:

- *3 cups mixed cooked beans*
- *2 cups chopped tomatoes*
- *1tbsp. yeast extract*
- *2 squares very dark chocolate*
- *1 tbsp. red chili flakes*

Direction: Preparation Time: 15 minutes Cooking Time: 35 minutes Servings: 2

✓ *Combine all the ingredients in your Instant Pot, cook for 35 minutes.*
✓ *Release the pressure naturally and serve.*

Nutrition: Calories: 240 Carbohydrates: 20g Fat: 3g

791) *Garlic and Herb Carrots*

Ingredients:

- *2 tbsp. butter*
- *1 lb. baby carrots*

- *1 cup water*
- *1 tsp. fresh thyme or oregano*
- *1 tsp. minced garlic*
- *Black pepper*
- *Coarse sea salt*

Direction: Preparation Time: 2 minutes Cooking Time: 18 minutes Servings: 3

✓ *Fill water into the inner pot of the Instant Pot, and then put it in a steamer basket.*

✓ *Layer the carrots into the steamer basket.*

✓ *Close and seal the lid, with the pressure vent in the "Sealing" position.*

✓ *Select the "Steam" setting and cook for 2 minutes on high pressure.*

✓ *Quickly, release the pressure and then carefully remove the steamer basket with the steamed carrots, discarding the water.*

✓ *Add butter to the inner pot of the Instant Pot and allow it to melt on the "Sauté" function.*

✓ *Add garlic and sauté for 30 seconds, and then add the carrots. Mix well.*

✓ *Stir in the fresh herbs, and cook for 2–3 minutes.*

✓ *Season with salt and black pepper, and then transfer to a serving bowl.*

✓ *Serve warm and enjoy!*

Nutrition: Calories: 122 Carbohydrates: 12g Fat: 7g

792) *Cilantro Lime Drumsticks*

Ingredients:

- *1 tbsp. olive oil*
- *6 chicken drumsticks*
- *4 minced garlic cloves*
- *½ cup low-sodium chicken broth*
- *1 tsp. cayenne pepper*
- *1 tsp. crushed red peppers*
- *1 tsp. fine sea salt*
- *1 lime, juiced*

To Serve:

- *tbsp. chopped cilantro*
- *Extra lime zest*

Direction: Preparation Time: 5 minutes Cooking Time: 15 minutes Servings: 6

✓ *Pour olive oil into the Instant Pot and set it on the "Sauté" function.*

✓ *Once the oil is hot adding the chicken drumsticks, and season them well.*

✓ *Using tongs, stir the drumsticks and brown the drumsticks for 2 minutes per side.*

✓ *Add the lime juice, fresh cilantro, and chicken broth to the pot.*

✓ *Lock and seal the lid, turning the pressure valve to*

"Sealing."

✓ *Cook the drumsticks on the "Manual, High Pressure" setting for 9 minutes.*

✓ *Once done let the pressure release naturally.*

✓ *Carefully transfer the drumsticks to an aluminum-foiled baking sheet and broil them in the oven for 3–5 minutes until golden brown.*

✓ *Serve warm, garnished with more cilantro and lime zest.*

Nutrition: Calories: 480 Carbohydrates: 3.3g

793) *Eggplant Spread*

Ingredients:

- *4 tbsp. extra-virgin olive oil*
- *2 lbs. eggplant*
- *4 skin-on garlic cloves*
- *½ cup water*
- *¼ cup pitted black olives*
- *3 sprigs fresh thyme*
- *1 lemon, juiced*
- *1 tbsp. tahini*
- *1 tsp. sea salt*
- *Fresh extra-virgin olive oil*

Direction: Preparation Time: 5 minutes Cooking Time: 18 minutes Servings: 5

✓ *Peel the eggplant in alternating stripes, leaving some areas with skin and some with no skin.*

✓ *Slice into big chunks and layer at the bottom of your Instant Pot.*

✓ *Add olive oil to the pot, and on the "Sauté" function, fry and caramelize the eggplant on one side, about 5 minutes.*

✓ *Add in the garlic cloves with the skin on.*

✓ *Flip over the eggplant and then add in the remaining uncooked eggplant chunks, salt, and water.*

✓ *Close the lid, ensure the pressure release valve is set to "Sealing."*

✓ *Cook for 5 minutes on the "Manual, High Pressure" setting.*
Once done, carefully open the pot by quickly releasing the pressure through the steam valve.

✓ *Discard most of the brown cooking liquid.*

✓ *Remove the garlic cloves and peel them.*

✓ *Add the lemon juice, tahini, cooked and fresh garlic cloves, and pitted black olives to the pot.*

✓ *I was using a hand-held immersion blender, process all the ingredients until smooth.*

✓ *Pour out the spread into a serving dish and season with fresh thyme, whole black olives, and some extra-virgin olive oil, prior to serving.*

Nutrition: Calories: 155 Carbs: 16.8g Fat: 11.7g

794)   *Carrot Hummus*

Ingredients:

- *chopped carrot*
- *2 oz. cooked chickpeas*
- *1 tsp. lemon juice*
- *1 tsp. tahini*
- *1 tsp. fresh parsley*

Direction: Preparation Time: 15 minutes Cooking Time: 10 minutes Servings: 2

✓ *Place the carrot and chickpeas in your Instant Pot.*

✓ *Add a cup of water, seal, cook for 10 minutes on Stew.*

✓ *Depressurize naturally. Blend with the remaining ingredients.*

Nutrition: Calories: 58 Carbohydrates: 8g Fat: 2g

795)   *Garlic Sautéed Spinach*

Ingredients:

- *1 ½ tbsp. olive oil*
- *4 cloves minced garlic*
- *6 cups fresh baby spinach*
- *Salt and pepper*

Direction: Preparation Time: 5 minutes Cooking Time: 10 minutes Servings: 4

✓ *Heat up oil in a huge skillet over medium-high heat.*

✓ *Add the garlic and cook for 1 minute.*

✓ *Stir in the spinach and season with salt and pepper.*

✓ *Sauté for 1 to 2 minutes until just wilted. Serve hot.*

Nutrition: Calories: 60 Carbohydrates: 2.6g Fat: 1.1g

796)   *Creamy Creamed Corn*

Ingredients:

- *16 oz. frozen corn kernels*
- *1 tsp. salt and*
- *½ tsp. ground black pepper*
- *1 tbsp. honey*
- *½ cup vegetarian butter, unsalted*
- *8 oz. cream cheese, softened*
- *½ cup almond milk*

Direction: Preparation Time: 2 hours Cooking Time: 2 hours Servings: 5

✓ *Using a 6-quart slow cooker, brush it with a non-stick cooking spray and put ingredients in it. Stir properly and cover the top.*

✓ *Plug in the slow cooker; set the cooking time to 4 hours and cook on low heat setting.*

✓ *Serve right away.*

Nutrition: Calories: 120 Carbs: 28g Protein: 2g

797)   *Savory Squash & Apple Dish*

Ingredients:

- *8 oz. dried cranberries*
- *4 medium-sized apples*
- *3 lb. butternut squash*
- *Half of a medium-sized white onion*
- *1 tbsp. ground cinnamon*
- *1 ½ tsp. ground nutmeg*

Direction: Preparation Time: 15 minutes Cooking Time: 4 hours Servings: 6

✓ *With a 6-quart slow cooker, spray it with a non-stick cooking spray and situate the ingredients in it. Stir properly and cover the top.*

✓ *Turn on the slow cooker; set cooking time to 4 hours then cook at low heat setting. Serve.*

Nutrition: Calories: 210 Carbohydrates: 11g Fat: 3g

798)   *Spicy Cajun Boiled Peanuts*

Ingredients:

- *5 lb. peanuts, raw and in shells*
- *6 oz. dry crab boil*
- *4 oz. jalapeno peppers, sliced*
- *2 oz. vegetable broth*

Direction: 1 Preparation Time: 15 minutes Cooking Time: 8 hours Servings: 15

✓ *Take a 6-quart slow cooker place the ingredients in it and cover it with water. Stir properly and cover the top.*

✓ *Plug in the slow cooker; adjust the cooking time to 8 hours and let it cook on the low heat setting or until the peanuts are soft and floats on top of the cooking liquid.*
Drain the nuts and serve right away.

Nutrition: Calories: 309 Carbohydrates: 5g Fat: 26g

799)   *Wonderful Steamed Artichoke*

Ingredients:

- *8 medium-sized artichokes, stemmed and trimmed*
- *2 tsp. salt*
- *4 tbsp. lemon juice*

Direction: Preparation Time: 5 minutes Cooking Time: 4 hours Servings: 4

✓ *Cut 1-inch part of the artichoke from the top and place it in a 6-quarts slow cooker, facing an upright position. Using a bowl, place the lemon juice and pour in the salt until it mixes properly.*

✓ *Pour this mixture over the artichoke and add the water to cover at least*

✓ *¾ of the artichokes.*

✓ *Cover the top, switch on the slow cooker; place the cooking time to 4 hours then cook at a high heat setting. Serve immediately.*

Nutrition: Calories: 78 Carbs: 17g Protein: 5g

800) *Creamy Garlic Cauliflower Mashed Potatoes*

Ingredients:

- 30 oz. cauliflower head, cut into florets
- 6 garlic cloves, peeled
- 1 tsp. salt
- ¾ tsp. ground black pepper
- 1 bay leaf
- 1 tbsp. vegetarian butter, unsalted
- 3 cups water

Direction: Preparation Time: 1 hour Cooking Time: 2 hours Servings: 6

✓ *In a 6-quart slow cooker, grease it with a non-stick cooking spray. Position the cauliflower florets into it. Except for the butter, stir in the remaining ingredients then mix it properly.*

✓ *Cover the top, turn on the slow cooker; adjust the cooking time to 3 hours then cook at a high heat setting. When done, open the slow cooker, remove the bay leaf and garlic cloves.*

✓ *Drain the cooking liquid, add the butter and let it melt. Then using an immersion blender, mash the cauliflower or until it gets creamy. Add the seasoning and serve.*

Nutrition: Calories: 66 Carbohydrates: 6g Fat: 3g

801) *Healthy Pumpkin Risotto*

Ingredients:

- 2 tbsp. olive oil
- ½ cup chopped white onion
- 1 tbsp. minced garlic
- 2 tsp. salt
- 1 tsp. ground black pepper
- 2 tsp. dried sage
- 1 ½ cups short grain rice
- 2 cups roasted pumpkin
- 32 fluid ounce vegetable broth

Direction: Preparation Time: 45 minutes Cooking Time: 1 hour Servings: 4

✓ *Place a medium-sized non-stick skillet pan over an average temperature of heat, add and let it heat. Then add the onion, garlic, sage and heat it for 5 minutes or until it gets softened. Pour in the rice and continue cooking for 3 minutes.*

✓ *Transfer this mixture to a 6-quart slow cooker and add the remaining ingredients except for pumpkin*

seeds. Stir properly and cover the top.

✓ *Plug in the slow cooker; adjust the cooking time to 1 hour 30 minutes and let it cook on the high heat setting or until the rice gets soft. Serve right away.*

Nutrition: Calories: 190 Carbs: 11g Protein: 12g

802) *Flavorful Roasted Peppers*

Ingredients:

- 5 medium-sized red bell pepper, cored and halved

Direction: Preparation Time: 20 minutes Cooking Time: 3 hours Servings: 5

✓ *Take a 6-quart slow cooker, grease it with a non-stick cooking spray and add the peppers.*

✓ *Cover the top, plug in the slow cooker; set the cooking time to 3 hours, and cook on the high heat setting, stirring halfway through.*
When done, remove the peppers from the cooker and let them cool off completely.

✓ *Then remove the pepper peels by tugging them from the edge or with a paring knife.*

✓ *Serve as desired.*

Nutrition: Calories: 5 Carbohydrates: 1g Fat: 0.2g

803) *Comforting Spinach and Artichoke Dip*

Ingredients:

- 8 oz. frozen spinach, thawed and squeezed
- 8 oz. diced water chestnuts
- 28 oz. cooked artichoke hearts, chopped
- 1 tsp. minced garlic
- 1 tsp. salt
- ¾ tsp. ground black pepper
- 2 tbsp. nutritional yeast
- 1 cup cashew, raw
- tsp. wholegrain mustard paste
- 2 tbsp. lemon juice
- 2 tbsp. soy-mayonnaise
- 1 cup almond milk, unsweetened

Direction: Preparation Time: 25 minutes Cooking Time: 2 hours Servings: 8

✓ *Using a food processor, place the cashews and pulse them until the mixture looks like flour, while ensuring not to over-blend.*

✓ *Add the garlic, salt, mustard paste, lemon juice, almond milk and mash it for 2 minutes or until it gets smooth. Place this mixture into a 6-quart slow cooker, add the remaining ingredients except for the mayonnaise and stir properly.*
Cover the top, plug in the slow cooker; put the

cooking time to 4 hours then cook on a high heat setting. Once done, open the slow cooker and pour in and stir the mayonnaise properly.

✓ Add the seasoning and serve.

Nutrition: Calories: 83 Carbs: 16g Protein: 4g

804) *Healthy Coconut Basil Tofu*

Ingredients:

- 12 oz. firm tofu, pressed and drained
- 4 cups baby bok choy, rinsed
- 8 oz. mushrooms, sliced
- 1 medium-sized white onion, peeled and sliced
- 1 tsp. minced garlic
- 1 ½ tbsp. grated ginger
- 1 tsp. salt
- 1tbsp. coconut sugar
- ½ tsp. crushed red pepper flakes
- ¼ cup cornstarch
- ¾ cup chopped basil
- 2 tbsp. tamari sauce
- tbsp. apple cider vinegar
- 1 tbsp. fish sauce
- 1 cup vegetable broth
- 14 oz. coconut milk, unsweetened

Direction: Preparation Time: 5 minutes Cooking Time: 4 hours Servings: 5

✓ Cut the tofu into large strips, halve bok choy, onion and cut it into large chunks.

✓ Using a bowl pour in and stir the ginger, basil, vinegar, tamari sauce, vinegar, fish sauce, and the vegetable broth.

✓ Pour this mixture into a 6-quart slow cooker and add the remaining ingredients except for the cornstarch.

✓ Toss to cover and then cover the top
Plug in the slow cooker; adjust the cooking time to 3 hours 30 minutes and let it cook on the high heat setting.

✓ Then stir in the cornstarch and continue cooking for another 30 minutes.

✓ Add the seasoning and serve.

Nutrition: Calories: 20 Carbs: 2g Protein: 3g

805) *Amazing Brussels Sprouts*

Ingredients:

- 2 lb. Brussels sprouts, trimmed and halved
- 1 ½ tsp. salt
- 1 1tsp. ground black pepper
- 2 tbsp. brown sugar

- 2 tbsp. unsalted vegan butter, grated
- ½ cup apple cider vinegar
- 2 tbsp. olive oil
- ¼ cup grated vegetarian Parmesan cheese

Direction: Preparation Time: 20 minutes Cooking Time: 4 hours Servings: 6

✓ Place a small saucepan over an average temperature of heat, add the vinegar, sugar stir, and boil the mixture.

✓ Switch the heat to a medium-low and let it cook for 6 to 8 minutes or until the sauce reduces by half. Thereafter let it cool off completely. Place the Brussels sprouts in a 4-quart slow cooker, add the salt, black pepper, oil, and then top it with the butter.

✓ Cover the top, plug in the slow cooker; adjust the cooking time to 2 hours and let it cook on the high heat setting.

✓ When done, sprinkle it with the prepared vinegar sauce and toss it to coat. Garnish it with cheese and serve.

Nutrition: Calories: 46 Carbs: 10g Protein: 3.2g

806) *Scrumptious Baked Potatoes*

Ingredients:

- 8 potatoes
- Salt to taste for serving
- Ground black pepper to taste for serving

Direction: Preparation Time: 10 minutes Cooking Time: 8 hours Servings: 8

✓ Rinse potatoes until clean, wipe dry and then prick with a fork.

✓ Wrap each potato in aluminum foil and place in a 6 to 8 quarts slow cooker.

✓ Cover with the lid, and then plug in the slow cooker and let cook on low heat setting for 8 hours or until tender.
When the cooking time is over, unwrap potatoes and prick with a fork to check if potatoes are tender or not.

✓ Sprinkle potatoes with salt, black pepper, and your favorite seasoning and serve.

Nutrition: Calories: 93 Carbs: 3g Protein: 3g

807) *Fantastic Butternut Squash & Vegetables*

Ingredients:

- ½ cups corn kernels
- pounds' butternut squash
- 1 medium-sized green bell pepper
- 14-½ oz. diced tomatoes

- ½ cup chopped white onion
- ½ tsp. minced garlic
- ½ tsp. salt
- ¼ tsp. ground black pepper
- 1 tbsp. and 2 tsp. tomato paste
- ½ cup vegetable broth

Direction: Preparation Time: 15 minutes Cooking Time: 4 hours Servings: 6

✓ Peel, centralize the butternut squash and dice, and place it into a 6-quart slow cooker. Create a hole on the green bell pepper, then cut it into ½- inch pieces and add it to the slow cooker.

✓ Add the remaining ingredients into the slow cooker except for tomato paste, stir properly and cover it with the lid.

✓ Turn on the slow cooker and cook on a low heat setting for 6 hours. When 6 hours of the cooking time is done, remove ½ cup of the cooking liquid from the slow cooker. Then pour the tomato mixture into this cooking liquid, stir properly and place it in the slow cooker.

✓ Stir properly and continue cooking for 30 minutes or until the mixture becomes slightly thick. Serve right away.

Nutrition: Calories: 134 Carbs: 23g Protein: 6g

808) *Fabulous Glazed Carrots*

Ingredients:

- 1 lb. carrots
- 2 tsp. chopped cilantro
- ¼ tsp. salt
- ¼ cup brown sugar
- ¼ tsp. ground cinnamon
- ⅛ tsp. ground nutmeg
- 1 tbsp. cornstarch
- 1 tbsp. olive oil
- 2 tbsp. water
- 1 large orange, juiced and zested

Direction: Preparation Time: 20 minutes Cooking Time: 2 hours Servings: 5

✓ Peel the carrots, rinse, cut them into ¼-inch-thick rounds and place them in a 6-quart slow cooker. Add the salt, sugar, cinnamon, nutmeg, olive oil, orange zest, juice, and stir properly.

✓ Cover, cooker in the slow cook on high heat setting for 2 hours. Stir the cornstarch and water properly until it blends well. Thereafter, add this mixture to the slow cooker.

✓ Continue cooking for 10 minutes or until the sauce in the slow cooker gets slightly thick. Sprinkle the cilantro over carrots and serve.

Nutrition: Calories: 160 Carbs: 40g Protein: 1g

809) *Flavorful Sweet Potatoes with Apples*

Ingredients:

- 3 medium-sized apples, peeled and cored
- 6 medium-sized sweet potatoes, peeled and cored
- ¼ cup pecans
- ¼ tsp. ground cinnamon
- ¼ tsp. ground nutmeg
- 2 tbsp. vegan butter, melted
- ¼ cup maple syrup

Direction: Preparation Time: 2 hours Cooking Time: 3 hours Servings: 6

✓ Cut the sweet potatoes and the apples into ½-inch slices. Grease a 6- quart slow cooker with a non-stick cooking spray and arrange the sweet potato slices in the bottom of the cooker.

✓ Top it with the apple slices; sprinkle it with the cinnamon and nutmeg, before garnishing it with butter. Cover it with the lid, using the slow cooker cook at low heat setting for 4 hours.

✓ When done, sprinkle it with pecan and continue cooking for another 30 minutes. Serve right away.

Nutrition: Calories: 120 Carbs: 24g Protein: 1g

810) *Wonderful Glazed Root Vegetables*

Ingredients:

- 6 medium-sized carrots
- 4 medium-sized parsnips
- 1 pound of sweet potatoes
- 2 medium-sized red onions
- 1 tbsp. olive oil
  1 tsp. salt
- ½ tsp. ground black pepper
- 5 tsp. chopped thyme
- 3 tbsp. honey
- 1 tbsp. apple cider vinegar

Direction: Preparation Time: 20 minutes Cooking Time: 4 hours Servings: 6

✓ Peel the carrots, parsnip, sweet potatoes, onions, and cut them into 1- inch pieces.

✓ Grease a 6 quarts slow cooker with a non-stick cooking spray, place the carrots, parsnip, onion in the bottom and then top it with the sweet potatoes.

✓ Using a bowl whisk the salt, black pepper, 2 tsp. of thyme, honey, and oil properly.
Pour this mixture over on the vegetables and toss it to coat.

✓ Close, then turn on the slow cooker and cook on a low heat setting for 4 hours or until the vegetables get tender.

✓ *When cooked, pour in the vinegar, stir, sprinkle it with the remaining thyme and serve.*

Nutrition: Calories: 137 Carbs: 26g Protein: 2g

811) <u>*Almond Cheesecake Bites*</u>

Ingredients:

- *½ cup reduced-fat cream cheese, soft*
- *½ cup almonds, ground fine*
- *¼ cup almond butter*
- *2 drops liquid stevia*

Direction: Preparation Time: 5 minutes Cooking Time: 0 minutes Servings: 6

✓ *In a large bowl, beat cream cheese, almond butter, and stevia on high speed until the mixture is smooth and creamy. Cover and chill for 30 minutes.*

✓ *Use your hands to shape the mixture into 12 balls. Place the ground almonds on a shallow plate. Roll the balls in the nuts completely covering all sides. Store in an airtight container in the refrigerator.*

Nutrition: Calories: 68 Protein: 5g Fat 5g

812) <u>*Almond Coconut Biscotti*</u>

Ingredients:

- *1 egg, room temperature*
- *1 egg white, room temperature*
- *½ cup margarine, melted*
- *2 ½ cup flour*
- *1/3 cup unsweetened coconut, grated*
- *¾ cup almonds, sliced*
- *2/3 cup Splenda*
- *2 tsp. baking powder*
- *1 tsp. vanilla*
- *½ tsp. salt*

Direction: Preparation Time: 5 minutes Cooking Time: 51 minutes Servings: 16

✓ *Heat oven to 350°F. Line a baking sheet with parchment paper.*

✓ *In a large bowl, combine dry ingredients.*

✓ *In a separate mixing bowl, beat other ingredients together. Add to dry ingredients and mix until thoroughly combined.*

✓ *Divide dough in half. Shape each half into a loaf measuring 8x2 ¾- inches. Place loaves on pan 3 inches apart.*

✓ *Bake 25–30 minutes or until set and golden brown. Cool on wire rack 10 minutes.*

✓ *With a serrated knife, cut the loaf diagonally into ½-inch slices. Place the cookies, cut side down, back on the pan, and bake another 20 minutes, or*

until firm and nicely browned. Store in an airtight container. The serving size is 2 cookies.

Nutrition: Calories: 234 Protein: 5g Fat 18g

813) <u>*Almond Flour Crackers*</u>

Ingredients:

- *½ cup coconut oil, melted*
- *1 ½ cups almond flour*
- *¼ cup Stevia*

Direction: Preparation Time: 5 minutes Cooking Time: 15 minutes Servings: 8

✓ *Heat oven to 350°F. Line a cookie sheet with parchment paper.*

✓ *In a mixing bowl, combine all ingredients and mix well.*

✓ *Spread dough onto a prepared cookie sheet, ¼-inch thick. Use a paring knife to score into 24 crackers. Bake 10–15 minutes or until golden brown.*

✓ *Separate and store in an air-tight container.*

Nutrition: Calories: 281 Protein: 4g Fat 23g

814) <u>*Asian Chicken Wings*</u>

Ingredients:

- *24 chicken wings*
- *6 tbsp. soy sauce*
- *6 tbsp. Chinese 5 spice*
- *Salt and pepper*
- *Nonstick cooking spray*

Direction: Preparation Time: 5 minutes Cooking Time: 30 minutes Servings: 3

✓ *Heat oven to 350°F. Spray a baking sheet with cooking spray.*

✓ *Combine the soy sauce, 5 spice, salt, and pepper in a large bowl. Add the wings and toss to coat. Pour the wings onto the prepared pan. Bake 15 minutes. Turn the chicken over and cook another 15 minutes until the chicken is cooked through.*

✓ *Serve with your favorite low-carb dipping sauce.*

Nutrition: Calories: 178 Protein: 12g Fat 11g

815) <u>*Banana Nut Cookies*</u>

Ingredients:

- *1 ½ cup banana, mashed*
- *2 cup oats*
- *1 cup raisins*
- *1 cup walnuts*
- *1/3 cup sunflower oil*

- *1 tsp. vanilla*
- *½ tsp. salt*

Direction: Preparation Time: 10 minutes Cooking Time: 15 minutes Servings: 18

✓ *Heat oven to 350°F.*

✓ *In a large bowl, combine oats, raisins, walnuts, and salt.*

✓ *In a medium bowl, mix banana, oil, and vanilla. Stir into oat mixture until combined. Let rest 15 minutes.*

✓ *Drop by rounded tbsp. full onto 2 ungreased cookie sheets. Bake 15 minutes, or until a light golden brown. Cool and store in an airtight container. The servings size is 2 cookies.*

Nutrition: Calories: 148 Protein: 3g Fat: 9g

816) *BLT Stuffed Cucumbers*

Ingredients:

- *3 slices bacon, cooked crisp and crumbled*
- *1 large cucumber*
- *½ cup lettuce, diced fine*
- *½ cup baby spinach, diced fine*
- *¼ cup tomato, diced fine*

What you'll need from the store cupboard:

- *1 tbsp. + ½ tsp. fat-free mayonnaise*
- *¼ tsp. black pepper*
- *⅛ tsp. salt*

Direction: Preparation Time: 15 minutes Cooking Time: 15 minutes Servings: 4

✓ *Peel the cucumber and slice it in half lengthwise. Use a spoon to remove the seeds.*

✓ *In a medium bowl, combine the remaining ingredients and stir well.*
Spoon the bacon mixture into the cucumber halves.

✓ *Cut into 2-inch pieces and serve.*

Nutrition: Calories: 95 Protein: 6g Fat: 6g

817) *Buffalo Bites*

Ingredients:

- *1 egg*
- *½ head cauliflower, separated into florets*
- *1 cup panko bread crumbs*
- *1 cup low-fat ranch dressing*
- *½ cup hot sauce*
- *½ tsp. salt*
- *½ tsp. garlic powder*
- *Black pepper*
- *Nonstick cooking spray*

Direction: Preparation Time: 6 minutes Cooking Time: 11 minutes Servings: 4

✓ *Heat oven to 400°F. Spray a baking sheet with cooking spray.*

✓ *Place the egg in a medium bowl and mix in the salt, pepper, and garlic. Place the panko crumbs into a small bowl.*

✓ *Dip the florets first in the egg then into the panko crumbs. Place in a single layer on the prepared pan.*

✓ *Bake 8–10 minutes, stirring halfway through, until cauliflower is golden brown and crisp on the outside.*

✓ *In a small bowl stir the dressing and hot sauce together. Use for dipping.*

Nutrition: Calories: 132 Protein: 6g Fat: 5g

818) *Candied Pecans*

Ingredients:

- *1 ½ tsp. butter*
- *½ cup pecan halves*
- *2 ½ tbsp. Splenda, divided*
- *1 tsp. cinnamon*
- *¼ tsp. ginger*
- *⅛ tsp. cardamom*
- *⅛ tsp. salt*

Direction: Preparation Time: 5 minutes Cooking Time: 11 minutes Servings: 6

✓ *In a small bowl, stir together 1 ½ tsp. Splenda, cinnamon, ginger, cardamom, and salt. Set aside.*

✓ *Melt butter in a medium skillet over med-low heat. Add pecans, and 2 tbsp. Splenda. Reduce heat to low and cook, occasionally stirring, until sweetener melts, about 5 to 8 minutes.*

✓ *Add spice mixture to the skillet and stir to coat pecans. Spread mixture to parchment paper and let cool for 10–15 minutes. Store in an airtight container. The servings size is ¼ cup.*

Nutrition: Calories: 173 Protein: 2g Fat: 16g

819) *Cauliflower Hummus*

Ingredients:

- *3 cup cauliflower florets*
- *3 tbsp. fresh lemon juice*
- *5 garlic cloves, divided*
- *5 tbsp. olive oil, divided*
- *2 tbsp. water*
- *1 ½ tbsp. Tahini paste*
- *1 ¼ tsp. salt, divided*
- *Smoked paprika and extra olive oil for serving*

Direction: Preparation Time: 6 minutes Cooking Time: 15 minutes Servings: 6

- ✓ In a microwave-safe bowl, combine cauliflower, water, 2 tbsp. oil, ½ tsp. salt, and 3 whole garlic cloves. Microwave on high for 15 minutes, or until cauliflower is soft and darkened.
- ✓ Transfer mixture to a food processor or blender and process until almost smooth. Add tahini paste, lemon juice, remaining garlic cloves, remaining oil, and salt. Blend until almost smooth.
- ✓ Place the hummus in a bowl and drizzle lightly with olive oil and a sprinkle or 2 of paprika. Serve with your favorite raw vegetables.

Nutrition: Calories: 107 Protein: 2g Fat 10g

820)   Cheese Crisp Crackers

Ingredients:

- 4 slices pepper Jack cheese, quartered
- 4 slices Colby Jack cheese, quartered
- 4 slices cheddar cheese, quartered

Direction: Preparation Time: 6 minutes Cooking Time: 11 minutes Servings: 4

- ✓ Heat oven to 400°F. Line a cooking sheet with parchment paper.
- ✓ Place cheese in a single layer on the prepared pan and bake for 10 minutes, or until cheese gets firm.
- ✓ Transfer to paper towel line surface to absorb excess oil. Let cool, cheese will crisp up more as it cools.
- ✓ Store in an airtight container, or Ziploc bag. Serve with your favorite dip or salsa.

Nutrition: Calories: 253 Protein: 15g Fat: 20g

821)   Cheesy Onion Dip

Ingredients:

- 8 oz. low-fat cream cheese, soft
- 1 cup onions, grated
- 1 cup low-fat Swiss cheese, grated
- 1 cup lite mayonnaise

Direction: Preparation Time: 6 minutes Cooking Time: 5 minutes Servings: 8

- ✓ Heat oven to broil.
- ✓ Combine all the ingredients in a small casserole dish. Microwave on high, stirring every 30 seconds until cheese is melted and ingredients are combined.Place under the broiler for 1–2 minutes until the top is nicely browned. Serve warm with vegetables for dipping.

Nutrition: Calories: 158 Protein: 9g Fat: 11g

822)   Cheesy Pita Crisps

Ingredients:

- ½ cup mozzarella cheese
- ¼ cup margarine, melted
- 4 whole-wheat pita pocket halves
- 3 tbsp. reduced-fat parmesan
- ½ tsp. garlic powder
- ½ tsp. onion powder
- ¼ tsp. salt
- ¼ tsp. pepper
- Nonstick cooking spray

Direction: Preparation Time: 6 minutes Cooking Time: 15 minutes Servings: 8

- ✓ Heat oven to 400°F. Spray a baking sheet with cooking spray.
- ✓ Cut each pita pocket in half. Cut each half into 2 triangles: place, rough side up, on prepared pan. In a small bowl, whisk together margarine, parmesan, and seasonings. Spread each triangle with the margarine mixture. Sprinkle mozzarella over top.
- ✓ Bake 12–15 minutes or until golden brown.

Nutrition: Calories: 131 Protein: 4g Fat: 7g

823)   Cheesy Taco Chips

Ingredients:

- 1 cup Mexican blend cheese, grated
- 2 large egg whites
- 1 ½ cup crushed pork rinds
- 1 tbsp. taco seasoning
- ¼ tsp. salt

Direction: Preparation Time: 16 minutes Cooking Time: 41 minutes Servings: 6

- ✓ Heat oven to 300°F. Line a large baking sheet with parchment paper.
- ✓ In a large bowl, whisk egg whites and salt until frothy. Stir in pork rinds, cheese, and seasoning and stir until thoroughly combined.
- ✓ Turn out onto the prepared pan. Place another sheet of parchment paper on top and roll out very thin, about 12x12-inches. Remove top sheet of parchment paper, and using a pizza cutter, score dough in 2-inch squares, then score each square in half diagonally.
- ✓ Bake 20 minutes until they start to brown. Turn off the oven and let them sit inside the oven until they are firm to the touch, about 10–20 minutes.
- ✓ Remove from oven and cool completely before breaking apart. Eat them as is or with your favorite dip.

Nutrition: Calories: 260 Protein: 25g Fat: 17g

824) *Chewy Granola Bars*

Ingredients:

- 1 egg, beaten
- 2/3 cup margarine, melted
- 3 ½ cup quick oats
- 1 cup almonds, chopped
- ½ cup honey
- ½ cup sunflower kernels
-
  ½ cup coconut, unsweetened
- ½ cup dried apples
- ½ cup dried cranberries
- ½ cup Splenda brown sugar
- 1 tsp. vanilla
- ½ tsp. cinnamon
- Nonstick cooking spray

Direction: Preparation Time: 11 minutes Cooking Time: 35 minutes Servings: 36

✓ Heat oven to 350°F. Spray a large baking sheet with cooking spray.

✓ Spread oats and almonds on a prepared pan. Bake 12–15 minutes until toasted, stirring every few minutes.

✓ In a large bowl, combine egg, margarine, honey, and vanilla. Stir in the remaining ingredients. Stir in oat mixture. Press into a baking sheet and bake 13–18 minutes, or until edges are light brown.

✓ Cool on a wire rack. Cut into bars and store in an airtight container.

Nutrition: Calories: 201; Total fat: 10g; Saturated fat: 1g; Protein: 5g; Carbs: 26g; Sugar: 9g; Fiber: 5g; Cholesterol: 16mg; Sodium: 8mg

825) *Chili Chicken Wings*

Ingredients:

- 2 lbs chicken wings
- 1/8 tsp. paprika
- 1/2 cup coconut flour
- 1/4 tsp. garlic powder
- 1/4 tsp. chili powder

Direction: Preparation Time: 10 minutes Cooking Time: 1 hour 10 minutes Servings: 4

✓ Preheat the oven to 400 F/ 200 C.

✓ In a mixing bowl, add all ingredients except chicken wings and mix well.
Add chicken wings to the bowl mixture and coat well and place on a baking tray.

✓ Bake in preheated oven for 55-60 minutes.

✓ Serve and enjoy.

Nutrition: Calories 440 Fat 17.1 g, Carbs 1.3 g, Sugar 0.2 g, Protein 65.9 g, Cholesterol 202 mg

826) *Garlic Chicken Wings*

Ingredients:

- 12 chicken wings
- 2 garlic clove, minced
- 3 tbsp. ghee
- 1/2 tsp. turmeric
- 2 tsp. cumin seeds

Direction: Preparation Time: 10 minutes Cooking Time: 55 minutes Servings: 6

✓ Preheat the oven to 425 F/ 215 C.

✓ In a large bowl, mix together 1 teaspoon cumin, 1 tbsp. ghee, turmeric, pepper, and salt.

✓ Add chicken wings to the bowl and toss well.

✓ Spread chicken wings on a baking tray and bake in preheated oven for 30 minutes.

✓ Turn chicken wings to another side and bake for 8 minutes more.
Meanwhile, heat the remaining ghee in a pan over medium heat.

✓ Add garlic and cumin to the pan and cook for a minute.

✓ Remove pan from heat and set aside.

✓ Remove chicken wings from oven and drizzle with ghee mixture/

✓ Bake chicken wings for 5 minutes more.

✓ Serve and enjoy.

Nutrition: Calories 378 Fat 27.9 g, Carbs 11.4 g, Sugar 0 g, Protein 19.7 g, Cholesterol 94 mg

827) *Spinach Cheese Pie*

Ingredients:

- 6 eggs, lightly beaten
- 2 boxes frozen spinach, chopped
- 2 cup cheddar cheese, shredded
- 15 oz. cottage cheese
- 1 tsp. salt

Direction: Preparation Time: 10 minutes Cooking Time: 40 minutes Servings: 8

✓ Preheat the oven to 375 F/ 190 C.

✓ Spray an 8*8-inch baking dish with cooking spray and set aside.

✓ In a mixing bowl, combine together spinach, eggs, cheddar cheese, cottage cheese, pepper, and salt. Pour spinach mixture into the prepared baking dish and bake in preheated oven for 10 minutes.

✓ Serve and enjoy.

Nutrition: Calories 229 Fat 14 g, Carbs. 5.4 g, Sugar 0.9 g, Protein 21 g, Cholesterol 157 mg

828) *Tasty Harissa Chicken*

Ingredients:

- 1 lb. chicken breasts, skinless and boneless
- 1/2 tsp. ground cumin
- 1 cup harissa sauce
- 1/4 tsp. garlic powder
- 1/2 tsp. kosher salt

Direction: Preparation Time: 10 minutes Cooking Time: 4 hours 10 minutes Servings: 4

✓ Season chicken with garlic powder, cumin, and salt.
✓ Place chicken in the slow cooker.
✓ Pour harissa sauce over the chicken.
  Cover slow cooker with lid and cook on low for 4 hours.
✓ Remove chicken from the slow cooker and shred using a fork.
✓ Return shredded chicken to the slow cooker and stir well.
✓ Serve and enjoy.

Nutrition: Calories 232 Fat 9.7 g, Carbs 1.3 g, Sugar 0.1 g, Protein 32.9 g, Cholesterol 101 mg

829) *Roasted Balsamic Mushrooms*

Ingredients:

- 8 oz. mushrooms, sliced
- 1/2 tsp. thyme
- 2 tbsp. balsamic vinegar
- 2 tbsp. extra virgin olive oil
- 2 onions, sliced

Direction: Preparation Time: 10 minutes Cooking Time: 50 minutes Servings: 4

✓ Preheat the oven to 375 F/ 190 C.
✓ Line baking tray with aluminum foil and spray with cooking spray and set aside.
✓ In a mixing bowl, add all ingredients and mix well.
✓ Spread mushroom mixture onto a prepared baking tray.
  Roast in preheated oven for 45 minutes.
✓ Season with pepper and salt.
✓ Serve and enjoy.

Nutrition: Calories 96 Fat 7.2 g, Carbohydrates 7.2 g, Sugar 3.3 g, Protein 2.4 g, Cholesterol 0 mg

830) *Roasted Cumin Carrots*

Ingredients:

- 8 carrots, peeled and cut into 1/2 inch thick slices
- 1 tsp. cumin seeds
- 1 tbsp. olive oil
- 1/2 tsp. kosher salt

Direction: Preparation Time: 10 minutes Cooking Time: 45 minutes Servings: 4

✓ Preheat the oven to 400 F/ 200 C.
✓ Line baking tray with parchment paper.
✓ Add carrots, cumin seeds, olive oil, and salt in a large bowl and toss well to coat.
  Spread carrots on a prepared baking tray and roast in preheated oven for 20 minutes.
✓ Turn carrots to another side and roast for 20 minutes more.
✓ Serve and enjoy.

Nutrition: Calories 82 Fat 3.6 g, Carbohydrates 12.2 g, Sugar 6 g, Protein 1.1 g, Cholesterol 0 mg

831) *Tasty & Tender Brussels Sprouts*

Ingredients:

- 1 lb. Brussels sprouts, trimmed cut in half
- ¼ cup balsamic vinegar
- 1 onion, sliced
- 1 tbsp. olive oil

Direction: Preparation Time: 10 minutes

Cooking Time: 35 minutes Servings: 4

✓ Add water in a saucepan and bring to boil.
✓ Add Brussels sprouts and cook over medium heat for 20 minutes. Drain well.
✓ Heat oil in a pan over medium heat.
  Add onion and cook until softened. Add sprouts and vinegar and stir well and cook for 1-2 minutes.
✓ Serve and enjoy.

Nutrition: Calories 93 Fat 3.9 g, Carbohydrates 13 g, Sugar 3.7 g, Protein 4.2 g, Cholesterol 0 mg

832) *Sautéed Veggies*

Ingredients:

- 1/2 cup mushrooms, sliced
- 1 zucchini, diced
- 1 squash, diced
- 2 1/2 tsp. southwest seasoning
- 3 tbsp. olive oil

Direction: Preparation Time: 10 minutes Cooking Time: 15 minutes Servings: 4

✓ In a medium bowl, whisk together southwest seasoning, pepper, olive oil, and salt.
✓ Add vegetables to a bowl and mix well to coat.
✓ Heat pan over medium-high heat.
  Add vegetables in the pan and sauté for 5-7

minutes.

✓ *Serve and enjoy.*

Nutrition: Calories 107, Fat 10.7 g, Carbs 3.6 g, Sugar 1.5 g, Protein 1.2 g, Cholesterol 0 mg

833)   *Mustard Green Beans*

Ingredients:

- *1 lb. green beans, washed and trimmed*
- *1 tsp. whole grain mustard*
- *1 tbsp. olive oil*
- *2 tbsp. apple cider vinegar*
- *1/4 cup onion, chopped*

Direction: Preparation Time: 10 minutes Cooking Time: 20 minutes Servings: 4

✓ *Steam green beans in the microwave until tender.*

✓ *Meanwhile, in a pan heat olive oil over medium heat.*

✓ *Add the onion in a pan sauté until softened.*

✓ *Add water, apple cider vinegar, and mustard in the pan and stir well.*
  Add green beans and stir to coat and heat through.

✓ *Season green beans with pepper and salt.*

✓ *Serve and enjoy.*

Nutrition: Calories 71 Fat 3.7 g, Carbohydrates 8.9 g, Sugar 1.9 g, Protein 2.1 g, Cholesterol 0 mg

834)   *Zucchini Fries*

Ingredients:

- *1 egg*
- *2 medium zucchini, cut into fries shape*
- *1 tsp. Italian herbs*
- *1 tsp. garlic powder*
- *1 cup parmesan cheese, grated*

Direction: Preparation Time: 10 minutes Cooking Time: 40 minutes Servings: 4

✓ *Preheat the oven to 425 F/ 218 C.*

✓ *Spray a baking tray with cooking spray and set it aside.*

✓ *In a small bowl, add egg and lightly whisk it.*
  In a separate bowl, mix together spices and parmesan cheese.

✓ *Dip zucchini fries in egg then coat with parmesan cheese mixture and place on a baking tray.*

✓ *Bake in preheated oven for 25-30 minutes. Turn halfway through.*

✓ *Serve and enjoy.*

Nutrition: Calories 184 Fat 10.3 g, Carbs 3.9 g, Sugar 2 g, Protein 14.7 g, Cholesterol 71 mg

835)   *Broccoli Nuggets*

Ingredients:

- *2 cups broccoli florets*
- *1/4 cup almond flour*
- *2 egg whites*
- *1 cup cheddar cheese, shredded*
- *1/8 tsp. salt*

Direction: Preparation Time: 10 minutes Cooking Time: 25 minutes Servings: 4

✓ *Preheat the oven to 350 F/ 180 C.*

✓ *Spray a baking tray with cooking spray and set it aside.*

✓ *Using a potato masher break the broccoli florets into small pieces.*

✓ *Add remaining ingredients to the broccoli and mix well.*
  Drop 20 scoops onto the baking tray and press lightly into a nugget shape.

✓ *Bake in preheated oven for 20 minutes.*

✓ *Serve and enjoy.*

Nutrition: Calories 148 Fat 10.4 g, Carbs 3.9 g, Sugar 1.1 g, Protein 10.5 g, Cholesterol 30 mg

836)   *Zucchini Cauliflower Fritters*

Ingredients:

- *2 medium zucchini, grated and squeezed*
- *3 cups cauliflower florets*
- *1 tbsp. coconut oil*
- *1/4 cup coconut flour*
- *1/2 tsp. sea salt*

Direction: Preparation Time: 10 minutes Cooking Time: 15 minutes Servings: 4

✓ *Steam cauliflower florets for 5 minutes.*

✓ *Add cauliflower into the food processor and process until it looks like rice.*

✓ *Add all ingredients except coconut oil to the large bowl and mix until well combined.*
  Make small round patties from the mixture and set them aside.

✓ *Heat coconut oil in a pan over medium heat.*

✓ *Place patties in a pan and cook for 3-4 minutes on each side.*

✓ *Serve and enjoy.*

Nutrition: Calories 68 Fat 3.8 g, Carbs 7.8 g, Sugar 3.6 g, Protein 2.8 g, Cholesterol 0 mg

837)   *Roasted Chickpeas*

Ingredients:

- *15 oz. can chickpeas, drained, rinsed, and pat*

dry
- *1/2 tsp. paprika*
- *1 tbsp. olive oil*
- *1/2 tsp. pepper*
- *1/2 tsp. salt*

Direction: Preparation Time: 10 minutes Cooking Time: 30 minutes Servings: 4

✓ *Preheat the oven to 450 F/ 232 C.*
✓ *Spray a baking tray with cooking spray and set it aside.*
✓ *In a large bowl, toss chickpeas with olive oil, paprika, pepper, and salt.*
  Spread chickpeas on a prepared baking tray and roast in preheated oven for 25 minutes. Stir every 10 minutes.
✓ *Serve and enjoy.*

Nutrition: Calories 158 Fat 4.8 g, Carbs 24.4 g, Sugar 0 g, Protein 5.3 g, Cholesterol 0 mg

838)   *Peanut Butter Mousse*

Ingredients:
- *1 tbsp. peanut butter*
- *1 tsp. vanilla extract*
- *1 tsp. stevia*
- *1/2 cup heavy cream*

Direction: Preparation Time: 10 minutes

Cooking Time: 10 minutes Servings: 2

✓ *Add all ingredients into the bowl and whisk until soft peak forms.*
✓ *Spoon into the serving bowls and enjoy.*

Nutrition: Calories 157 Fat 15.1 g, Carbohydrates 5.2 g, Sugar 3.6 g, Protein 2.6 g, Cholesterol 41 mg

839)   *Pumpkin & Banana Ice Cream*

Ingredients:
- *15 oz. pumpkin puree*
- *4 bananas, sliced and frozen*
- *1 tsp. pumpkin pie spice*
- *Chopped pecans*

Direction: Preparation Time: 5 minutes Cooking Time: 10 minutes Servings: 4

✓ *Add pumpkin puree, bananas, and pumpkin pie spice in a food processor.*
✓ *Pulse until smooth.*

✓ *Chill in the refrigerator.*
✓ *Garnish with pecans.*

Nutrition: Calories: 71 Carbs: 18g Protein: 1.2g

840)   *Coffee Mousse*

Ingredients:
- *4 tbsp. brewed coffee*
- *16 oz. cream cheese, softened*
- *1/2 cup unsweetened almond milk*
- *1 cup whipping cream*
- *2 tsp. liquid stevia*

Direction: Preparation Time: 10 minutes

Cooking Time: 20 minutes Servings: 8

✓ *Add coffee and cream cheese in a blender and blend until smooth.*
✓ *Add stevia, and milk and blend again until smooth.*
✓ *Add cream and blend until thickened.*
  Pour into the serving glasses and place in the refrigerator.
✓ *Serve chilled and enjoy.*

Nutrition: Calories 244 Fat 24.6 g, Carbs 2.1 g, Sugar 0.1 g, Protein 4.7 g,

841)   *Brulee Oranges*

Ingredients:
- *4 oranges, sliced into segments*
- *1 tsp. ground cardamom*
- *6 tsp. brown sugar*
- *1 cup nonfat Greek yogurt*

Direction: Preparation Time: 5 minutes Cooking Time: 10 minutes Servings: 4

✓ *Preheat your broiler.*
✓ *Arrange orange slices in a baking pan.*
✓ *In a bowl, mix the cardamom and sugar.*
  Sprinkle mixture on top of the oranges. Broil for 5 minutes.
✓ *Serve oranges with yogurt.*

Nutrition: Calories: 168 Carbohydrates: 26.9g Protein: 6.8g

VEGETARIAN

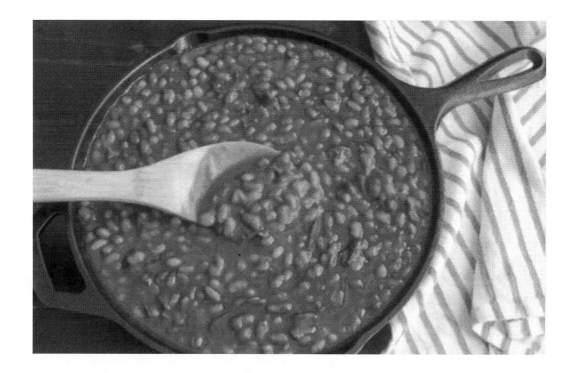

842)   Baked Beans

Ingredients:

- ¼ pound dry lima beans, soaked overnight and drained
- ¼ pound dry red kidney beans, soaked overnight and drained
- 1¼ tablespoons olive oil
- 1 small onion, chopped
- 4 garlic cloves, minced
- 1 teaspoon dried thyme, crushed
- ½ teaspoon ground cumin
- ½ teaspoon red pepper flakes, crushed
- ¼ teaspoon paprika
- 1 tablespoon balsamic vinegar
- 1 cup homemade tomato puree
- 1 cup low-sodium vegetable broth
- Ground black pepper, as required
- 2 tablespoons fresh parsley, chopped

Direction: Preparation Time: 15 minutes Cooking Time: 2 hours 10 minutes Servings: 4

- ✓ In a large pan of boiling water, add the beans over high heat and bring to a boil.
- ✓ Now, reduce the heat to low and simmer, covered for about 1 hour. Remove from the heat and drain the beans well.
- ✓ Preheat the oven to 325 degrees F. In a large ovenproof pan, heat the oil over medium heat and cook the onion for about 8-9 minutes, stirring frequently.
- ✓ Add the garlic, thyme and red spices and sauté for about 1 minute.
  Add the cooked beans and remaining ingredients and immediately remove from the heat.
- ✓ Cover the pan and transfer into the oven. Bake for about 1 hour. Serve with the garnishing of cilantro.

Meal Prep Tip:

- ✓ Transfer the beans mixture into a large bowl and set aside to cool. Divide the mixture into 4 containers evenly. Cover the containers and refrigerate for 1-2 days. Reheat in the microwave before serving.

Nutrition: Calories 136 Total Fat 4.3 g Saturated Fat 0.9 g Cholesterol 0 mg Total Carbs 19 g Sugar 4.7 g Fiber 4.6 g Sodium 112 mg Potassium 472 mg Protein 5.7 g Spicy

843)   Black Beans

Ingredients:

- 4 cups filtered water
- 1½ cups dried black beans, soaked for
- 8 hours and drained

- ½ teaspoon ground turmeric
- 3 tablespoons olive oil
- 1 small onion, chopped finely
- 1 green chili, chopped
- 1 (1-inch) piece fresh ginger, minced
- 2 garlic cloves, minced
- 1-1½ tablespoons ground coriander
- 1 teaspoon ground cumin
- ½ teaspoon cayenne pepper Sea salt, as required
- 2 medium tomatoes, chopped finely
- ½ cup fresh cilantro, chopped

Direction: Preparation Time: 15 minutes Cooking Time: 1½ hours Servings: 6

- ✓ In a large pan, add water, black beans and turmeric and bring to a boil on high heat.
- ✓ Now, reduce the heat to low and simmer, covered for about 1 hour or till the desired doneness of beans. Meanwhile, in a skillet, heat the oil over medium heat and sauté the onion for about 4-5 minutes.
- ✓ Add the green chili, ginger, garlic, spices and salt and sauté for about 1-2 minutes. Stir in the tomatoes and cook for about 10 minutes, stirring occasionally.
  Transfer the tomato mixture into the pan with black beans and stir to combine.
- ✓ Increase the heat to medium-low and simmer for about 15-20 minutes. Stir in the cilantro and simmer for about 5 minutes.
- ✓ Serve hot.

Meal Prep Tip:

- ✓ Transfer the beans mixture into a large bowl and set aside to cool. Divide the mixture into 6 containers evenly. Cover the containers and refrigerate for 1-2 days. Reheat in the microwave before serving.

Nutrition: Calories 160 Total Fat 8 g Saturated Fat 1 g Cholesterol 0 mg Total Carbs 17.9 g Sugar 2.4 g Fiber 6.2 g Sodium 50 mg Protein 6 g

844)   Lentils Chili

Ingredients:

- 2 teaspoons olive oil
- 1 large onion, chopped 3 medium carrot, peeled and chopped
- 4 celery stalks, chopped
- 2 garlic cloves, minced
- 1 jalapeño pepper, seeded and chopped
- ½ tablespoon dried thyme, crushed
- 1 tablespoon chipotle chili powder

- *½ tablespoon cayenne pepper*
- *1½ tablespoons ground coriander*
- *1½ tablespoons ground cumin*
- *1 teaspoon ground turmeric*
- *Ground black pepper, as required*
- *1 tomato, chopped finely*
- *1 pound lentils, rinsed*
- *8 cups low-sodium vegetable broth*
- *6 cups fresh spinach*
- *½ cup fresh cilantro, chopped*

Direction: Preparation Time: 15 minutes Cooking Time: 2 hours 20 minutes Servings: 8

- ✓ *In a large pan, heat the oil over medium heat and sauté the onion, carrot and celery for about 5 minutes.*
- ✓ *Add the garlic, jalapeño pepper, thyme and spices and sauté for about 1 minute.*
- ✓ *Add the tomato paste, lentils and broth and bring to a boil.*
- ✓ *Now, reduce the heat to low and simmer for about 2 hours.*
  Stir in the spinach and simmer for about 3-5 minutes. Stir in cilantro and remove from the heat.
- ✓ *Serve hot.*

Meal Prep Tip:

- ✓ *Transfer the chili into a large bowl and set aside to cool. Divide the chili into 8 containers evenly.*
- ✓ *Cover the containers and refrigerate for 1-2 days. Reheat in the microwave before serving.*

Nutrition: Calories 259 Total Fat 2.3 g Saturated Fat 0.3 g Cholesterol 0 mg Total Carbs 41 g Sugar 3.6 g Fiber 19 g Sodium 118 mg Potassium 856 mg Protein 18.2 g

845) *Quinoa in Tomato*

Ingredients:

- *2 tablespoons olive oil*
- *1 cup quinoa, rinsed*
- *1 green bell pepper, seeded and chopped*
- *1 medium onion, chopped finely*
- *3 garlic cloves, minced*
- *2½ cups filtered water*
- *2 cups tomatoes, crushed finely*
- *1 teaspoon red chili powder*
- *¼ teaspoon ground cumin*
- *¼ teaspoon garlic powder*
- *Ground black pepper, as required*

Direction: Sauce Preparation Time: 15 minutes Cooking Time: 40 minutes Servings: 4

- ✓ *In a large pan, heat the oil over medium-high heat and cook the quinoa, onion, bell pepper and garlic*

for about 5 minutes, stirring frequently.
- ✓ *Stir in the remaining ingredients and bring to a boil.*
- ✓ *Now, reduce the heat to medium-low. Cover the pan tightly and simmer for about 30 minutes, stirring occasionally. Serve hot.*
- ✓ **Meal Prep Tip:**
- ✓ *Transfer the quinoa mixture into a large bowl and set aside to cool.*
- ✓ *Divide the chili into 4 containers evenly.*
- ✓ *Cover the containers and refrigerate for 1-2 days. Reheat in the microwave before serving.*

Nutrition: Calories 260 Total Fat 10 g Saturated Fat 1.4 g Cholesterol 0 mg Total Carbs 36.9 g Sugar 5.2 g Fiber 5.4 g Sodium 16 mg Protein 7.7 g

846) *Grains Combo*

Ingredients:

- *¾ cup amaranth 1 cup quinoa, rinsed*
- *¼ cup wild rice*
- *4¼ cups filtered water*
- *2 teaspoons ground cumin*
- *½ teaspoon paprika Salt, as required*
- *1¼ cups boiled chickpeas*
- *2 medium carrots, peeled and grated*
- *1 garlic clove, minced*
- *Ground black pepper, as required*

Direction: Preparation Time: 15 minutes Cooking Time: 35 minutes Servings: 6

- ✓ *In a large pan, add the amaranth, quinoa, wild rice, water, and spices over medium-high heat and bring to a boil.*
- ✓ *Now, reduce the heat to medium-low and simmer, covered for about 20-25 minutes.*
- ✓ *Stir in remaining ingredients and simmer for about 3-5 minutes. Serve hot.*

Meal Prep Tip:

- ✓ *Transfer the grains mixture into a large bowl and set aside to cool. Divide the mixture into 6 containers evenly.*
- ✓ *Cover the containers and refrigerate for 1 day. Reheat in the microwave before serving.*

Nutrition: Calories 365 Total Fat 5.6 g Saturated Fat 0.6 g Cholesterol 0 mg Total Carbs 64 g Sugar 5.8 g Fiber 12 g Sodium 58 mg Protein 16.4 g

847) *Barley Pilaf*

Ingredients:

- *½ cup pearl barley*
- *1 cup low-sodium vegetable broth*
- *2 tablespoons olive oil, divided*

- *2 garlic cloves, minced finely*
- *½ cup onion, chopped*
- *½ cup eggplant, sliced thinly*
- *½ cup green bell pepper, seeded and chopped*
- *½ cup red bell pepper, seeded and chopped*
- *2 tablespoons fresh cilantro, chopped*
- *2 tablespoons fresh mint leaves, chopped*

Direction: Preparation Time: 20 minutes Cooking Time: 1 hour 5 minutes Servings: 4

✓ *In a pan, add the barley and broth over medium-high heat and bring to a boil. Immediately, reduce the heat to low and simmer, covered for about 45 minutes or until all the liquid is absorbed. In a large skillet, heat 1 tablespoon of oil over high heat and sauté the garlic for about 1 minute.*

✓ *Stir in the cooked barley and cook for about 3 minutes. Remove from heat and set aside. In another skillet, heat the remaining oil over medium heat and sauté the onion for about 5-7 minutes. Add the eggplant and bell peppers and stir fry for about 3 minutes. Stir in the remaining ingredients except for walnuts and cook for about 2-3 minutes. Stir in barley mixture and cook for about 2-3 minutes.*

✓ *Serve hot.*

Meal Prep Tip:

✓ *Transfer the pilaf into a large bowl and set aside to cool. Divide the pilaf into 4 containers evenly. Cover the containers and refrigerate for 1 day. Reheat in the microwave before serving.*

Nutrition: Calories 168 Total Fat 7.4 g Saturated Fat 1.1 g Cholesterol 0 mg Total Carbs 23.5 g Sugar 1.9 g Fiber 5 g Sodium 22 mg Protein 3.6 g

848)   Baked Veggies Combo

Ingredients:

- *2 large zucchinis, sliced*
- *1 large yellow squash, sliced*
- *3 cups fresh broccoli florets*
- *1-pound fresh asparagus, trimmed*
- *2 garlic cloves, minced*
- *1 tablespoon fresh rosemary, minced*
- *1 tablespoon fresh thyme, minced*
- *½ teaspoon ground cumin*
- *½ teaspoon red pepper flakes, crushed*
- *¼ teaspoon cayenne pepper*
- *2 tablespoons olive oil*
- *Salt, as required*

Direction: Preparation Time: 15 minutes Cooking Time: 40 minutes Servings: 8

✓ *Preheat the oven to 400 degrees F. Line 2 large baking sheets with aluminum foil. In a large bowl, add all ingredients and toss to coat well.*

✓ *Divide the vegetable mixture onto prepared baking sheets and spread in a single layer. Roast for about 35-40 minutes. Remove from oven and serve.*

Meal Prep Tip:

✓ *Remove from oven and set the veggies aside to cool completely.*

✓ *Transfer the veggie mixture into 8 containers and refrigerate for 2-3 days.*

✓ *Reheat in microwave before serving.*

Nutrition: Calories 77 Total Fat 4 g Saturated Fat 0.6 g Cholesterol 0 mg Total Carbs 9.4 g Sugar 3.8 g Fiber 3.8 g Sodium 45 mg Protein 3.8 g

849)   Mixed Veggie Salad

Ingredients:

For Dressing:

- *1/3 cup olive oil ½ cup fresh lemon juice*
- *1 tablespoon fresh ginger, grated*
- *2 teaspoons mustard 4-6 drops liquid stevia*
- *¼ teaspoon salt*

For Salad:

- *2 avocados, peeled, pitted and chopped*
- *2 tablespoons fresh lemon juice*
- *2 cups fresh baby spinach, torn 1 cup red cabbage, shredded*
- *1 cup purple cabbage, shredded*
- *2 large carrots, peeled and grated*
- *1 small orange bell pepper, seeded and sliced into matchsticks*
- *1 small yellow bell pepper, seeded and sliced into matchsticks*
- *½ cup fresh parsley leaves, chopped*
- *1 cup walnuts, chopped*
- *2 cups small broccoli florets*

Direction: Prep Time: 20 minutes Servings: 8

✓ *For dressing: in a food processor, add all ingredients and pulse until well combined. In a large bowl, add the avocado slices and drizzle with lemon juice.*

✓ *Add the remaining vegetables and mix. Place the dressing and toss to coat well. Serve immediately.*

Meal Prep Tip:

✓ *Transfer dressing into a small jar and refrigerate for 1 day. In 8 containers, divide avocado and remaining vegetables.*

✓ *Refrigerate for 1 day. Before serving, drizzle each portion with dressing and serve.*

Nutrition: Calories 314 Total Fat 28.1 g Saturated Fat 4 g Cholesterol 0 mg Total Carbs 14.1 g Sugar 4.3g Fiber 6.9 g Sodium 113 mg Potassium 642 mg Protein 6.8 g

850) *Tofu with Brussels Sprout*

Ingredients:

- 1 tablespoon olive oil, divided
- 8 ounces extra-firm tofu, drained, pressed and cut into slices
- 2 garlic cloves, chopped
- 1/3 cup pecans, toasted and chopped
- 1 tablespoon unsweetened applesauce
- ¼ cup fresh cilantro, chopped
- ¾ pound Brussels sprouts, trimmed and cut into wide ribbons

Direction: Preparation Time: 15 minutes Cooking Time: 15 minutes Servings: 4

✓ In a skillet, heat ½ tablespoon of the oil over medium heat and sauté the tofu and for about 6-7 minutes or until golden brown.

✓ Add the garlic and pecans and sauté for about 1 minute. Add the applesauce and cook for about 2 minutes.

✓ Stir in the cilantro and remove from heat. Transfer tofu into a plate and set aside In the same skillet, heat the remaining oil over medium-high heat and cook the Brussels sprouts for about 5 minutes. Stir in the tofu and remove from the heat. Serve immediately.

Meal Prep Tip:

✓ Remove the tofu mixture from heat and set aside to cool completely.

✓ In 4 containers, divide the tofu mixture evenly and refrigerate for about 2 days. Reheat in microwave before serving.

Nutrition: Calories 204 Total Fat 15.5 g Saturated Fat 1.8 g Cholesterol 0 mg Total Carbs 11.5 g Sugar 3 g Fiber 4.8 g Sodium 27 mg Potassium 468 mg Protein 9.9 g

851) *Beans, Walnuts & Veggie Burgers*

Ingredients:

- ½ cup walnuts
- 1 carrot, peeled and chopped
- 1 celery stalk, chopped
- 4 scallions, chopped
- 5 garlic cloves, chopped
- 2¼ cups cooked black beans
- 2½ cups sweet potato, peeled and grated
- ½ teaspoon red pepper flakes, crushed
- ¼ teaspoon cayenne pepper
- Salt and ground black pepper, as required

Direction: **Preparation Time: 20 minutes Cooking Time: 25 minutes Servings: 8**

✓ Preheat the oven to 400 degrees F. Line a baking sheet with parchment paper. In a food processor, add walnuts and pulse until finely ground. Add the carrot, celery, scallion and garlic and pulse until chopped finely.

✓ Transfer the vegetable mixture into a large bowl. In the same food processor, add beans and pulse until chopped. Add 1½ cups of sweet potato and pulse until a chunky mixture forms.

✓ Transfer the bean mixture into the bowl with vegetable mixture. Stir in the remaining sweet potato and spices and mix until well combined. Make 8 patties from mixture. Arrange the patties onto prepared baking sheet in a single layer. Bake for about 25 minutes. Serve hot.

Meal Prep Tip:

✓ Remove the burgers from oven and set aside to cool completely. Store these burgers in an airtight container, by placing parchment papers between the burgers to avoid the sticking.

✓ These burgers can be stored in the freezer for up to 3 weeks. Before serving, thaw the burgers and then reheat in microwave.

Nutrition: Calories 177 Total Fat 5 g Saturated Fat 0.3 g Cholesterol 0 mg Total Carbs 27.6 g Sugar 5.3 g Fiber 7.6 g Sodium 205 mg Potassium 398 mg Protein 8 g

MEASUREMENT CONVERSIONS

Volume Equivalent (Liquid)

US STANDARD	US STANDARD (OUNCES)	METRIC (APPROXIMATE)
2 tablespoons	1 fl. oz.	30 mL
¼ cup	2 fl. oz.	60 mL
½ cup	4 fl. oz.	120 mL
1 cup	8 fl. oz.	240 mL
1½ cups	12 fl. oz.	355 mL
2 cups or 1 pint	16 fl. oz.	475 mL
4 cups or 1 quart	32 fl. oz.	1 L
1 gallon	128 fl. oz.	4 L

Volume Equivalent (Dry)

US STANDARD	METRIC (APPROXIMATE)
⅛ teaspoon	0.5 mL
¼ teaspoon	1 mL
½ teaspoon	2 mL
¾ teaspoon	4 mL
1 teaspoon	5 mL
1 tablespoon	15 mL
¼ cup	59 mL

⅓ cup	79 mL
½ cup	118 mL
⅔ cup	156 mL
¾ cup	177 mL
1 cup	235 mL
2 cups or 1 pint	475 mL
3 cups	700 mL
4 cups or 1 quart	1 L
½ gallon	2 L
1 gallon	4 L

Oven Temperatures

FAHRENHEIT (F)	CELSIUS (C) (APPROXIMATE)
250°F	120°C
300°F	150°C
325°F	165°C
350°F	180°C
375°F	190°C
400°F	200°C
425°F	220°C
450°F	230°C

30 Day Meal Plan

Day	Breakfast	Lunch	Dinner	Snacks
1	Reduced Carb Berry Parfaits	Curried Carrot Soup	Grilled Tuna Steaks	Tabbouleh-Arabian Salad
2	Whole-Grain Breakfast Cookies	Beef and Mushroom Barley Soup	Red Clam Sauce & Pasta	Roasted Portobello Salad
3	Granola With Fruits	Tomato and Guaca Salad	Cobb Salad	Shredded Chicken Salad
4	Scrambled Turmeric Tofu	Coconut-Lentil Curry	Mussels in Tomato Sauce	Spinach Shrimp Salad
5	Rolls with Spinach	Chicken Vera Cruz	Tabbouleh-Arabian Salad	Sweet Potato and Roasted Beet Salad
6	Whole-Grain Pancakes	Lighter Shrimp Scampi	Greek Broccoli Salad	Potato Calico Salad
7	Paleo Breakfast Hash	Maple-Mustard Salmon	Dijon Salmon	Mango and Jicama Salad
8	Strawberry Coconut Bake Sprouted	Cider Pork Stew	Strawberry Spinach Salad	Tenderloin Grilled Salad
9	Toast with Creamy Avocado and Sprouts	Lemony Salmon Burgers	Cauliflower Mac & Cheese	Barley Veggie Salad

10	Veggie Breakfast Wrap	Lemon Cauliflower & Pine Nuts	Easy Egg Salad	Broccoli Salad
11	Breakfast Egg and Ham Burrito	Sweet Potato, Kale, and White Bean Stew	Shrimp in Garlic Butter	Cherry Tomato Salad
12	Turkey Sausages and Egg Casserole	Lighter Eggplant Parmesan	Beef Chili	Tuna Salad
13	Chicken and Egg Salad	Stuffed Portobello with Cheese	Stuffed Mushrooms	Arugula Garden Salad
14	Whole Egg Baked Sweet Potatoes	Pasta Salad	Vegetable Soup	Supreme Caesar Salad
15	Healthy Avocado Toast	Spanish Stew	Misto Quente	Sunflower Seeds and
16	Muffins of Savory Egg	Chicken with Caprese Salsa	Garlic Bread	Chicken Salad in Cucumber Cups
17	Parfaits of Yogurt, Honey, and Walnut	Creamy Taco Soup	Bruschetta	Scallop Caesar Salad
18	Yogurt And Kale Smoothie	Ham and Egg Cups	Cheesy Cauliflower Gratin	Chicken Avocado Salad
19	Greek-Yogurt Style	Balsamic- Roasted Broccoli	Blueberry Buns	Ground Turkey Salad
20	Peach and Pancakes with Blueberry	Hearty Beef and Vegetable Soup	Baked Chicken Legs	California Wraps

21	Bulgur Porridge Breakfast	Cauliflower Muffin	French toast in Sticks	Asian Cucumber Salad
22	Buckwheat Grouts	Cauliflower Rice with Chicken	Muffins Sandwich	Shredded Chicken Salad
23	Breakfast Bowl	Pork Chop Diane	Bacon BBQ	Tuna Salad
24	Peach Muesli Bake	Turkey with Fried Eggs	Stuffed French toast	Roasted Portobello Salad
25	Steel-Cut Oatmeal Bowl with Fruit and Nuts	Sweet Potato, Kale, and White Bean Stew	Lean Lamb and Turkey Meatballs with Yogurt	Cauliflower Tofu Salad
26	Whole-Grain Dutch Baby Pancake	Slow Cooker Two-Bean Sloppy Joes	Scallion Sandwich	Mango and Jicama Salad
27	Cranberry & Almond Granola Bars	Lighter Eggplant Parmesan	Tuna Salad Recipe 1	Sweet Potato and Roasted Beet Salad
28	Breakfast Quesadilla	Orange-Marinated Pork Tenderloin	Cherry Tomato Salad	Cauliflower Tofu Salad
29	Blackberry-Mango Shake	Lime-Parsley Lamb Cutlets	Shredded Chicken Salad	Spinach Shrimp Salad
30	Green Goddess Bowl with Avocado Cumin Dressing	Roasted Beef with Peppercorn Sauce	Ground Turkey Salad	Potato Calico Salad

Conclusion

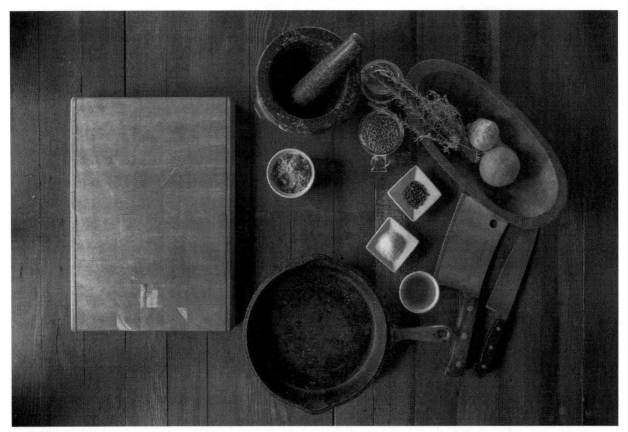

Thank you for making it to the end. The warning symptoms of diabetes type 1 are the same as type 2; however, in type 1, these signs and symptoms tend to occur slowly over months or years, making them harder to spot and recognize. Some of these symptoms can even occur after the disease has progressed.

Each disorder has risk factors that when found in an individual, favor the development of the disease. Diabetes is no different.

However, Most of the risk factors can be minimized by taking action. For example, developing a more active lifestyle, taking care of your habits, and lowering your blood glucose sugar by restricting your sugar intake. If you staIn addition, if to notice you are predi Recent studies show that developing healthy eating habits and following diets that are low in carbs, losing excess weight and leading an active lifestyle can help to protect you from developing diabetes, especially diabetes type 2, by minimizing the risk factors of developing the disorder.

You can also have an oral glucose tolerance test in which you will have a fasting glucose test first and then be given a sugary drink and then have your blood glucose tested 2 hours after that to see how your body responds to glucose meals. In healthy individuals, blood glucose should drop 2 hours post sugary meals again due to insulin action.

Another indicative test is the HbA1C. This test reflects the average of your blood glucose level over the last 2 to 3 months. It is also a test to see how well you manage your diabetes. When your body is low on sugars, it will be forced to use a subsequent molecule to burn for energy, in that case, this will be fat. The burning of fat will lead you to lose weight.

I hope you have learned something!

Recipe Index

Made in the USA
Monee, IL
21 March 2022

93258858R00146